Building Your Resilience
Finding Meaning in Adversity

Molly Birkholm

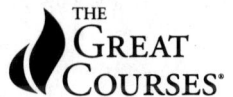

Published by

The Great Courses

Corporate Headquarters

4840 Westfields Boulevard | Suite 500 | Chantilly, Virginia | 20151-2299

Phone 1.800.832.2412 | Fax 703.378.3819 | www.thegreatcourses.com

Copyright © The Teaching Company, 2019

Printed in the United States of America

This book is in copyright. All rights reserved. Without limiting the rights under copyright reserved above, no part of this publication may be reproduced, stored in or introduced into a retrieval system, or transmitted, in any form, or by any means (electronic, mechanical, photocopying, recording, or otherwise), without the prior written permission of The Teaching Company.

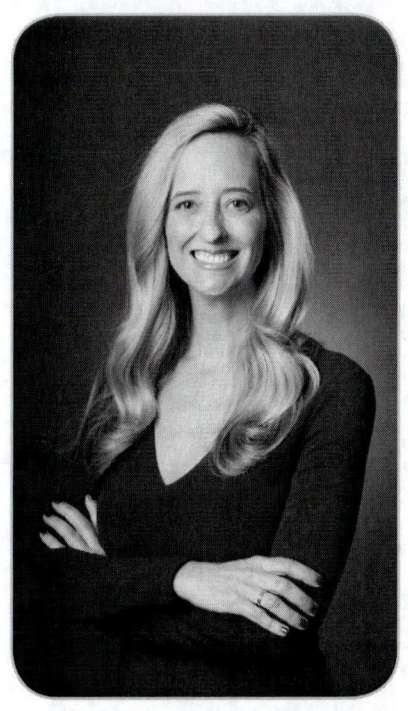

Molly Birkholm
Trauma Specialist

Molly Birkholm is a trauma specialist, a cofounder of Warriors at Ease, and the CEO of Molly Birkholm Inc. She has spent extended time living in ashrams and monasteries in India and Bhutan, where she studied yoga, meditation, Sanskrit, and Hindu and Buddhist philosophy. She is trained in iRest® Yoga Nidra, and she has also completed the Sivananda Yoga Vedanta Centre Advanced Teachers' Training Course.

As a yoga and meditation teacher and trainer, professional speaker, consultant, and writer, Ms. Birkholm inspires others to create meaningful life changes. Using research-based yoga and mindfulness meditation techniques, her stress management programs, resiliency training, corporate retreats, and trauma treatment programs are shared with leaders and top organizations around the world, including the US Department of Defense, McKinsey & Company, JPMorgan Chase, and the Young Presidents' Organization.

In addition to serving as a trainer for the iRest® Institute, Ms. Birkholm is a featured teacher for Yoga International and the host of a yearlong online course called Women's Empowerment Initiative. As a cofounder of Warriors at Ease, she helped pioneer evidence-based, trauma-sensitive yoga and meditation programs for people with post-traumatic stress disorder in the military and other communities affected by trauma, including human trafficking survivors, people in recovery, homeless individuals, youth, prisoners, and refugees. Ms. Birkholm has conducted innovative clinical research with the National Institutes of Health and the Department of Defense on these protocols, and each year, she offers public and private retreats and teacher trainings. She also actively supports human trafficking relief advocacy and education.

In addition to her work as a teacher, trainer, and retreat leader, Ms. Birkholm has published several audio and video products. Her iRest Yoga Nidra CDs and Sivananda Yoga & iRest Yoga Nidra DVD are distributed worldwide. She lives in South Florida with her son, Santiago, and her yellow Labrador, Cleo.

Ms. Birkholm's other Great Course is *iRest: Integrative Restoration Yoga Nidra for Deep Relaxation.* ●

Disclaimer

This series of lectures is intended to increase your understanding of the emotional and social lives of children and/or adults and is for educational purposes only. It is not a substitute for, nor does it replace, professional medical advice, diagnosis, or treatment of mental health conditions.

These lectures are not designed for use as medical references to diagnose, treat, or prevent medical or mental health illnesses or trauma, and neither The Teaching Company nor the lecturer is responsible for your use of this educational material or its consequences. Furthermore, participating in this course does not create a doctor-patient or therapist-client relationship. The information contained in these lectures is not intended to dictate what constitutes reasonable, appropriate, or best care for any given mental health issue and does not take into account the unique circumstances that define the health issues of the viewer. If you have questions about the diagnosis, treatment, or prevention of a medical condition or mental illness, you should consult your personal physician or other mental health professional. The opinions and positions provided in these lectures reflect the opinions and positions of the relevant lecturer and do not necessarily reflect the opinions or positions of The Teaching Company or its affiliates.

The Teaching Company expressly DISCLAIMS LIABILITY for any DIRECT, INDIRECT, INCIDENTAL, SPECIAL, OR CONSEQUENTIAL DAMAGES OR LOST PROFITS that result directly or indirectly from the use of these lectures. In states that do not allow some or all of the above limitations of liability, liability shall be limited to the greatest extent allowed by law. ●

Table of Contents

Introduction
Instructor Biography i

Disclaimer iii

Course Scope 1

Classes
1   The Foundation of Resilience 3

2   The Hero's Journey 22

3   The Resilient Human Spirit 41

4   The Consequences of Stress 59

5   Mastering Physical Resilience 79

6   Improving Emotional Resilience 98

7   Strengthening Mental Resilience 117

8   The Practice of Self-Care 136

9   The Rewards of Sleep 158

10   Finding Equanimity with Mindfulness 177

11	Understanding Trauma.............................197
12	Discovering Post-Traumatic Growth 217
13	Suzi Landolphi on Post-Traumatic Growth...........236
14	Cultivating Community and Connection............254
15	Finding Safety 272
16	Opening to Joy and Gratitude 293
17	Practice 1: Building Resilience.....................312
18	Practice 2: De-stressing with Your Breath 336
19	Practice 3: Promoting Sleep......................350
20	Practice 4: Relaxing Yoga for Self-Care 364
21	Practice 5: Practicing Mindfulness..................383
22	Practice 6: Evoking the Relaxation Response 392
23	Practice 7: Finding Safety with Yoga Nidra 412
24	Your Hero's Journey 423

Supplementary Material
Resilience Self-Evaluation Tool.........................438

Finding a Support Network 452

Bibliography and Additional Resources.................454

Course Scope

Whether you are healing from adversity or looking to prepare yourself for those inevitable moments of life when your resilience is tested, this course can help. Over 24 classes, this course explores the philosophical, scientific, and practical ways you can live a resilient, inspired life.

Classes investigate resilience from physical, mental, and emotional perspectives, and they discuss specific strategies you can use to rewire your brain and navigate life's challenges with more clarity and ease. You'll learn how stress and trauma affect the body and mind, and what you can do to reverse its potentially damaging effects. You'll also find out what tools really help to promote resilience, from the ancient archetype of the hero's journey to cutting-edge research on post-traumatic growth.

Along the way, true stories of resilience will provide inspiration and insight into people's ability to discover wisdom and meaning in adversity. The course also includes information on clinically researched coping skills and self-care techniques that can be used to build resilience.

You'll also be offered seven practice classes, giving you the opportunity to build your resilience in real time. The practice classes include resilience-building breathing exercises, movement practices, and guided meditations that will bring the teachings right into your home. The practice classes incorporate multilevel instruction, making them accessible for most people.

This guidebook also includes the course's Resilience Self-Evaluation Tool, which will help you explore how your strengths have successfully helped you surmount challenges in the past as well as discover areas for growth that may need some extra attention. Each facet of this course works together to help you evaluate your resilience, learn new skills, and apply newfound wisdom to your own life. ●

Class 1

The Foundation of Resilience

To get the most out of this course, it is strongly recommended that you use the Resilience Self-Evaluation Tool in the guidebook after viewing or listening to the first class. When you finish the course, go back and take the self-evaluation again to see what has changed, what you've learned, and if you see areas for future growth. You can take it as many times as you would like as you move through life. It provides a valuable way to check in with yourself several times a year to ensure you are staying resilient during the changing seasons of life.

The self-evaluation is centered on eight themes of resilience:

1. Core values and purpose.

2. Finding meaning in adversity.

3. Equanimity.

4. Self-care.

5. Healthy coping skills.

6. Having a positive sense of self.

7. Support and connection with others.

8. Having a proactive worldview.

These eight themes are the foundation of your brain and body's resilience. The remainder of this guidebook chapter provides an orientation regarding each.

Core Values and Purpose

Core values are the bedrock of resilience. If you haven't spent a lot of time thinking about what your core values are, try doing so. It can help to spend time really feeling why these values matter as well as how they are brought to life through your actions.

Living close to your core values can be a very clarifying and strengthening experience. It can also make life easier. Then next time you are faced with a big decision, you can use your core values as a touchstone: Which choice best honors your core values?

> Viewing adversity as an opportunity is what takes people out of the victim mentality and empowers them to be survivors and makers of change.

Core values can also help you define your purpose in life. They can empower the roles you play in life, whether as a parent, a community member, or an employee. For instance, if one of your core values is selfless love, being a parent is a beautiful place to practice this virtue.

Finding Meaning in Adversity

The next theme you will find throughout the course is the importance of finding meaning in adversity. Traumas in life are defined by a loss of control or a shattering of one's former paradigm.

However, struggles can force you to engage with life's most important questions. Your suffering can make you compassionate and give you the opportunity to care and feel deeply. Try sitting with a belief that instead of life happening to you, life is happening for you. Welcoming alleviates suffering.

Equanimity

The third theme you will find throughout this course is equanimity, which can be defined as "evenness of mind" or "mental composure." Ideally, you want to be able to maintain a state of mental calmness, even in the midst of challenging situations. The ability to maintain equanimity is something you can cultivate through practices like meditation, breathing, mindfulness, and yoga.

True equanimity is found in learning to ride the waves of life with a sense of openness and curiosity. Doing so requires learning to manage your emotional states and maintain a healthy connection between body and mind.

Self-Care

Self-care means maintaining your energy reserves by regularly taking care of your physical, emotional, and mental needs. This is essential to staying healthy and strong in an enduring way.

Self-care activities include exercise, breathing, meditation, eating healthy, taking time to relax, devoting time to your spiritual practice of choice, keeping a positive mindset, and sleep. Self-care can also include measures like spending time with loved ones, setting appropriate boundaries, and participating in activities that lift you up instead of holding you back.

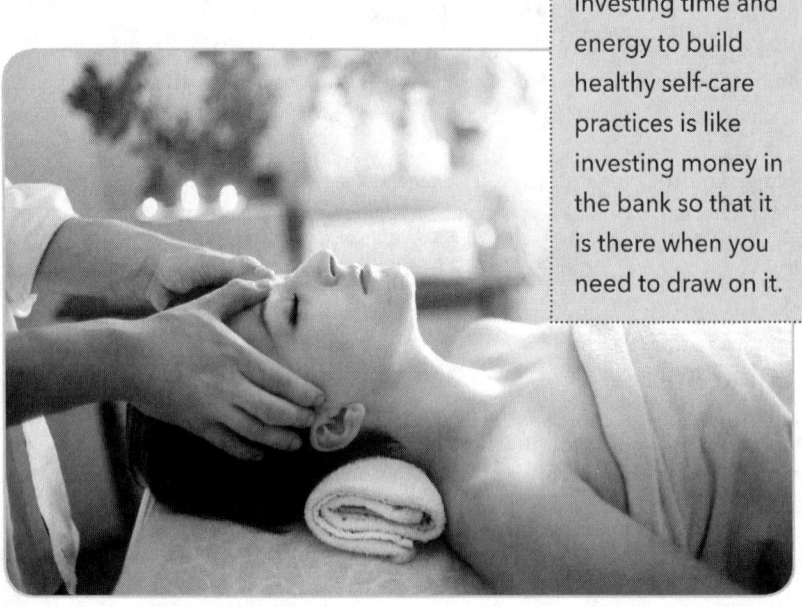

> Investing time and energy to build healthy self-care practices is like investing money in the bank so that it is there when you need to draw on it.

Healthy Coping Skills

Coping skills involve taking care of yourself in response to stress. Having a set of healthy coping skills includes measures like the aforementioned self-care practices. It also includes having trusted friends and advisors, using humor, deep breathing, and learning to observe your emotions, which are essential to navigating difficulties.

Typically, when people stop using healthy coping mechanisms, they start using unhealthy coping mechanisms, like drinking, smoking, drugs, gambling, or unhealthy sex habits. These unhealthy coping mechanisms can create more problems than the issues they are trying to resolve. If you find yourself turning to these unhealthy coping mechanisms, it's an important sign you need to amp up your self-care practices and start using some of your healthier coping skills.

Having a Positive Sense of Self

Having a positive sense of self is the next theme of resilience. Unfortunately, many people pin their identities on their outside persona, which is a vulnerable place to put one's sense of self-worth. For example, if someone ties her self-worth to her career, a professional setback could destroy her sense of self-worth.

Cultivating a healthy sense of self requires actively learning to listen to and love yourself. Having a healthy sense of self-worth is built upon understanding who you are on the inside, having a connection with yourself, and spending regular time cultivating that connection through activities like meditation and mindfulness.

Keep in mind that this does not mean thinking that you are better than others, which is a certain sign that someone suffers from a lack of confidence.

Support and Connection with Others

Having a support system and a healthy connection with others can strengthen nearly every aspect of resilience. Knowing you have people you can lean on for support and reaching out to them—both in good times and in moments when you need help—is essential for thriving amidst adversity.

Having people in your life you can trust can provide a tremendous sense of courage and freedom to step outside your comfort zone and try new things. A healthy community provides a sense of security and comfort in an uncertain world.

Sometimes, individuals want to only be the person who helps other people, but it is also extremely important to be someone who is authentic and vulnerable about the times when you need help. When you are honest about your reality, you open the door for others to be vulnerable and authentic as well. This is the place where true connection occurs. There is tremendous freedom in being honest and being able to both give and receive help.

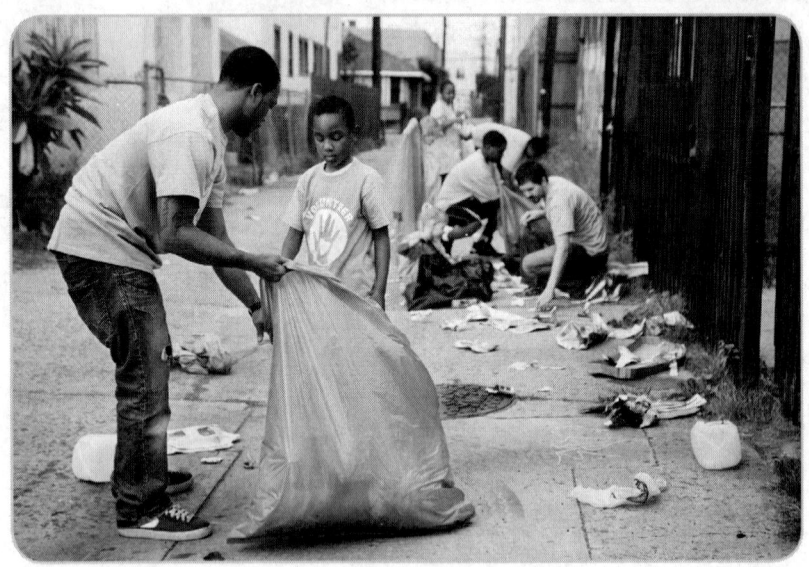

Having a Proactive Worldview

The eighth theme of resilience is having a proactive worldview. Though it can be easy to feel like a powerless victim in a massive, violent, confusing world, there is one thing you can affect: your perspective and state of mind. No one can take this away from you. You may not be able to change situations, but you always have the ability to change how you respond to situations.

It is important to be deeply grounded in your own personal truths while at the same time having psychological flexibility to adapt to changes that are constantly arising. A balance between the two can help you feel that you are safe in yourself and that you also have the ability to adapt and adjust in the face of new information. When you combine that with a sense of perseverance and determination, you can completely change the way you approach adversity in your life.

Suggested Reading

Graham, *Bouncing Back*.

Holiday, *The Obstacle Is the Way*.

Lynch, *Dancing in the Light*.

Sandberg and Grant, *Option B*.

Shatté and Reivich, *The Resilience Factor*.

Activities

- Contemplate what has helped you be more resilient in your life.
- Use the Resilience Self-Evaluation Tool.
- Complete Practice Class 1 (Class 17), titled "Building Resilience."

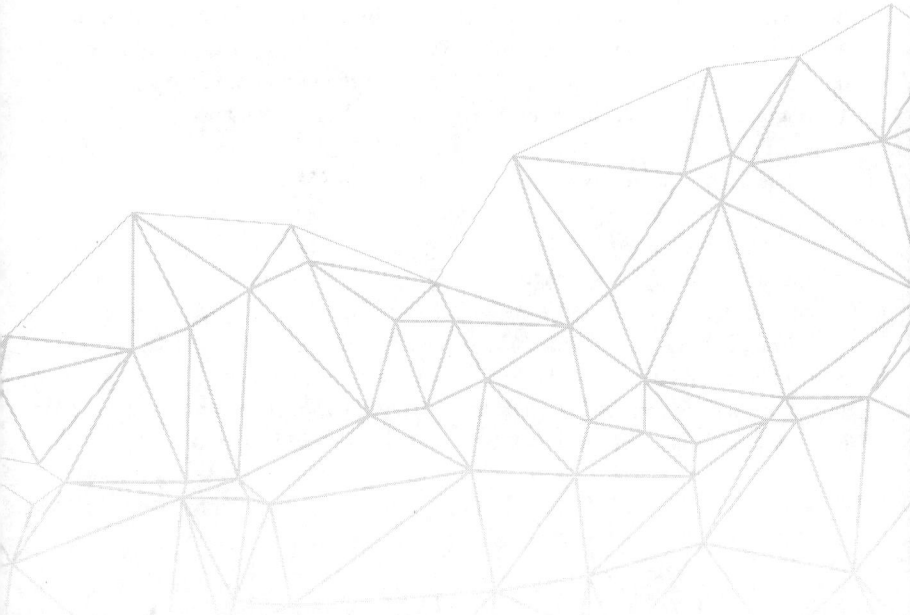

Class 1 Transcript

The Foundation of Resilience

"There is nothing you cannot do." That's the motto that 100-years-young Tao Porchon-Lynch lives by, and she's proved it to be true during a life filled with more adventures than an epic movie. Tao was born in India to an Indian mother and a French father. Her mother died when she was seven months old, and then her aunt and uncle raised her. Tao is one of the only remaining people on Earth who marched with Mahatma Gandhi and Martin Luther King.

In her early 20s, Tao left India and moved to Paris, where she became a well-known fashion model. Eventually, she found herself in the midst of World War II, where as a French Resistance fighter, she helped Jews escape imprisonment. After the war ended, she moved to Hollywood and became an actress. She was friends with Marilyn Monroe and dated many of the famous actors of the time. Throughout her life, she has been an advocate for human rights.

So, what keeps Tao so young? She's practiced yoga for 85 years, "But I only began teaching yoga about 45 years ago," she told me. I told her that's longer than I've been alive. After taking her yoga class, I can sincerely tell you that she can do more yoga poses than I can. Tao is also an award-winning ballroom dancer. At 96, she competed in *America's Got Talent* to standing ovations and great praise. When asked what brings longevity and resilience, she says, "Stay connected to the oneness, to the peace, within yourself. Love everyone you meet and treat them as yourself. Don't waste a second of your time hating anyone. It is better to light one candle than to curse the darkness of ignorance."

Tao Porchon-Lynch is a woman who embodies the essence of resilience. And I think her focus on our inner resources—what we all have within ourselves—is critically important. Like Tao, we all face challenges in our life. But we really do have reserves of inner strength that we can draw on, not only to meet those challenges, but to turn them into opportunities for growth. Our resilience is what defines whether we grow stronger from the experiences, or whether they cripple us.

There are few things that are certain in this life, but something we can know for sure is that life is always changing. It may be peaceful right now, but at some point, life is going to come at you swinging, and it's going to hit hard sometimes. It may be the death of a loved one, the sudden loss of a job, an accident or injury, the end of an important relationship, or it could be any number of a few million other things that can knock us off our balance in life. I say this not to scare you, but to acknowledge that our path through life is filled with adversity. It's not a question if challenges will come; it's really a matter of when.

So what can we do to prepare ourselves for this inevitability? Or what can we do to recover if we've already been knocked down? That's what this course is all about: building our resilience. Resilience is our ability to physically, emotionally, and mentally bounce back from adverse circumstances. Our ability to thrive in life depends upon our ability to embrace, transform, and transcend adversity. Which is another way of saying that our ability to thrive in life depends on our resilience.

The good news is that we know more about how we can proactively boost our resilience than we have at perhaps any time in history. The information and practices that I'll share with you in this course have the power to transform how you experience life and ride the big waves when challenges do arise. Throughout these 24 classes, we'll be exploring the philosophical, scientific, and also practical ways we can live resilient, inspired lives. In the first two-thirds of the course, I'll guide you through a series of topics that will give you a comprehensive understanding of what makes us bounce back from life's adversities. Then, in the final third of the course, I'll invite you to participate in practice classes, including movements, yoga, breathing, mindfulness, and meditation, as well as other activities that can help you boost your resilience. You are welcome to begin these practices right away and to practice as often as you would like.

My non-money back guarantee is that you will get far more out of this experience if you really make it your own. As information is presented, draw parallels to your own life. Experiment with what practices feel effective for you, taking special note of which classes make you feel relaxed or sleep better, which help you process emotions, and which empower you to feel stronger in the face of a challenge. The key to unlocking your resilience potential is to live it—to practice every single day. Every day we have opportunities to choose how we respond to challenges and setbacks. Those who learn to keep their peace amidst all the different experiences of life grow stronger, not in spite of the adversity, but because of it.

We will be looking at all sorts of tools we can use to improve our physical, emotional, and mental conditioning to withstand the stresses of life, as well as how we can affect our neuroplasticity, which is our brain's ability to rewire when presented with new information. To get the most out of this course, we strongly recommend taking the Resilience Self-Evaluation in the Guide Book after listening to this first class. Then when you finish the course, go back and take the Self-Evaluation again to see what has changed, what you've learned, and explore areas for future growth. You can take it as many times as you would like as you move through life. It provides a valuable touchpoint to check in with yourself several times a year to ensure you're staying resilient during the changing seasons of life.

The Resilience Evaluation tool is centered around eight themes of resilience: core values and purpose, finding meaning in adversity, equanimity, self-care, healthy coping skills, a positive sense of self, support and connection with others, and a proactive worldview. These eight themes are really the foundation of your brain and body's resilience. So what I'd like to do for the rest of this class is to introduce you to each theme, giving you a sort of high-level orientation to the key ideas that we will continue to develop throughout the course.

Let's start with the first theme, core values and purpose. If you think about historically what has given you strength and resilience during challenging times, I'm curious what arises. For many people, including myself, the real foundation of resilience is having a strong sense of the core values that you base your life upon. These are fundamental principles that we can turn to for strength in life. Are there certain core values that come to mind as I mention this? For me, they are truthfulness, non-violence, selfless love, and compassion. When I have a hard time making a decision or feel challenged in life, I feel like I can turn to these values and use them as a touchstone for making the right decision. The answers are usually clear when we're sincerely honest with ourselves. For some people, core values may originate in their religion, culture, organization, or family. Then as we move through life, they may change over time. Some may grow stronger; others may lose relevance.

I've done Resilience Training and Trauma Treatment programs and retreats with the US Military and US Department of Veterans Affairs since 2007 and have seen the way core values can sustain service members in moments of tremendous adversity. For example, the Marine Corps core values are honor, courage, and commitment. I asked a Marine friend, Jerry Bloomquist, to describe what those core values mean to him and this is what he said:

> The core values of the Marines—Honor, Courage, and Commitment—represent what we stand for as an organization and as individuals, in peace, battle, or [in] any place we find ourselves. We learn these values in boot camp and from there on out, those become our values that we live and die by. We all stand for the same values and that makes us stronger. We all come from the same cloth. It gives us one heartbeat. We're an organization on the same page.
>
> There is honor in how you conduct yourself, between each other, and for our country. There is honor in striving to be the best. To do that requires courage to be able to do the right things and make professional decisions, especially when no one is watching. It's part of a transformational process to push ourselves to the farthest extreme and [to] find our courage and strength in the midst of it. We believe in everyone to the left and right of us and commit to defending each other, even to our own death. That's a layer of commitment I don't think most

people can comprehend. That is the power of core values. They become what you are made of.

You can hear in his description the ways in which core values cultivate resilience. Our core values in many ways are the fabric of what we're made of. When we're put to the test, it is our core values that hold us, guide us, and give us strength. There is this feeling that even if we went down fighting, be it against a disease, an enemy at war, or something else, if we died living our core values, it would be the right way to end this sweet life.

Core values are the bedrock of resilience. If you haven't spent a lot of time lately thinking about what your core values are, it can really help to strengthen your resilience to spend time really feeling why these values matter, as well as how they are brought to life, not as a concept, but through your actions. Living close to your core values can be a very clarifying and strengthening experience. It can also make life easier. The next time you're faced with a big decision, you can use your core values as a touchstone. Which choice best honors your core values? Having determination to live your core values will give you faith in their ability to support you through adversity. I think of core values like a boat that you get on in a storm that can carry you through to the other side.

Our core values can also help define our purpose in life. They can empower the roles we play in life, whether that is as a parent, a community member, or an employee. Ideally, our purpose in life reflects our core values and gives us the opportunity to actively practice them. For instance, if one of your core values is selfless love, being a parent is a beautiful place to practice this virtue. Every day you'll be given opportunities to give it life. Or, perhaps your core value in life is integrity and your occupation as a manager of a department. All of your decisions can honor what it means to you to have integrity in your actions.

The next theme you will find throughout the course is the importance of finding meaning in adversity. Our traumas in life are defined by a loss of control or a shattering of our former paradigm. This can be an experience that destroys us. Or, this shattering of our former existence can break us open to find our authentic self and our inner strength that we may not have ever known even existed.

As human beings, we often tend to pull back from problems. In general, we seem to have a problem with problems. And actually, our biggest problem is that we think we shouldn't have them. But one of the things we're going to emphasize in this course is that, in reality, our problems are the path. Problems create our opportunities for growth and transformation. Believing that changes can make you stronger, finding wisdom in life's challenges, and taking the time to heal from past hardship and trauma, are the keys to unlocking your potential as a human being.

This is the importance of struggle; it forces us to engage with life's most important questions. Our suffering makes us compassionate. It makes us appreciate love. It gives us the opportunity to care and feel so deeply. It makes us able to feel the suffering of others and reach out to make a difference in their lives. Try sitting with a belief that instead of life happening to you, life is happening for you. Welcoming alleviates suffering. This shift from feeling limited by our problems to viewing adversity as an opportunity is what takes us out of the victim mentality and empowers us to be survivors and changemakers who take what we've learned from our own challenges and then use that wisdom to help others. We're going to explore this topic extensively in the class on Post-Traumatic Growth when we take a really deep look at this revolutionary paradigm for turning life's biggest challenges into opportunities for growth and evolution.

The third theme you'll find throughout our exploration of resilience is equanimity, which can be defined as evenness of mind or mental composure. Ideally, we want to be able to maintain a state of mental calmness, even in the midst of challenging situations. The ability to maintain equanimity is something we can cultivate through practices like meditation, breathing, mindfulness, and yoga. And of course, the most important place we can practice cultivating equanimity is in our day to day lives.

Oftentimes, people think that equanimity is something we will have when everything is perfect in life, and it's simply not true. Real equanimity arises from learning to welcome your entire experience, the good and the bad, and maintain your peace in the midst of it. Accepting and allowing yourself to feel all emotions, including uncomfortable ones, like fear and sadness, gives us the freedom to move through life without attachment to having everything be perfect, exactly as we want. Let's be real here. That day when everything is perfect? Most likely, it will never come, and even if it does, it will not last.

Equanimity also doesn't mean just going with the flow and never doing something to change the course of events in the world around us. Of course, sometimes life requires a fight. It requires creating boundaries. It requires taking action. If we can do this from a place of equanimity instead of a place of emotional reactivity, we will be far more effective in life. True equanimity is found in learning to ride the waves of life with a sense of openness and curiosity. Doing so requires learning to manage your emotional states and maintain a healthy connection between body and mind.

This brings us to our next theme of resilience, which is self-care. Maintaining your energy reserves by regularly taking care of your physical, emotional, and mental needs is essential to staying healthy and strong in an enduring way. It's interesting because oftentimes when I talk about self-care, people will say, "Oh, I already know all about how to take care of myself." The problem is that many of us know these concepts as a theory, but few actually put the concepts into practice. Self-care practices include things like exercise, breathing, meditation, eating healthy, taking time to relax, getting a massage, devoting time to your spiritual practice of choice, and keeping a positive mindset. Of course, this also include sleep. It can include things like spending time with loved ones, setting appropriate boundaries, and participating in activities that lift you up instead of holding you back.

Investing time and energy to build healthy self-care practices is like investing money in the bank. We want to save along the way by making monthly deposits into our savings account so that when we have an emergency, that money is there. In just the same way, when we care for ourselves on a regular basis, we're working to ensure our bodies and minds are healthy when the day comes—which it will—when our resilience is tested.

Self-care is really about routinely taking care of your needs, whereas coping skills, our fifth theme of resilience, involves taking care of yourself in response to stress. Having a set of healthy coping skills includes things like using our self-care practices, but it also includes having trusted friends and advisors, using humor, deep breathing, and learning to observe our emotions, which are essential to navigating difficulties.

Typically, when people stop using healthy coping mechanisms, they start using unhealthy coping mechanisms, like drinking, smoking, drugs, gambling, or unhealthy sex habits. This life isn't easy, and it is our innate tendency to want to relieve suffering. The problem is these unhealthy coping mechanisms can create more problems than the issues they're trying to resolve. If you find yourself turning to these unhealthy coping mechanisms, it's an important sign you need to amp up your self-care practices and start using some of your healthier coping skills.

The more you learn to cultivate awareness about the state of your body and mind, the sooner you can recognize when you're stressed, and then lean into your healthy coping skills to consciously respond to stress. And let me just note in passing that hope, gratitude, faith, and optimism are some of the greatest coping skills we can cultivate. We'll talk more about that in another class as well.

Having a positive sense of self is the next theme of resilience, and while it might seem obvious, it is unfortunately a subject that's either taken for granted or simply glossed over. There's an interesting story that illustrates this about the Dalai Lama when he was first exposed to Western culture. During an interview at a conference, someone asked the Dalai Lama, "What can we do about low self-esteem?" The Dalai Lama looked blank and he said, "What?" The interviewer replied, "Well, what if you don't like yourself? And you think you're worthless?" The Dalai Lama looked even more blank, and he asked his interpreters what the interviewer was talking about.

There is no term for *low self-esteem* in Tibetan, so the translator tried to describe what that phrase meant. The Dalai Lama responded, "I think very rare. Very rare." Then the interviewer turned to the audience and said, "Who here ever suffers from low self-esteem and self-hatred?" They all put up their hands. The Dalai Lama was shocked because that was not how he understood people, especially Westerners, who appeared so confident. The experience led to him revising his ideas about how to teach. Despite what outer facades we may present, there's an epidemic of low self-esteem and lack of self-worth in our society today, as we can see in the skyrocketing suicide rates, even amongst celebrities, people who supposedly have it all.

If we look at the origins of the word *personality*, it comes from the Latin word *persona,* which originally meant, "a mask." In the Greek and Roman theaters, actors always appeared wearing a mask of their character. It isn't so different than how we live today. Most people pin their identities on their outside persona, which is a vulnerable place to put your sense of self-worth. If anything negative happens to any of your perceived sources of self-worth, such as your career, family, income, or social status, suddenly your identity falls apart. We can see this in the way that many people speak about themselves in such a critical way. Really, if we spoke about others the way many of us speak about ourselves, we wouldn't have any friends.

Cultivating a healthy sense of self requires coming home to yourself and really actively learning to listen to yourself and love yourself. Having a healthy sense of self-worth is built upon understanding who you are on the inside, having a connection with yourself, and spending regular time cultivating that connection through things like meditation and mindfulness. Keep in mind, this does not mean thinking that you are better than others, which is a certain sign that someone suffers from a lack of confidence. We will spend a lot of time in future classes talking about how we can cultivate self-compassion and develop a sense of trust in our abilities to accomplish tasks and reach our goals.

Nearly every aspect of resilience can be strengthened by the next theme we'll explore in the course, having a support system and healthy connection with others. Knowing you have people you can reach out to for support and reaching out to them, both in good times and in moments when you need help, is essential for thriving amidst adversity. Having people in your life whom you can trust can provide a tremendous sense of courage and freedom to step outside your comfort zone and try new things. Healthy community provides a sense of security and comfort in an uncertain world. Sometimes we want to only be the person who helps other people, but it's also extremely important to be someone who is authentic and vulnerable about the times when you need help. When we're honest about our reality, we open the door for others to be vulnerable and authentic as well. This is the place where true connection occurs. There is tremendous freedom in being honest and being able to both give and receive help.

My son Santiago and I regularly feed a small group of homeless people who live near our house. As we have gotten to know them, we've learned all about their community, which is a small group of eight people who live together in a parking lot behind a restaurant. It is fascinating to watch how they look out for each other. They protect each other's belongings. They share with each other and care for each other. Honestly, they are far closer to their neighbors than I am to mine. It's interesting to think about.

As humans, we innately gravitate towards community. This goes back to our prehistoric ancestors, who realized they were safer living in groups than alone. Naturally, as your relationship with your community deepens, you will start to cultivate a sense of compassion and empathy for those around you. It's easiest to feel connected to people who are like us, but it's just as important to connect with people who are different than us. One of the ways we can do this is by giving back to our community through things like volunteer work; devoting time to friends, family, strangers in need; and donating to good causes. Helping others ultimately helps us just as much—sometimes even more. In reality, we are stronger together.

This brings us to our eighth theme of resilience, which is having a proactive worldview. It is easy in a world filled with violence, hatred, and 24-hour news cycles to feel like we're powerless victims of a world where we can't affect anything. There is one thing, though, that we can affect, and that's our perspective and state of mind. No one can take this away from us. We may not be able to change situations, but we always have the ability to change how we respond to situations. As we've seen in the treatment of prisoners of war, the fastest way to break a person is to make them feel like they don't have any options. And don't think any of us are immune from this. We can see the same philosophies applied in things like marketing and politics—any place where people play on our vulnerability to affect an outcome.

We can improve our resilience in every moment by knowing that we always have options for how we can respond to a situation. It is important to be deeply grounded in your own personal truths while at the same time having psychological flexibility to adapt to changes that are constantly arising. A balance between the two can help us feel that we are safe in ourselves, and that we also have the ability to adapt and adjust in the face of new information. When we combine that with a sense of perseverance and determination, we completely change the way we approach adversity in our lives.

This is the power and importance of a proactive worldview where we're engaged with meeting life on life's terms and taking actions necessary to live the life we want to live. We can choose how we respond to stress. We can choose the people we surround ourselves with. We can choose the practices we do to care for ourselves. We can choose how we give back. We can choose how we spend our time. Ultimately, when we're each living as the fullest and healthiest expression of ourselves, we will be able to create the most good in this world. Our state of mind affects every single person we come into contact with. We constantly have the ability to positively or negatively affect our surroundings. As Marianne Williamson so eloquently said, "Our deepest fear is not that we are inadequate. Our deepest fear is that we are powerful beyond measure."

So those are the eight key themes we'll be developing in the coming classes. From staying in touch with our core values to cultivating a proactive worldview, we'll equip ourselves with the tools, the habits, and the mindset that will empower us to bounce back from adversity and thrive in the face of life's challenges. This journey through resilience can truly be a life-changing one, if you let it. I'm reminded of a powerful story about an old Cherokee who was teaching his grandson about life.

He said to the boy, "A fight is going on inside me. It is a terrible fight, and it is between two wolves. One is evil; he is anger, envy, sorrow, regret, greed, arrogance, self-pity, guilt, resentment, inferiority, lies, false pride, superiority, and ego." He continued, "The other is good; he is joy, peace, love, hope, serenity, humility, kindness, benevolence, empathy, generosity, truth, compassion, and faith. The same fight is going on inside of you—and inside every other person, too." The grandson thought about it for a minute and then asked his grandfather, "Which wolf will win?" The old Cherokee simply replied, "The one you feed."

Class 2

The Hero's Journey

The hero's journey—a storytelling structure that can be seen in countless stories and screenplays—is essentially a blueprint for developing resilience. With this blueprint of the hero's journey in hand, you can see your personal journey through life in a new way.

There are several different versions of the steps involved in the hero's journey. Joseph Campbell originally identified 17 stages, but this class follows the model that Christopher Vogler develops in his book *The Writer's Journey*, which distills the monomyth down to 12 steps. You can also think of the hero's journey as having three actions: the separation, the initiation, and the return. Keep in mind that these phases may occur externally or internally for the hero. They may be physical, emotional, spiritual, or all three.

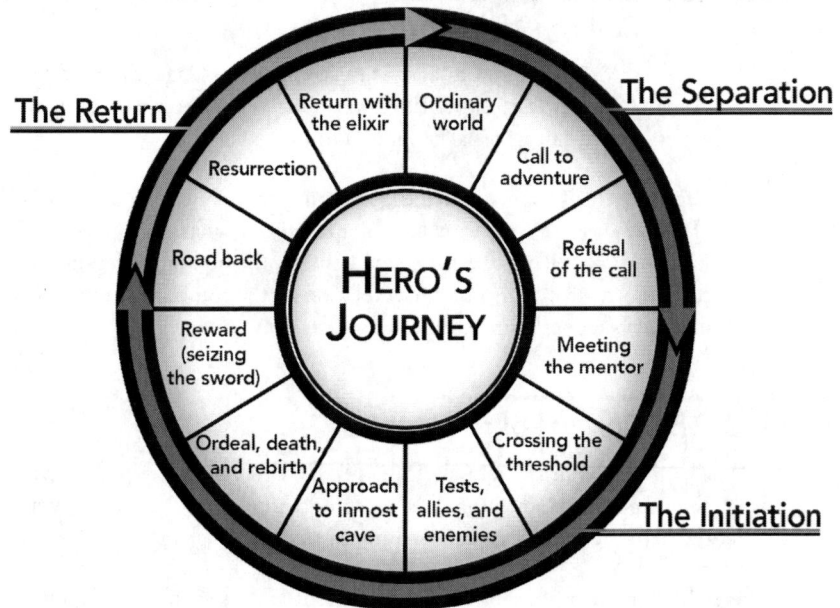

Step 1: The Ordinary World

- The first step is called the ordinary world. It begins amidst everyday life, with the hero unaware of the adventures that wait ahead.

- This context is necessary to understand the hero, as it often includes a glimpse into what day-to-day life is like as well as a general understanding of the hero's personality. The humanity of the hero is present, which includes an honest reflection of both their strengths and their limitations.

- Amidst this experience of the hero's normal life, there is often a sense of foreboding. The problem is not yet evident, but it can be felt on the horizon.

Step 2: The Call to Adventure

- The next step is the call to adventure. During this stage, the need to change becomes clear either through a shift in perspective or a direct call to action. Life as usual cannot continue.

- Often, the call to adventure is something traumatic, like a sudden life change, accident, threat, loss of a loved one, change in career, or something that jeopardizes the well-being of the hero, their family, or community. It can also be the revelation of the source of a problem that has been bothering the hero for some time.

Step 3: The Refusal of the Call

- The third step is the refusal of the call. Here, the hero is apprehensive about the call to adventure. Fears begin to arise, regardless of whether the hero is excited for the adventure or resistant to change.

- The hero may start to question himself or herself, or have second thoughts about the life changes. Feelings may arise of not wanting to leave the comforts of life, home, or the familiar.

Step 4: Meeting the Mentor

- The fourth stage involves meeting the mentor, which serves as an empowering moment in the story. What might have seemed impossible alone suddenly seems possible with the guidance and wisdom of someone who has walked the path before.

- The mentor may serve many roles. The mentor may see possibilities in the hero that the hero cannot see, which creates a bridge for the hero to walk across. The mentor may have practical tools that the hero can use on their journey. They may offer training, insights, or wisdom for the journey ahead. The mentor often has a unique way of seeing life that shifts the hero's worldview.

Step 5: Crossing the Threshold

- With the empowerment given by the mentor, the hero is able to find enough peace and strength amidst their fears to embark on the next step: crossing the threshold. The threshold symbolizes leaving behind the world the hero is comfortable with and stepping into the unknown ahead.

- Sometimes, the hero will have no choice. Other times, the hero will bravely, yet with some reluctance, begin from his or her own initiative. With this step, the hero commits to the quest, knowing it will not be easy. However, the hero also knows it is not possible to go back to life as it was before. The hero must let go of some of their questions to move on.

Step 6: Tests, Allies, and Enemies

- The sixth step—tests, allies, and enemies—involves the hero beginning to feel out their new reality. They have fully emerged out of their former life and into the next phase, where they are inevitably confronted with tests that challenge their previous perceptions. It may be that they have to unlearn what they knew before so that they can then learn something new.

- Here, the hero's former self is being challenged. Obstacles are thrown at the hero. Amidst the process of navigating these challenges, the hero attempts to discover who their allies and enemies are. Both the allies and the enemies teach the hero lessons of some kind, which become part of what prepares them for the future.

- In this phase of the hero's journey, each obstacle prepares the hero in some way for what is to come. The hero learns about their unique skills and gains a deeper wisdom about how they can affect change in the world around them.

Step 7: The Approach to the Inmost Cave

- During the seventh step, the approach to the inmost cave, the hero feels like they are approaching the place of greatest threat or evil. The cave represents everything that the hero fears most. Symbolically, it is clear that the biggest threats of all are the fears they bring with them into the cave. Here, the hero often learns the hard way that anger, fear, and aggression must be abandoned in order to keep growing.

- This phase often involves some self-reflection to use the lessons learned along the journey to confront their original fears and to uncover the courage they will need for what is to come. Innately, the hero knows they will be tested in a way they never have been before.

Step 8: The Ordeal, Death, and Rebirth

- During the eighth stage—the ordeal, death, and rebirth—the hero encounters a difficult foe and learns that there is no fast or easy way out. They must uncover a deeper belief in themselves than they have ever had before to win this battle.

- Often they must put down the tools they thought would help them, including the tools they have used in the past, when they find that they are useless against this, their biggest challenge. Winning this battle requires something new.

- The challenge in the ordeal stage can be an internal struggle against the hero's biggest fear. It can be a physical test or a confrontation with their biggest enemy. It may even be a combination of these.

- All of the resources, wisdom, and skill that the hero has collected along the journey are needed to make it through the ordeal. The former self of the hero must die in order for the new version of the self to come forth.

Step 9: The Reward

- The ninth step is the reward stage. Here, the hero transcends their lower self to reach a higher state of being. They rise with renewed power, intuition, and strength, along with deeper wisdom and a broadened view of possibilities.

- Often, the hero comes out of their battle with a prize or reward for their efforts. This prize can take many forms, depending upon the nature of the battle. It can be a greater sense of peace, purpose, and meaning in their life. It might be a deeper relationship with a loved one, a new career, a romance, or a new chance at life. The reward is in some way the missing piece they need to return again to the ordinary world.

Step 10: The Road Back

- The next step involves walking the road back home and over the threshold crossed when the journey began. Think back to the fear present as the hero left the familiarity of their former life as they made their way into the unknown. Now, they are walking back across the threshold in the other direction with a sense of triumph and a renewed sense of excitement and enthusiasm for life.

- On the road back, the hero must evaluate how they return to life so that they do not slip back into the way things used to be. The hero must integrate their new insights into the ordinary world—a world that may not have changed at all while they themselves have changed so profoundly.

Step 11: Resurrection

- In the penultimate step—resurrection—the biggest challenge yet arises, even though the hero may have thought that the return would be filled with triumph and ease. The hero must face the ultimate encounter with their biggest fears and even the possibility of their own death, which includes the death of their former self.

- The hero, who was born amidst the adventure and who has now earned new merits, dies if they return to the life they led before. The hero cannot keep their new wisdom just for themselves, or they will suffer tremendously. The wisdom dies if not kept alive through the hero's thoughts, words, and deeds. The hero must shed their former skin and fully embrace the expansiveness of their new reality.

Step 12: The Return with the Elixir

- During the final step, the return with the elixir, the hero steps fully into their new truth and embodies it in the ordinary world. It is a world that no longer seems as ordinary as the hero had once thought it to be.

- During this phase, the hero realizes the full value of what he or she has gained. The hero then empowers other people to confront their demons, hardships, and bullies. The hero also learns from the people they are helping, finding that the hero doesn't always have to go into the proverbial cave to find the dragon. The hero can find the dragon any place they still discover their own selfishness, anger, greed, hatred, or jealousy.

- To be a true hero, one must recognize that the story is ultimately not about the hero being the hero. The ultimate hero's journey teaches the hero how to transcend the self. A hero comes back from their journey with the same name and form, but the hero lets the work of their heart flow through them instead of thinking it is about them.

- The true hero does not attach to their heroicness. The more the person is able to release the sense that they are the hero who is helping other people, the more the person will be able alleviate suffering and experience peace in their own heart and mind. The hero does the work that needs to be done while renouncing attachment to the outcome.

Conclusion

- The hero's journey provides an archetype to understand the truths that you can only discover by leaving your ordinary world and undertaking your own journey of separation, initiation, and return. Whether your hero's journey occurs in the office of a good therapist, or on a soul-searching adventure around the world, or while healing in the cancer unit of a hospital, the quest to find your true self is a universal quest that everyone has to walk in their own way.

- Each time you navigate through the hero's journey, you receive the opportunity to strengthen resilience by discovering new vibrancy in life, new sources of wisdom and meaning, and a deeper embodiment of your authentic, true self. You are in the midst of your own hero's journey now. Consciously understanding it will unlock new sources of resilience in you.

Suggested Reading

Campbell, *The Hero with a Thousand Faces*.

Vogler, *The Writer's Journey*.

Activities

- Create your definition of a hero.

- Once you've created your definition, ask several other people how they define a hero.

- Look for the steps of the hero's journey throughout your life. If it is helpful, you can write out the 12 steps and document the phases of your life in each step. You can also write out a diagram of multiple hero's journey stories you have navigated throughout your life, and see how they intertwine together and connect with each other.

- You are welcome to go to Class 24 and do the hero's journey guided meditation as many times as is helpful.

Class 2 Transcript

The Hero's Journey

I have a question for you, because you are the person this class is really about. What is your definition of a hero? Spend a moment thinking about your response. After this class, try asking some of the people you know the same question. It is interesting to see how each of us perceives heroes.

For example, I asked a Special Operations service member what his definition of *hero* is, and here's what he told me: "A hero is someone who gives themselves to the well-being of other people regardless of the outcome. In the process, they discover the difference between right and wrong." My friends at Boulder Crest Retreat use this definition in their Post-Traumatic Growth programs: "A hero is a person who survives an extraordinary experience and returns to share important truths about life that they learned so that they can enrich the lives of others." Since I'm asking you to come up with your own definition, I'll share mine as well. To me, "A hero is someone who is willing to go to the dark places in themselves and in the world in order to create harmony while harvesting the wisdom along the way to come back and share with others."

Now take a moment to consider the people you consider to be your heroes. Perhaps Mother Theresa, Martin Luther King, Gandhi, or Harriet Tubman—or it could be a family member, a friend, a teacher, or even a group of people, like the first responders who rushed into the World Trade Center knowing they would not come out alive. Part of what makes someone a hero is the adversity they go through in their lives. The challenges they experience are, in some way, the cost of admission of living a life of purpose and meaning. It is also what builds resilience. What's fascinating is that if you look at the process through adversity that so many heroes have navigated, there are many common experiences that begin to arise. It's not just the common experiences of heroes like Abraham Lincoln or Marie Curie; it's also the shared experience of the teachers, doctors, parents, and grandparents who every day in their own way find challenge, meaning, and purpose in the world around them while making a difference in the lives of others.

Today, I'm going to suggest that every person's life can be a hero's journey simply by finding opportunities for growth and wisdom in the challenges we face every day. The hero's journey feels like a good name for this lifelong experience because it gives our struggle the sense of importance it deserves so it doesn't feel so painful or impossible to endure and transcend the challenges in our life.

So how will the hero's journey help us be more resilient? The hero's journey *is* a story of resilience. It is essentially a blueprint for developing resilience. And with this blueprint of the hero's journey in hand, we can see our own personal journey through life in a new way. The archetype gives us renewed energy and clarity to confront the challenges at hand, knowing many have come before us and made it through to the other side stronger and wiser than when they began.

As we navigate our own process, we can look to real-life heroes and the heroes in mythology and movies to help us understand our experience and transcend the limits of what we thought was possible. When we do this, we don't feel alone. The archetype helps give us a sense of purpose as we make our way through this roadmap that so many have traveled before. It reminds us that there is a long-term payoff that perhaps we can't see, but is always there.

Sometimes we may consider the notion of a *hero* and think, "Well, that's not me; I'm just a normal mom from Fort Lauderdale." But we don't have to be perfect in every way to walk the hero's journey. Quite the opposite. Oftentimes it is our imperfections that set us on our journey. It would be pretty boring if the hero realized they had all the answers at the beginning of the story and everything in their lives was already perfect. Everyone's story has meaning. Everyone's story is important. When we understand our story, we're more empowered to be the person we've always wanted to be. Whatever your story is up to this point, there is meaning present. Understanding that story will help create a meaningful future by helping you see that challenges are an important part of helping you grow as a human being. Then, next time you encounter a challenging situation, you can apply this model to help you on your journey.

We are now going to go through the stages of the hero's journey. And as we go along, these stages will probably sound familiar, partially because you've been living it, and also because it's the archetype of many of the most famous books and movies, from *Star Wars* to *Harry Potter* to *Lord of the Rings*. The story line is known as the monomyth, the one story that we all share.

I really don't want this to be just another lecture. I invite you to consider each stage of the hero's journey and notice if you find your own story in it. As we walk through this journey together, ask yourself, "What is my hero's journey story? What lessons did I learn through moments of adversity and deep self-inquiry? Can I find where I am in the process of this journey or identify these stages in another chapter of my life?" To give you a model for this, I'm going to share a piece of my own story for each stage of the hero's journey.

If you draw a circle, you have to go all the way around and then end at the starting point to complete the circle. There is no shortcut. We have to go through a cycle that starts and ends in our ordinary world. During our unique quest, we have to pass through a special world that challenges all of our perceptions.

There are several different versions of the steps involved in the hero's journey. Joseph Campbell originally identified 17 stages. But we're going to follow the model that Christopher Vogler develops in his book *The Writer's Journey*, which distills the monomyth down to 12 steps. You can also think of the hero's journey as having three actions: the separation, the initiation, and the return. Keep in mind that these phases may occur externally or internally for the hero. They may be physical, emotional, spiritual, or all of the above.

The first step is called the ordinary world. It begins amidst everyday life, with the hero unaware of the adventure that awaits ahead. This context is necessary to understand the hero, as it often includes a glimpse into what day-to-day life is like, as well as a general understanding of the hero's personality and details about their life. The humanity of the hero is present, which includes both an honest reflection of both their strengths and their limitations. Amidst the experience of the hero's normal life, there is often a sense of foreboding present where the problem is not yet evident, but you can feel it on the horizon.

My hero's journey began not long after I graduated from University. I accepted a job as an investment banking analyst and was making the transition to working for a big bank. I found myself in New York City, sharing a teeny, tiny one-room apartment with two dear friends from college. I had just started my great job and was determined to be successful in my career. I worked long hours all week and partied long hours on the weekends.

The next step is the call to adventure. During this stage, the need to change becomes clear either through a shift in perspective or a direct call to action. Either way, it becomes evident that life as usual cannot continue. Oftentimes the call to adventure is something traumatic, like a sudden life change, accident, threat, loss of a loved one, change in career, or something that jeopardizes the well-being of the hero, their family, or community. It can also be the coming to light of something that has been bothering the hero for some time, though now they can see the source of the problem.

My call to adventure came suddenly. On May 3rd, 2000, I hopped into a taxi. Minutes later came the crash. For a moment, I felt myself leave my body. When I realized what was happening, I reached down and felt like I grabbed my life. It was as if I could hear myself screaming, "No! I'm not leaving! I worked so hard to get where I'm at! My life has just begun!" I felt like I came crashing back down into my body, a place where I found excruciating pain. There was a lifeless cab driver crushed in the front seat, and I was trapped in the car with him. I was in and out of consciousness for the hour it took them to get me out of the car.

The third step is the refusal of the call. Here we find the hero apprehensive about the call to adventure. Fears begin to arise, regardless of whether the hero is excited for the adventure or resistant to change. The hero may start to question themselves or have second thoughts about their life changes. Feelings may arise of not wanting to leave the comforts of life, home, or the familiar that, even if it isn't perfect, is a known entity.

In my case, my accident left me with a fractured skull, spine, and sternum. I wanted my old life back, though I knew it would never be the same. Once I could return to work, I poured myself into it, working late hours and trying to avoid thinking about the trauma of witnessing the cab driver's death and the incredible pain my body was experiencing. I was diagnosed with PTSD—post-traumatic stress disorder—and had every single symptom: flashbacks, nightmares, insomnia, hypervigilance, depression, and anxiety.

The fourth stage involves meeting the mentor, which serves as an empowering moment in the story. What might have seemed impossible alone suddenly seems possible with the guidance and wisdom of someone who has walked the path before. The mentor may serve many roles. Oftentimes the mentor will see possibilities in the hero that they themselves cannot see, which creates a bridge for the hero to walk across. The mentor may have practical tools that the hero can use on their journey. They may offer training, insights, or wisdom for the journey ahead. The mentor often has a unique way of seeing life that shifts the hero's worldview.

In the years that followed my accident, I met many mentors. My yoga and meditation teachers were the most influential. I dove headfirst into the practices and spent every spare minute of my life studying yoga philosophy and practicing. My therapist and some career mentors also helped me find my way into the next phase of what I wanted to do in life. Amidst all the studies, I kept working and also simultaneously navigating a lengthy lawsuit over my car accident.

With the empowerment given by the mentor, the hero is able to find enough peace and strength amidst their fears to embark on the next step, crossing the threshold. The threshold symbolizes leaving behind the world the hero is comfortable with and stepping into the unknown ahead. Sometimes the hero will have no choice, while other times the hero will bravely, yet with some reluctance, begin from their own initiative. With this step, the hero commits to the quest, knowing it will not be easy, but also knowing it is not possible to go back to life as it was before. The hero must let go of some of their questions to move on.

I crossed the threshold four years after my car accident, when the lawsuit finally settled and I had the financial freedom to take the trip to Asia I had been intricately planning for a long time. A month after receiving the settlement, I was on a plane to India. It was not easy to leave everyone I loved, and my family was not happy about the decision. Yet, I knew in every cell of my body that it was the right decision. I had to find my core, the part of me that was unchanging.

We refer to the sixth step as tests, allies, and enemies. Here, the hero begins to feel out their new reality. They have fully emerged out of their former life and into the next phase where they are inevitably confronted with tests that challenge their previous perceptions. It may be that they have to unlearn what they knew before so that they can then learn something new. Here we see the hero's former self being challenged. Obstacles get thrown at the hero. Amidst the process of navigating these challenges, the hero attempts to discover who their allies and enemies are. Oftentimes they are wrong before they are right, which can cause an internal questioning of themselves. Both the allies and the enemies teach the hero lessons of some kind, which become part of what prepares them for the future.

In this challenging sixth stage, the hero's intuition, faith, and strength get tested. Oftentimes they get knocked down and must find their way up again, giving them greater insights into who they are as a person and the nature of the world around them. Amidst the adversity, we see how the projections of the mind affect the situation, and often the hero is forced to step out of previous perceptions to find the solution from a new point of view.

What is interesting in this phase of the hero's journey is that each obstacle prepares the hero in some way for what is to come. The hero learns about their unique skills and gains a deeper wisdom about how they can affect change in the world around them. As I made my way through ten countries in southeast Asia over many months, I was confronted with tests I could have never imagined. I put myself in the sacred crucible of these ancient lands, willing to sacrifice anything to discover what was real. The journey led me through ancient temples and pilgrimage sites, austere ashrams and Himalayan monasteries, impoverished orphanages and refuges for women, drought-stricken deserts and jungle monsoons.

During the seventh step, the approach to the inmost cave, the hero feels like they are approaching the place of greatest threat or evil. The cave represents everything that the hero fears most, and symbolically, it is clear that the biggest threats of all are the fears they bring with them into the cave. Here the hero often learns the hard way that anger, fear, and aggression must be abandoned in order to keep growing. This phase often involves some self-reflection to use the lessons learned along the journey to confront their original fears and to uncover the courage they will need for what is to come. Innately, the hero knows they will be tested in a way they have never been before.

In my own journey to the East, I learned invaluable lessons about the true depths of suffering, shattering my perceptions and softening my heart. While I had always tried to be a compassionate person, I quickly realized that I had no clue about the full breadth of suffering in the world. Opportunities for service constantly arose, and I questioned how to use my abilities and resources for the greatest good.

During the eighth stage, the ordeal, the hero steps into the ring with the dragon, so to speak. Here the hero learns that there is no fast or easy way out. They must uncover a deeper belief in themselves than they have ever had before to win this battle. Often they must put down the tools they thought would help them, including the tools they have used in the past, when they find they are useless against this, their biggest challenge. Winning this battle requires something new.

The challenge in the ordeal stage can be an internal struggle against the hero's biggest fear, or it can be a physical test or a confrontation with their biggest enemy. It may be a combination of these. All of the resources, wisdom, and skill that the hero has collected along their journey is needed to make it through the ordeal stage. The former self of the hero must die in order for the new version of the self to come forth. To do so, they must risk everything they find most important and are most afraid to lose. The dragon must be slain for them to reach the next phase, and so slay the dragon they do. The moment comes when you just can't let that dragon haunt you anymore.

As I rediscovered the universality of human experience through selfless service, a feeling of true interconnectedness occurred where there was no longer a *me* and a *them*. There was only *us*. The hunger of every starving person, the loneliness of every abandoned child, the silent suffering of the oppressed, and the joy of every soul given an opportunity for something better all felt like it was happening inside of me. There was no choice except to serve.

The ninth step is the reward, or the seizing of the sword. Here we see the hero transcend their lower self to reach a higher state of being. They rise with renewed power, intuition, and strength, along with a deeper wisdom and a broadened view of possibilities. Oftentimes the hero comes out of their battle with a prize or reward for their efforts. This prize can take many forms, depending on the nature of the battle. It can be a greater sense of peace, purpose, and meaning in their life. Or, it can be deeper relationship with a loved one, a new career, a romance born from their heart's deepest desire, or a new chance at life. The reward is in some way the missing piece they need to return again to the ordinary world.

I seized my reward after a long retreat in a Buddhist monastery high in the Himalayas in Bhutan. That's when my mind finally settled, and I found the part of me that was unchanging. The stillness that is always present, but that we just can't hear when the mind is so busy telling its stories. I had found my core. Towards the end of my retreat, my marching orders arose in the form of one sentence: "Go teach those who are suffering the most on this Earth how to find true peace and happiness inside of themselves.

The tenth step involves walking the road back home and over the threshold crossed when the journey began. Think back to the fear present as the hero left the familiarity of their former life, as they made their way into the unknown. Now they are walking back across the threshold the other direction with a sense of triumph and a renewed sense of excitement and enthusiasm for life. On the road back, the hero must evaluate how they return to life so that they do not slip back into the way it was. The hero must integrate their new insights into the ordinary world—a world that may not have changed at all while they themselves have changed so profoundly.

When I finally returned to the United States, I quickly realized the impossibility of fitting into my former life. The existence I had left behind seemed like it belonged to an entirely different person. I did my best to find my place again and settle into former relationships, but my attempts felt forced and compromising. My head kept trying to convince me of one thing while my heart was saying the opposite.

During the 11th step, resurrection, just when the hero thought that the return would be filled with triumph and ease, the biggest challenge yet arises. The hero must face the ultimate encounter with their biggest fears and even the possibility of their own death, which includes the death of their former self.

The hero, who was born amidst the adventure and who has now earned their new merits, dies if they return to the life they led before. The hero cannot keep their new wisdom just for themselves, or they will suffer tremendously. The wisdom dies if not kept alive through the hero's thoughts, words, and deeds. This pain becomes a teacher showing what wants to change and what needs to take life through them. If they listen to the pain as a teacher, they can find their path through to the next stage of life. To resurrect, the hero must shed that former skin and fully embrace the expansiveness of their new reality. If the hero shares their newfound wisdom, they succeed in remaining a hero and growing more heroic through each life they change with the meaning they discovered. This is the ultimate resurrection—when the light of the hero shines out into the world to light other lives.

In January of 2007, I flew down to Miami for a visit. I spent several months sleeping too much, going to the beach, doing little else. I felt depressed and lost. After so much inspiration and adventure in Asia, life seemed, well, lifeless. Then one day, a doctor friend asked if I would teach some wheelchair yoga classes at the Miami Department of Veterans Affairs hospital. Given that I had no plans for the rest of my life, I agreed.

During the final stage, the return with the elixir, the hero steps fully into their new truth and embodies it in the ordinary world—a world that no longer seems as ordinary as they had once thought it to be. During this phase, the hero realizes the full value of what they have gained. They then empower other people to confront their demons, hardships, and bullies. The hero also learns from the people they're supposedly helping. They find that they don't have to go to the proverbial cave to find the dragon. They can find the dragon anyplace they still discover their own selfishness, anger, greed, hatred, or jealousy.

To be a true hero, however, one must recognize that the story is ultimately not about them being the hero. The ultimate hero's journey teaches the hero how to transcend the self. Then there is a person who comes back from their journey with the same name and form, but they're letting the work of their heart flow through them instead of thinking it is about them. They don't attach to it. They see that the more they are able to release any sense of doership—a sense that they are the supposed hero who's helping these other people out there—the more they will be able to alleviate suffering and experience peace in their own hearts and minds.

So you see, the story really isn't about the hero, and it never was. It's about dissolving the notion of self and the ego that separates the hero from their ultimate reality. The story is about interconnectedness with the whole. When the hero feels this, it becomes impossible to do anything but alleviate suffering because any sense of separation dissolves. The hero remains a part of the whole, feeling everything, and in some way untouched by any of it. The hero does the work that needs to be done while renouncing attachment to the outcome. Here the hero discovers resilience as they begin living out their ultimate destiny. There is nothing, perhaps, that builds more resilience than knowing why you were put on this earth.

This final phase of the hero's journey for me was really the beginning of a whole new one. Within months of teaching veterans, my classes expanded throughout the VA. Soon we were doing clinical research with the Department of Defense and the National Institutes of Health. Eventually, I was a part of developing the clinically-based yoga and meditation programs that are now used throughout the Department of Defense and VA. Together with three other women, we founded Warriors at Ease, a non-profit that has trained hundreds of teachers who teach both Resilience and Trauma Treatment programs at dozens of military bases and veterans hospitals.

I always say that I learned the basics of yoga and meditation in Asia, but it was the veterans who taught me the true meaning of peace. It takes someone who has been to the depths of sorrow to truly know the meaning of peace. There is a feeling that life is living through me now. I show up, I work hard, but it's not at all about me. It's about living and sharing these teachings that can alleviate the root cause of our suffering. When we learn to connect and abide in the part of ourselves that is unchanging, we discover true resilience.

The hero's journey provides us all with an archetype to understand the truths that we can only discover by leaving our ordinary world and undertaking our own journey of separation, initiation, and return. Whether your hero's journey occurs in the office of a good therapist, or on a soul-searching adventure around the world, or while helping in the cancer unit of a hospital, the quest to find your true self is a universal quest that we all have to walk in our own way. It is the initiation to discover our resilience—the wisdom and inner strength that can help us meet, greet, welcome, and respond to whatever we face in life. Each time we navigate our way through the hero's journey, we give ourselves the opportunity to strengthen our resilience by discovering new vibrancy in life, new sources of wisdom and meaning, and a deeper embodiment of our authentic, true selves.

You are in the midst of your own hero's journey now. Consciously understanding it will unlock new sources of resilience in you. During Class 24, there is a guided meditation that will take you on more of a meditative journey through the process I've just described here today. You are welcome to skip to that class next to have an experiential exploration of the hero's journey. Thank you.

Class 3

The Resilient Human Spirit

There are universal principles to strengthen resilience that span centuries, continents, and cultures. These principles are a part of people's individual and collective histories. They can be found in human physiology and throughout societies. While you may have been immersed in these elements your entire life, you can strengthen your resilience by understanding this inheritance that has been passed down through the ages and that still provides support today.

Instinct

- Instinct plays a role in dealing with adversity. Your instincts involve your inborn behaviors, thought patterns, and ways of being that are not learned.

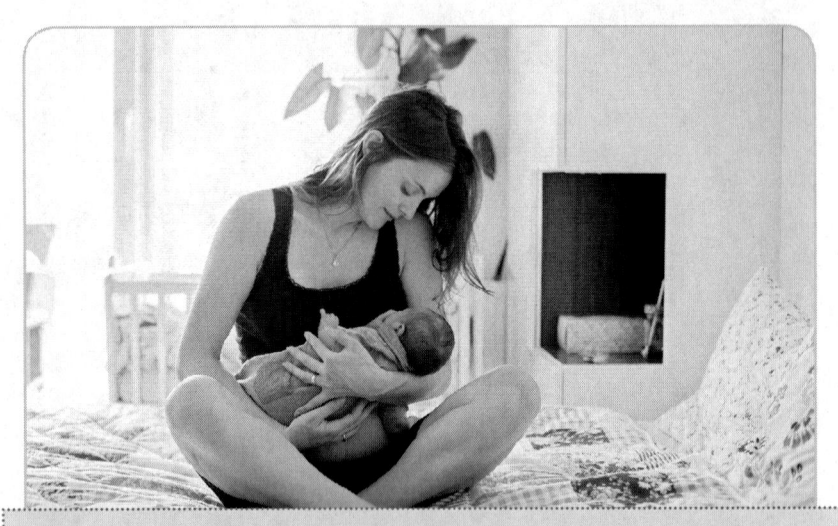

When a baby comes out of the womb, the baby already knows how to nurse. This is a survival instinct that is carried through genetic material.

- You also have instincts that alert you to danger. People have an instinctual nature that has been honed over time to sense potential threats. However, it often takes going through a trauma to remind someone that this strong instinct is always available.

- Another example of instincts comes from shaking: After animals go through something challenging, they physically shake off the trauma. Humans sometimes do this too. People shake with fear in the moment, but they can also proactively shake the body as a means of helping to somatically release the trauma from the body.

- Trauma release exercises, or TRE, can reconnect people with the instinctual nature to shake off something challenging that occurred. Shaking or vibrating the body can be a highly effective means of calming the nervous system and releasing muscular tension brought on by stress or trauma.

- Instinct also extends to the way people communicate and interact with each other. People have an inborn knowing of how to communicate and feel the messages others are sending, even if they are not verbal.

- When a problem arises, for many people, their perception of the problem is the biggest obstacle. People know how to deal with adversity, but they may have forgotten or have narrowed their perspective to such a degree that they can't see the big picture.

- When you calm your brain down and learn to be present and mindful in the moment, you can learn to connect with a deeper instinct of how you are feeling and how those around you are feeling as well. The natural answer of what you need to do in each moment is always present if you are able to get perspective and listen for the answer.

- A potential stumbling point is intellect. Though people value intellect highly, it can sometimes override or block what helps a person feel connected to himself or herself and the world. Intellect is important, but it is not the entire story.

Deep Listening

- Cultures that are not deeply involved in technology show many interesting ways to deal with adversity—ways that you can adapt to your circumstances in a world of smartphones, social networks, and 24-hour news cycles. One such culture is that of the Australian Aboriginals, who anthropologists estimate have lived in relatively the same way for approximately the past 35,000 years.

- The Australian Aboriginals have a word, *dadirri,* that translates as "deep listening." It is based upon the notion that people are constantly trying to create balance and harmony both inside themselves and in the surrounding world. The Aboriginals practice *dadirri* both as a meditation and as an approach to ordinary interactions in daily life, constantly aiming to bring balance between the inner world and outer world.

- The Aboriginals do not see themselves as separate beings. If there is disharmony outside of them, in their family or tribe, they assume that there must also be disharmony inside of them. They see how the individual affects the whole and how the whole affects the individual. *Dadirri* is a means of listening and feeling for what will create harmony and connection where there was separation or imbalance.

- When the Aboriginals have a problem, they listen for the answer. When they perceive illness or emotional upset in themselves, another person, or the world around them, they look for where they are not connecting with the whole to discover where disharmony or unease is occurring. They then listen for how they can help bring balance to the situation and let their actions reflect this.

> **The Golden Rule**
> As you seek to create balance between yourself and the world around you, the golden rule of treating others as you want to be treated is the perfect place to start.

Rites of Passage

- The use of rites of passage is one of the most important ways humans have navigated adversity. Both traditionally and still to the present day, unique stages and transitions in life—including birth, adolescence, marriage, and death—are marked by ceremonies or rituals. Ideally, these rites of passage are used as a means of supporting an individual or group as they embark on a new phase of life.

- Native Americans use rites of passage in very powerful ways. For example, when Native Americans went to war, the hero's journey was laid out. It is fascinating how these ancient cultures realized the importance of community and support to empower someone to navigate adversity.

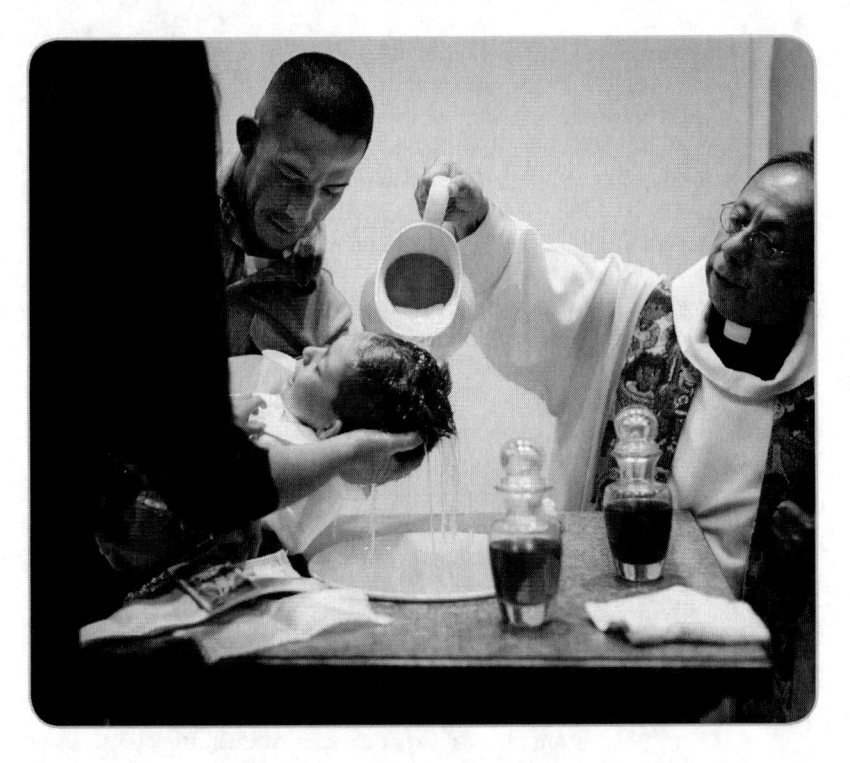

- When the warriors were preparing to go into battle, tribes would create elaborate ceremonies. Members of the tribe would wear colorful and symbolic ceremonial dress. Likewise, the warriors would don war paint, decorate themselves, and prepare their weapons. The ceremonial ways in which they were dressed symbolized the plan for the battle ahead.

- The tribe would chant and play drums, whistles, and rattles in the traditional ways they had been taught by their ancestors. Together, they would dance as they called upon their ancestors and Mother Earth for protection and strength, often through symbolism and offerings. The warriors would then go off to fight their battle.

- When some tribes, including the Lakota, were returning from war, they would paint their faces black, which symbolized victory. In many tribal cultures, the returning warriors would stay on the outskirts of the village for some time. Some tribes used fasting, sweat lodges for purification, and different ceremonies to release the war. When they returned to the village, wounds were dressed with plants and herbal remedies, often as a part of a ceremony.

- Science is now showing that many of the techniques that the Native American tribes were using are in fact ways that the body integrates traumatic or stressful experiences. Hearing voice and sound modulation through chant and music, experiencing physical touch, repetitive movements such as rhythmic dance, and supportive community are all essential ways that people process adverse experiences and return to harmony.

Faith

- Faith plays a crucial role in infusing these ceremonies with life. Otherwise, they are just empty motions. Any mundane action can be made special when you infuse it with conscious intention. When many people think back to what has carried them through times of adversity, faith is often a part of it.

- Faith in something is what sustains people through times of adversity. That can include faith in yourself, a partner, or a teacher. It can also include faith in love, faith things will get better, faith in a country or cause, faith in science, or faith in a higher power. Faith is what gets people out of bed in the morning to try again.

- Ultimately, what you have faith in is what you will see unfolding in your life in one way or another. That is because your actions will reflect where your faith resides.

- Religions are a collection of values and beliefs that people follow, but even if one does not participate in a religion, everyone can have values and beliefs that they lean into as they move through life. Faith in these values is what gives the values life.

- For instance, if a person does not have faith that he or she can accomplish something, it is likely the person won't even try. However, with even the smallest seed of faith inside, then he or she will find the aspiration to get up and begin again. Without faith, no one would have traveled to space, set sail across an ocean, or fallen in love after their hearts had been broken.

Suggested Reading

Frank, *The Diary of a Young Girl*.

Gilbran, *The Prophet*.

Morgan, *Mutant Message Down Under*.

Activities

- Spend some time thinking about your genetic and cultural inheritances that keep you resilient. This can include aspects of your physiology, religion, rites of passage, family traditions, or any other factors that have been passed down to you.

- Think about what traits of resilience you want to pass to the next generation.

- It may also be helpful during this time to reconnect and deepen your connection with the aspects of your resilience inheritance that you would like to increase, such as your faith.

Class 3 Transcript

The Resilient Human Spirit

There are universal principles to strengthen our resilience that span centuries, continents, and cultures. These principles that help us rise and thrive are a part of our individual and collective histories. They can be found in our human physiology and also throughout our societies. While we may have been immersed in these elements our entire lives, we can strengthen our resilience by understanding this inheritance that has been passed down through the ages and that still supports us to this day.

While much of what you will learn in this course reflects what modern science has to share about resilience, this class emphasizes several of the elements that have been essential to transcending adversity for thousands of years—the things that science can't exactly measure, but that have been essential parts of how we build our resilience. These elements include things like human instinct, a universal golden rule, rites of passage, and faith. And by exploring them, we're really uncovering the deepest roots of what makes the human spirit so resilient.

From an historical and philosophical perspective, *Homo sapiens* have had to find a way to deal with challenges and learn from their experiences. Certain traditions and patterns formed over time, enabling humans to cope with the inevitable adversity we all face in life. One of the crucial differences between *Homo sapiens* and other species is our ability to selectively place our attention on certain elements of our environment that we want to focus on while ignoring other elements that do not seem as important. Resilient people have an ability not just to recognize existing patterns, but to create new patterns in a way that helps them find meaning, gratitude, and joy, even in the face of incredible hardship. In other words, resilient people can create new stories when the ones they're already living no longer work for them. Over time, these traits of resilience get passed down through our genes from generation to generation as we discover what helps us survive.

Resilience requires tapping into our inborn sources of strength and natural patterns—the part of ourselves that instinctively knows both when something is wrong and how to heal. Resilience also includes the ability to create healthy new patterns as we gain information and when the old patterns aren't working any longer. Let's start by discussing the role instinct plays in dealing with adversity. Our instincts involve our inborn behaviors, thought patterns, and ways of being that are not learned. Immediately when a baby comes out of the womb, they already know how to nurse. Where does this deeper knowing come from? That's a survival instinct that is carried through our genetic material that has been refined and affirmed over hundreds of thousands of years.

We also have instincts that alert us to danger. Indeed, we have an instinctual nature that's been honed over time to sense potential threats. Over the years of working with all types of trauma, I've heard people say countless times, "I just knew something was about to happen" or "I just knew something was wrong with me." Yet, in many ways in modern society, we've come to value the intellect more highly than instinct or intuition. We've forgotten how to listen deeply to the inner voice that knows. Oftentimes it takes us going through a trauma to be reminded that this strong instinct is always available inside of us. Oftentimes trauma reunites us with that instinct.

Given we are discussing this primordial part of ourselves that we call instinct, let's briefly look at the animal kingdom to see how they deal with adversity. In many ways, animals deal with trauma much more easily than we do. They don't take anything that happens to them personally. Animals do not ask, "why me" when something bad happens to them. Instead, they do what they need to do to survive, and then they move on with their lives.

My dear friend Suzi Landolphi, who you will be meeting later in the course, is the founder of Big Heart Ranch in Malibu, which is a very special place where people and animals go to heal each other. Big Heart has a blind mustang named

Tennie who got the name because he only had a 10% chance of living when he was born. He could barely walk, couldn't see, and had a whole slew of other problems. The interesting thing about this sweet horse is that he doesn't seem to know he has a problem. He doesn't mope around feeling bad for himself. If he tries to jump and falls down, he doesn't say to himself, "I'm such an idiot! Why did I fall? I'm so broken! Somebody should have helped me. Look at everything that's wrong with me. I'm worthless." He doesn't say any of that. If he falls, he gets up, shakes himself off, and tries again.

But speaking of Tennie shaking himself off, have you noticed that after animals go through anything challenging, they always shake their bodies? They physically shake off the trauma. As humans we sometimes find ourselves doing this too. We shake with fear in the moment, but we can also proactively shake the body as a means of helping us somatically release the trauma from our body. Trauma release exercises, or TRE, can reconnect us with our instinctual nature to shake off something that's challenging that occurred. Shaking or vibrating the body can be a highly effective means of calming the nervous system and releasing muscular tension brought on by stress or trauma.

Instinct also extends to the way we communicate and interact with each other. We have an inborn knowing of how to communicate and feel the messages others are sending, even if they're not verbal. Tennie is interesting in this respect, too, because horses primarily communicate visually with their eyes, but Tennie is blind and always has been. One of the ways horses warn each other to get away is to pin their ears back. Tennie has never seen another horse do this, but when one of the horses messes with him, he instantly pins his ears back as a warning. It's his instinct, and he has his own way of knowing how to survive—not because someone taught him or because he is particularly physically strong, but because that instinct was born inside of him, passed down through thousands of years of genetic material.

Most of the time, our perception of the problem is our biggest obstacle. We know how to deal with adversity, but in many ways, we've forgotten or have narrowed our perspective to such a degree that we can't see the big picture. When we calm our brains down and learn to really be present and mindful in the moment, we can learn to connect with a deeper instinct of how we are feeling, and how those around us are feeling as well. The natural answer of what we need to do in each moment is always present if we're able to get perspective and really listen for the answer. Think about it: You survived even your worst moments.

If we look at ourselves from a human development perspective, the human brain developed very big, very quickly relative to the other parts of the body, which resulted in us having stronger intellects and in many ways forgetting all about our inborn instincts. In some ways, moving past just our instinctual nature is why *Homo sapiens* have evolved as a species, but as we see now with the ailments facing modern society, including anxiety, depression, addiction, and so many more, our loss of connection with our inborn instincts is also causing tremendous suffering. The intellect that we value so highly, sometimes to the point of worship, can sometimes override or block what helps us feel connected to ourselves and the world around us. It's not to say that the intellect is not important. It's just to say that the intellect is not the whole story.

So, instinct is one of the elements that has supported human resilience across the history of our species. Other elements can be discerned by looking at traditional cultures. Cultures that are not technologically involved show many interesting ways to deal with adversity—ways that we can adapt to our circumstances in a world of smartphones, social networks, and 24-hour news cycles. One such culture is that of the Australian Aboriginals, who anthropologists estimated have lived in relatively the same way for approximately the past 35,000 years.

The Aboriginals have a word, *dadirri*, that translates as "deep listening." It is based on the notion that we are constantly trying to create balance and harmony both inside of ourselves and in the world around us. The Aboriginals practice *dadirri* both as we would meditation and as an approach to ordinary interactions in daily life, constantly aiming to bring balance between the inner and outer worlds. The Aboriginals do not see themselves as separate as often as we do. If there is disharmony outside of them, in their family or tribe, they assume that there must also be disharmony inside of them, too. They see how the individual affects the whole and how the whole affects the individual. *Dadirri* is a means of listening and feeling for what will create harmony and connection where there was separation or imbalance. Passed down from one generation to the next, *dadirri* practice is a means of living in wholeness. When the Aboriginals have a problem, they listen for the answer. When they perceive illness or emotional upset in themselves, another person, or the world around them, they look for where they are not connecting with the whole to discover where disharmony or dis-ease is occurring. They then listen for how they can bring balance to the situation and let their actions reflect this.

It's interesting because when I learned about that, I immediately thought about a daily struggle that occurs between my son Santiago and me. Our lives are full, and I often move extremely quickly trying to balance family, work, home, and spiritual practice. He likes to move slowly, taking his own sweet time at a snail's pace. So I thought, what would happen if I brought myself into balance—if I slowed down to a normal, balanced pace. Yeah, maybe not everything on my to-do list would get done, but if it eliminated me having to say, "Come on, buddy, hurry up!" ten times a day, it may be worth it. It took a few days of me slowing down for Santiago to start moving at a normal pace. It was amazing what occurred. And then when I start moving too quickly again, Santiago slows me down and reminds me. It's unconscious, but we are seeking to bring each other into balance. If we both stay balanced, our home feels more harmonious.

It's fascinating; in some ways, we are all innately trying to balance each other out in our homes, our communities, our offices, and the world as a whole. You can see it all around us. When one political voice starts screaming too loud and moves too far to one side, another voice starts screaming louder and moves farther towards the other extreme. Nature is the same too. Nature naturally moves towards creating balance or equilibrium. We all are. The most important thing we can do to bring balance to the world is to bring our own lives into balance.

As we seek to create balance between ourselves and the world around us, the golden rule of treating others as we want to be treated is the perfect place to start. The golden rule is a principle that we can find in every culture and religion around the world. Christianity says, "Love thy neighbor as thyself." Judaism says, "What is hateful to you, do not do to your fellow humans." Islam says, "Hurt no one so that no one may hurt you." Hinduism says, "This is the sum of duty: to do nothing to others which would cause them pain." Buddhists call it karma and say, "What you do to others will be done to you." The Shawnee Tribe says, "Do not kill or injure your neighbor, for it is not he or she that you injure; you injure yourself." The golden rule is really about imagining how someone else feels and acting in a way that is respectful of that.

We might be quick to say, "Yeah, it's nice that all of these religions put forth this belief, but in the meantime they're all killing each other." The degree to which this exists feels like a powerful call to action to return to what unites us instead of what makes us different. If we look to the leaders who have shaped history, we can see many situations where it has been practiced, whether through protecting people who are unable to protect themselves, as we saw in the Holocaust, or through Abolition and Civil Rights campaigns. The golden rule isn't just a theory; it's meant to be a practice that we live out in modern life when something is causing suffering, be it a personal problem or a social issue. You can practice for whatever suffering you feel or perceive. It's especially powerful when two adversarial sides both practice. The practices only become real when we live them in our own unique way.

To me, loving my neighbor as myself includes feeling their pain as if it was my own, wishing for their freedom from suffering, taking whatever actions I can to alleviate it, and sending them love. It's similar to the way I love my child, only I try to extend the quality of selfless love out to all beings, which is easier said than done. The practice that has best helped me do this, especially in challenging situations, is actually a Buddhist practice called *tonglen*. *Tonglen* means "giving and receiving." It comes from a beautiful genre of texts called *lojong* that teach you how to cultivate compassion. Regardless of what spiritual path the practice comes from, *tonglen* feels to me similar to what Jesus was doing when he cured the sick, multiplied the loaves of bread and fish to feed the hungry and poor, and expressed his humility by washing the feet of those who came to him in devotion to show all were equal. It seems as if it is also what he was doing when he took on the sins of humankind as he died. It is a very powerful practice for cultivating compassion and truly understanding the suffering of others, including your "enemies."

For those interested, here's a very basic description of the practice of *tonglen*. It's a much larger practice than this, but even practiced in very basic form, it can be really powerful. So here goes: You practice by visualizing a situation where adversity is present. This can include a person who is challenging you, the illness of someone, or a problem existing in the world, like hunger or war. You breathe the pain and suffering into your heart. As you breathe it in, you visualize the suffering being destroyed. Then you breathe out, sending love and light to all affected by the situation. Do this for a while—several minutes at least. Think and feel deeply into the root cause of the suffering while trying to feel the pain as if it's your own. If it's hard, well, that's why they call it a practice. Keep in mind, feeling it does not excuse the situation. Feeling it helps you understand it.

You can also do the practice with your own pain and suffering. Breathe the pain into your heart and breathe out, sending yourself love and light. This can also apply in relationships and so many other contexts. If you would like to learn more about *tonglen*, there are many good descriptions and guided practices online. Personally, I like Jetsunma Tenzin Palmo's teachings on the subject. Links are included in the guidebook.

Keep in mind that doing this practice does not make okay the hurtful actions of another. It is a means of understanding why they are the way they are, or why you are the way you are; cultivating compassion; and not being personally crippled by anger, hatred, fear, or any state of mind that may cause a feeling of inaction or make you act in a way you may later regret. Personally, this practice helps me bring to life the golden rule, to love my neighbor as myself. *Tonglen* sometimes reveals actions we feel drawn to take as a result of the experience. Hopefully after practicing, that action arises from a deep ground of stillness and compassion instead of a place of impulsive reactivity. If we understand why someone feels the way they do and operate from a place of compassionate action grounded in being, we can be more proactive in our approach to dealing with it in a way that alleviates the root cause of the suffering and creates harmony in the situation.

The specific practice of *tonglen*, and more broadly, the practice of living out of the golden rule, is an empowering practice because it gives us a feeling for what we can do in the world instead of feeling crippled by it. And that's a crucial part of developing resilience. We may not be able to change the world around us, but we can always change ourselves. If we want people to treat us kindly, we should treat others with kindness. If we want others to tell us the truth, we should speak the truth to others. If we want people to help us when we're having a difficult time, we should help other people. Sometimes the simplest practices are the most overlooked and the most powerful. If we really practice the golden rule, especially when it's challenging, it will change the way we experience the world.

So we've looked at instinct, deep listening, and the golden rule. Let's turn now to one of the most important ways humans have navigated adversity, by using rites of passage. Both traditionally and still to the present day, unique stages and transitions in life, including birth, adolescence, marriage, and death, are marked by ceremonies or rituals. Ideally, these rites of passage are used as a means of supporting an individual or group as they embark on a new phase of life.

Native Americans use rites of passage in very powerful ways. When we look at the ways in which Native Americans went to war, we can see the hero's journey laid out in front of us. It's fascinating how these ancient cultures realized the importance of community and support to empower someone to navigate adversity. While many of us will never be going to war, we all navigate different life challenges and transitions, so it's useful to see the way collective support and ritual can sustain us during these times.

When the warriors were preparing to go into battle, tribes would create elaborate ceremonies. Members of the tribe would wear colorful and symbolic ceremonial dress. Likewise, the warriors would don war paint, decorate themselves, and prepare their weapons. The ceremonial ways in which they were dressed symbolized the plan for the battle ahead. The tribe would chant and play drums, whistles, and rattles in the traditional ways that had been taught to them by their ancestors. Together they would dance as they called upon their ancestors and Mother Earth for protection and strength, often through symbolism and offerings.

The warriors would then go off to fight their battle. When some tribes, including the Lakota, were returning from war, they would paint their faces black, which symbolized victory. In many tribal cultures, the returning warriors would stay on the outskirts of the village for some time. Some tribes used fasting, sweat lodges for purification, and different ceremonies to release the war. One legend recounts that, when the war had left the warriors, they would go down to the river to wash themselves clean before returning to the tribe.

When they returned to the village, wounds were dressed with plants and herbal remedies, oftentimes as part of a ceremony. Ceremonies including song, dance, and other rituals were performed. Many tribes would wear masks to invoke certain Gods and drive out evil spirits. Other tribes participated in healing medicine wheel ceremonies that sometimes would last for many days. Touch was also an important part of the ceremonies. Scars symbolized bravery and fortitude and were often touched by others in the tribe as a means of tapping into their strength. Warriors would tell their stories from the battlefield, and those stories would become a part of the collective legends of the tribe.

Science is now showing that many of the techniques that the Native American tribes were using are in fact ways that the body integrates traumatic or stressful experiences. Hearing voice and sound modulation through chant and music, experiencing physical touch, repetitive movements such as rhythmic dance, and supportive community are all essential ways that we process adverse experiences and return to harmony. We can also find ceremonial rites of passage throughout every religion. Whether the Bar and Bat Mitzvah in Judaism, Baptism in Christianity, or receiving an empowerment in Buddhism, ceremonies mark the threshold, the crossing from one stage of life into another. Similar to the way a lamp won't light unless you plug it into the wall, followers of religions feel that these rites of passage mark an infusion of energy where one is connected with God or a power larger than themselves in a new way. Many people feel that it supports them in the next phase of life.

Of course, faith plays a crucial role in infusing these ceremonies with life. Otherwise, they're just empty motions. Any mundane action can be made special when we infuse it with conscious intention. *Vi va sa* is a beautiful and potent Sanskrit word. *Vi va sa* translates literally as "breath," but it also carries a deeper connotation, which translates as "that by which one lives in faith" or "trust which carries you through life." In just the same way as the breath is always there silently carrying us through life, faith also does the same. If you think back to what has carried you through times of adversity, faith is almost always a part of it.

Faith in something is what sustains us through times of adversity. That something may include faith in ourselves, a partner, or teacher; faith in love; faith things will get better; faith in a country or cause; faith in science; or faith in a higher power. Faith is what gets us out of bed in the morning to try again. Ultimately, what we have faith in is what we will see unfolding in our life in one way or another because our actions will reflect where our faith resides. Religions are a collection of values and beliefs that people follow, but even if one does not participate in a religion, everyone can have values and beliefs that they lean into as they move through life. Our faith in these values is what gives them life. For instance, if we don't have faith that we can accomplish something, we won't even try, but if we have even the smallest seed of faith inside us, then we find the aspiration to get up and begin again. Without faith, no one would have traveled to space, set sail across an ocean, or fallen in love after their hearts had been broken.

Swami Sivananda once wrote a little piece about faith that I've read many times during moments of hardship. He said:

> Faith electrifies life. You waiver in your experience when your faith is wavering. Faith has the power to remove obstacles in a path. Faith gives enthusiasm and gives expression to aspiration. Be strong in faith and have the right faith enkindled in the heart. The delight of life is in the constant striving for actualizing the ideal. And unless we claim the touch of faith within us, we do not see the joy of a new creation, a new realization, a new life and a new dream.

Oh, I love that so much, I want to say it again. "The delight of life is in the constant striving for actualizing the ideal. And unless we claim the touch of faith within us, we do not see the joy of a new creation, a new realization, a new life, and a new dream."

May we all have faith that we can transcend our adversity, grow wiser in the process, and accomplish our unique dreams. Achieving our goals and dreams is the reward of resilience. As we learned in the hero's journey, you don't get to kiss the prince or princess until you've slain the dragon. The good news is that we are not alone in this journey. From our genetic inheritance to our cultural traditions, our resilience is inextricably connected to those who have come before us, and we are preparing the way for those who come long, long after we leave this precious human life. We never have been alone on this journey, and we never will be.

Class 4

The Consequences of Stress

The conditions of life change all the time. Stress is how the body responds to that change. Though stress is often thought of as a response to negative challenges, any time you adapt to change—such as starting a new job or hearing about a scary diagnosis from a loved one—your stress response activates, which keeps you motived and focused on what you need to do to adapt to the change. This class explores what stress is, what it does to the body and brain, how you can manage it, and how it can help or hurt your ability to be resilient.

What Is Stress?

- Stress has several effects on the body. The peripheral nervous system is the network of nerves that sends and receives messages between the central nervous system—that is, the brain and spinal cord—and the rest of the body. The peripheral nervous system is further broken down into the somatic nervous system and the autonomic nervous system, both of which play a role when it comes to stress.

- The somatic nervous system includes sensory neurons, which take information from the senses to the central nervous system, and motor neurons, which tell muscles how to move. The autonomic nervous system controls involuntary functions, like digestion and heartbeats.

- The autonomic nervous system is further broken down into the sympathetic nervous system and the parasympathetic nervous system. The sympathetic nervous system prepares the body to deal with stress. It speeds up the heart rate, dilates the pupils, and inhibits digestion, for example. The parasympathetic nervous system slows the body back down, and it is associated with rest and relaxation.

> **Fight, Flight, or Freeze**
> A term that is commonly associated with the activation of the sympathetic nervous system is *fight-or-flight*. When startled—for instance, by a clap—your body initially reacts as if it is life-threatening until your higher brain kicks in and recognizes what is actually going on. Relatively recent scientific findings have pointed to a third option: freezing, creating a fight-flight-or-freeze trio.

Causes of Stress

- Everyone experiences stress to some degree. Stress can be caused by financial obligations, social obligations, work, family, traffic, constant connection to the news, email and social media, and countless other demands.

- There are two main types of stress: acute and chronic. Acute stress occurs when an unexpected change to your environment provokes a short-term stress response. Acute stress is what happens when you cram to finish a paper or work assignment, or when your dog bolts out of the house and you have to go find him. This can result in short-term symptoms like headaches, digestive issues, muscle tension, difficulty sleeping, and emotional distress. This kind of stress is more or less manageable, and it actually gives good opportunities to practice resilience.

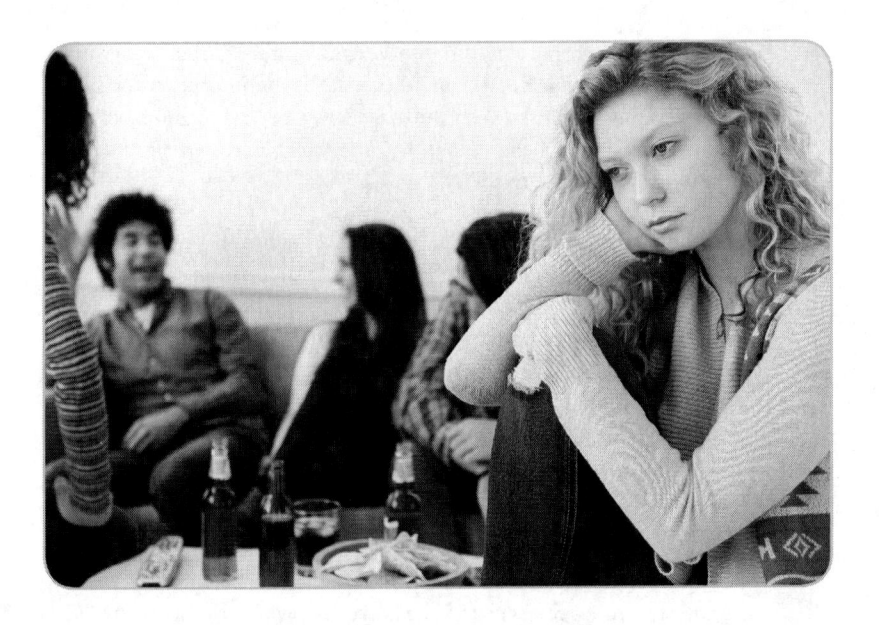

- Chronic stress, on the other hand, is often debilitating, and it can hinder your resilience when you don't intervene. Chronic stress occurs when you feel constant pressure or worry. It happens when someone hates their job, is stuck in an unhealthy marriage, has unstable housing, or is constantly short on money.

> According to the American Psychological Association, nearly 25 percent of Americans report experiencing regular high stress, and 50 percent report experiencing regular moderate stress.

- Sometimes, chronic stress happens as a result of trauma or other hardship from childhood, which leaves a lasting impact on the belief and nervous systems. When this happens, a person might experience hyperarousal and believe that no one can be trusted or that one shouldn't ever make mistakes.

- Chronic stress can lead to an abundance of health problems. Over time, it lowers the amount of serotonin and dopamine in the brain, which can lead to depression. High blood pressure, stroke, and cancer are other health problems that can stem from stress. Perhaps one of the most dire consequences of chronic stress is that it can leave a person feeling disconnected from themselves and others, and this disconnection can contribute to suicide and violence.

The Effects of Stress

- Stress changes the body and brain. For example, it changes the size of brain structures. Stress causes the amygdala, which is heavily involved in the experience of fear, to grow. Stress also causes the hippocampus, which enables people to form memories, to shrink. Stress also causes the prefrontal cortex, where people's most advanced thinking and problem solving occurs, to go offline. This can make it harder to think through one's actions and make decisions.

- Stress also makes people age faster. Research by Nobel Prize–winning biologist Elizabeth Blackburn has shown that the length of the telomeres has a direct correlation with the aging process. Telomeres are the protective structures at the end of chromosomes. The longer the telomeres, the slower the aging process. Stress shortens telomeres.

- Stress also tends to target weak spots. For example, if a person is prone to headaches, headaches become more likely during times of stress.

Reactions to Stress

- Stress can be a problem, but one's reaction to the stress can also be part of the problem. For example, if you become stressed about stress, the experience will become compounded. However, if you take away your stressful reaction to stress, you can immediately start to ease a layer of the negative effects caused by the stress.

- It also may help to change your perception of the stress. There are some situations where a certain amount of stress can keep you alert, motivated, and protected from outside threats. In these situations, you can view stress as something that may be helping you instead of hurting you. (This is not to say that you should stay in situations that are chronically stressful.)

> **Stress Management**
> Changing your relationship with stress is one tool that can help boost your ability to bounce back from life's challenges. The rest of this class explores other aspects of stress management so that you can give yourself the support you need to move through stress without ignoring why it's there and why you need it.

The Relaxation Response

- When you are stressed, your sympathetic nervous system is activated, so to de-stress, you want to activate your parasympathetic nervous system. In other words, you want to relax.

- When people are stressed, it is common to lean on consumables like wine or comfort food, but there is a much more effective way to relax: the relaxation response. The term *relaxation response* was originally coined by Herbert Benson of Harvard Medical School. Evoking the relaxation response is characterized by a reduction in the rate of breathing, heart rate, and metabolism.

- The relaxation response shifts the body from the fight-or-flight sympathetic nervous system to the rest-and-digest parasympathetic nervous system. Sometimes this shift happens naturally, but you can also train your body to evoke the relaxation response. There are many ways to access the relaxation response, like breathing techniques, qi gong, tai chi, progressive muscle relaxation, meditation, prayer, yoga, massage, and even activities like knitting.

Mind Training

- The emotional brain activates the stress response, which puts the logical brain, including the prefrontal cortex, in the background. With a stronger logical brain, you will have more control over your emotional brain, and therefore over your stress response. Yoga and meditation are two great tools for strengthening your logical brain.

- Sometimes mind training also requires retraining your thought patterns. For example, if you believe the world is a threatening place, you will likely feel stress most of the time.

- Psychotherapy and tools like iRest—a clinically adapted form of an ancient practice called Yoga Nidra—can be very effective in changing debilitating thought patterns. They create more access to positive thoughts and emotions, establishing feelings of safety, and accepting circumstances that are beyond your control.

Boundary Setting

- A huge piece of stress management is simply knowing what to take on and when. If you're working on a big project at work, it might be best not to take on an additional big project on top of that. Boundary setting also involves things like making sure you give yourself time for exercise, healthy food, and sleep—all of which are crucial for resilience.

- Boundary setting involves recognizing the aspects of stress that you can control. When you start to feel stressed—and it is not helpful stress—or when you're experiencing secondhand stress from others, try taking a moment to think about what is in your control. For example, if you start to recognize unhelpful feelings of stress while watching the news on TV, remember that you can always turn off the TV.

Social Support

- Another component of responding well to stress is social support. Stress is an interpersonal phenomenon. People can contribute to your stress, and you can contribute to theirs. Stress can even be contagious: If someone in your environment is stressed, that person can cause you or others in your environment to feel stressed, too.

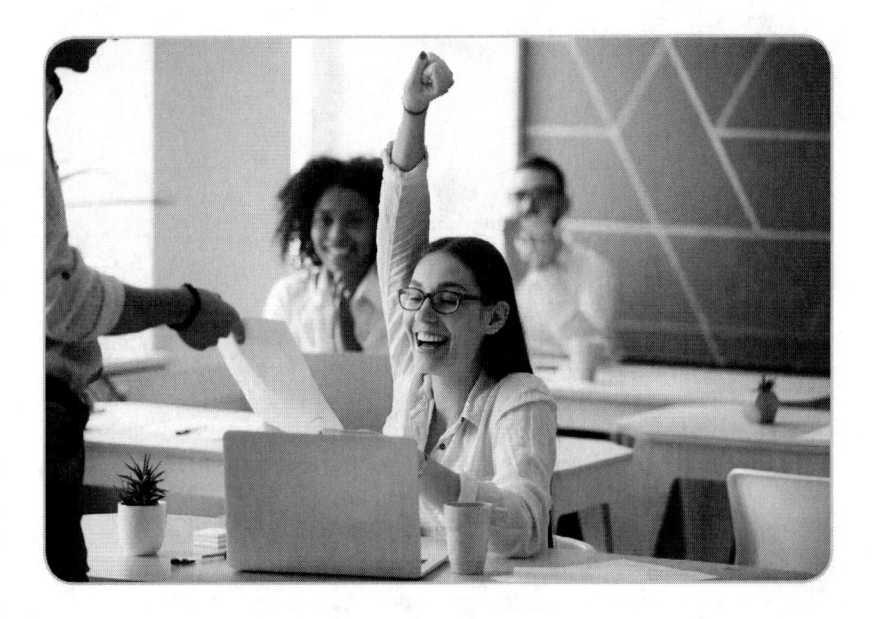

- However, just as stress can be contagious, so can your ability to de-stress. By actively working on managing your stress response and changing your relationship with stress, you can help those around you in a stressful situation rather than adding to all of the stress.

- Additionally, everyone has strengths and weaknesses, and because of that, support can be extremely beneficial in helping you bounce back from stress. There is always someone who can help in some form or another.

- Oxytocin is known as the love hormone. However, oxytocin is released in times of stress. This is your body encouraging you to find support during times of need, and stress is certainly a time of need. The physical benefits of oxytocin, like relaxing your blood vessels, are amplified when you get support from others. You can thank your stress response both for preparing you to take action and for encouraging you to connect with others.

Suggested Reading

Benson and Proctor, *Relaxation Revolution*.

Kabat-Zinn, *Wherever You Go, There You Are*.

Siegel and Bryson, *The Whole-Brain Child*.

Activities

- Answer the following questions:

    » What are your biggest stressors?

    » What aspects of your stress can you affect? Which are out of your control?

    » Can you shift how you are holding these experiences so that they seem less stressful?

    » How can you help alleviate the stress of someone else?

- Think about your favorite activities that evoke the relaxation response. Are there any new activities that evoke the relaxation response that you'd like to explore?

- Complete Practice Class 2 (Class 18), titled "De-Stressing with Your Breath."

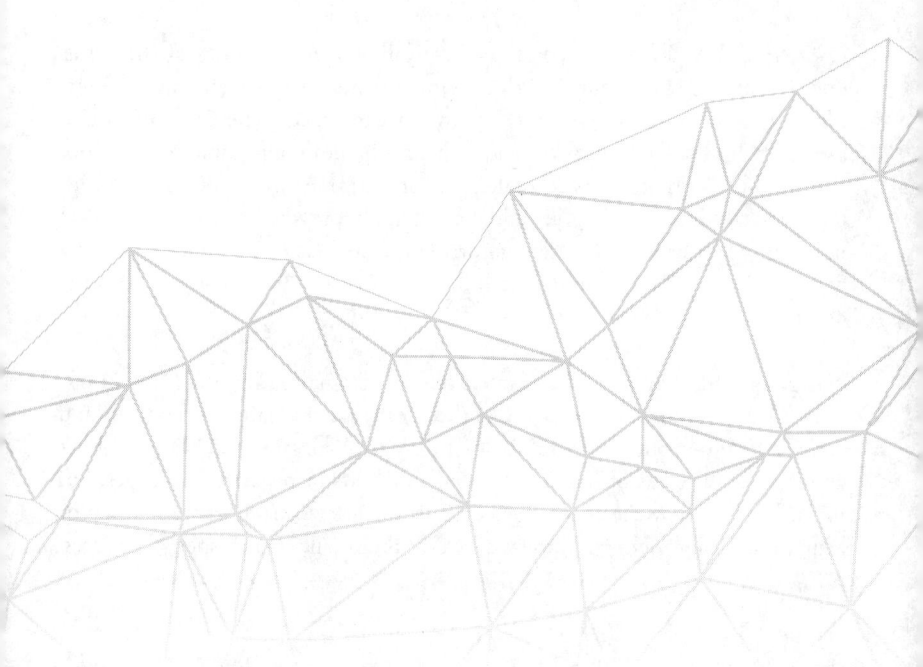

Class 4 Transcript

The Consequences of Stress

One of my favorite activities is ocean swimming. I live on the beach in Fort Lauderdale, and I try to go for a swim every day. It's interesting because every day I go in the ocean, it feels like it has a different personality. Some days it is perfectly flat, clear, and still, and I can swim around for hours enjoying all of the incredible sea life. The next day, a storm can roll in, and the waves are tossing me everywhere and pulling me under. Other days feel peaceful, and then a jellyfish comes to remind me of what pain feels like, or I spot a shark resting on the bottom of the ocean while swimming a little farther out than I probably should be.

Over time, I've come to experience these different personalities of the sea as powerful analogies for daily life. It's the same Atlantic Ocean every single day, yet it's always different, and you never know what to expect. The daily practice of swimming in the ocean provides me with a really meaningful point of reference that both holds me with its constancy and at the same time challenges me with its ever-changing personalities and potential. It provides me with countless new opportunities to cultivate comfort within periods of discomfort—to stay connected to a steadiness and peacefulness, no matter what is happening in the ocean that day.

Navigating the changing ocean waters is a lot like navigating the stress in our lives. The conditions of life, just like the ocean, are changing all the time, and stress is how our body responds to that change. A lot of times, we only think about stress in terms of how we respond to threats or negative challenges, but in truth, any time we're adapting to change, such as when we start a new job or hear a scary diagnosis from someone we care about, our stress response activates, which keeps us motivated and focused on whatever we need to do to adapt to the change. In this class, we're going to fully explore stress: what it is, what it does to our body and brain, and how we can manage it—how it can help or hurt our ability to be resilient.

Everyone knows what it feels like to be stressed. But do you know what exactly is going on in your body when you are stressed? Let's look at that. Our peripheral nervous system is the network of nerves that sends and receives messages between our central nervous system, or our brain and spinal cord, and the rest of our body. The peripheral nervous system is further broken down into the somatic nervous system and the autonomic nervous system, both of which come into play when we're looking at stress.

The somatic nervous system includes sensory neurons, which take information from our senses to our central nervous system, and motor neurons, which tell our muscles how to move. And the autonomic nervous system controls our involuntary functions, like our digestion and heartbeat. Our autonomic nervous system is further broken down into the sympathetic nervous system and the parasympathetic nervous system. Are you following me? The sympathetic nervous system prepares the body to deal with stress; it speeds up your heart rate, dilates your pupils, and inhibits your digestion, for example. The parasympathetic nervous system slows your body back down and is associated with rest and relaxation.

So let's see this all in action. If someone were to sneak up behind you right now and clap really loudly, your somatic nervous system would send sensory input from your ears to the central nervous system, which would send a message to your muscles, perhaps to brace yourself, duck, or turn around. At the same time, your sympathetic nervous system would be kicked into gear, flooding you with stress hormones, like adrenaline and cortisol, in order to prepare your body to deal with the unexpected change in its environment. You might notice your heart starts to race, or perhaps you start sweating a little.

A term that is commonly associated with the activation of the sympathetic nervous system is fight-or-flight. This fight-or-flight response is one of our oldest and most basic physiological functions, designed to, literally, keep us alive. So while obviously someone clapping behind you is not life-threatening, your body initially reacts to the unexpected sound, in a matter of split seconds, as if it were life-threatening—that is, until your higher brain kicks in and recognizes what is actually going on.

Due to relatively recent scientific findings included in the Polyvagal theory, we've been adding a third option to this response—not just fight-or-flight, but fight-flight-or-freeze. And it makes sense. A lot of times our body shuts down and freezes. I saw a frog do it the other day when my son was trying to catch it. My son was worried that he was dead because he suddenly stopped moving entirely, but then the second my son walked away, the frog hopped right off. Humans have the exact same response.

Everyone experiences stress to some degree. As I just said, we were designed to have a stress response. How much stress we experience varies widely, of course, but the majority of us experience at least moderate stress on a regular basis. Our stress can be caused by financial obligations; social obligations; work; family; traffic; constant connection to the news, email, and social media; and countless other demands we face. According to the American Psychological Association, almost 25% of Americans report experiencing regular high stress, and 50% report experiencing regular moderate stress.

An unexpected change to our environment that provokes a short-term stress response is known as acute stress. Acute stress is what happens when you cram to finish that paper or work assignment, or when your dog bolts out of the house and you have to go find him. Acute stress can result in short-term symptoms like headaches, digestive issues, muscle tension, difficulty sleeping, and emotional distress. This kind of stress is more or less manageable and actually gives us a good opportunity to practice our resilience.

Chronic stress, on the other hand, often debilitates us and can hinder our resilience when we don't intervene. With chronic stress, we're not just stressed; we're distressed. Chronic stress is when we feel constant pressure or worry. It happens when we hate our jobs, are stuck in an unhealthy marriage, when we have unstable housing, or never seem to have enough money. Sometimes chronic stress happens as a result of trauma or other hardship from our childhood, which leaves a lasting impact on our belief and nervous systems. When this happens, we might experience hyperarousal and believe that no one can be trusted, or that we shouldn't ever make mistakes. When we have beliefs like this, our stress response isn't only activated in response to an actual threat, but in response to perceived threats as well. And when we've experienced trauma, our spectrum of perceived threat can grow tremendously.

Chronic stress can lead to an abundance of health problems. Over time, it lowers the amount of serotonin and dopamine in our brains, which can lead to depression. High blood pressure, stroke, and cancer are other health problems that can stem from stress, too. Perhaps one of the most dire consequences of chronic stress is that it can leave us feeling disconnected from ourselves and others, and this disconnection can contribute to suicide and violence as well.

So we know that stress can contribute to an array of health problems. Now let's take a look at how stress is actually changing our body and brain. First of all, stress changes the size of brain structures. Stress causes the amygdala, which is heavily involved in our experience of fear, to grow. Stress also causes the hippocampus, which enables us to form memories, to shrink. When we go into fight-or-flight mode, we are primarily using the more primitive part of our brain, also known as our reptilian brain.

So in case growing amygdalae and shrinking hippocampi weren't enough, stress also causes the prefrontal cortex, where most of our advanced thinking and problem-solving occurs, to go offline. Not surprisingly, this can make it much harder for us to think through our actions and make decisions. When we are in immediate danger, this response can be very helpful because it ensures that our body is fully focused on fighting the threat or fleeing the scene. But when our stress response becomes activated while we're arguing with a loved one, for instance, the last thing we want is to make decisions without using our prefrontal cortex.

I've already mentioned how chronic stress can increase our risk for depression and cancer. This is because stress can upregulate, or turn on, stress genes. In addition to cancer and depression, these genes can contribute to conditions like heart disease and diabetes. Stress also makes us get older faster. Research by Nobel Prize-winning biologist Elizabeth Blackburn has shown that the length of our telomeres has a direct correlation with our aging process. Telomeres are the little protective structures on the end of our chromosomes that function much in the same way as the plastic tip at the end of a shoelace. The longer our telomeres, the slower our aging process. So guess the effect that stress has on our telomeres. That's right: It shortens them. Evoking the relaxation response, as we do during mindfulness or relaxing exercises, actually lengthens telomeres. The more I learn about what modern science has to say about these ancient practices, the more I want to get on my yoga mat and meditation cushion every single day.

Stress also tends to target our weak spots. If you're prone to headaches, you're more likely to get them during times of stress. If you have a history of a particular physical weakness, like back pain, stress can cause the muscles to tense and once again create the experience of pain in those challenging areas. If you struggle with emotional regulation, controlling yourself during times of stress will be even more challenging.

The effects of stress can change throughout lifespan, too. High stress in childhood can cause cognitive damage, as the stress hormone cortisol can be very harmful to the developing brain. And older adults are met with new types of stress, such as the loss of abilities, the loss of work and perceived purpose, and the frequent loss of friends and loved ones. Not only that, but they also tend to have less physical resilience to stress than when they were younger, causing disease and illness to get triggered more rapidly.

We now know that stress has a lot of negative effects, but this course is about resilience. It's about how we can push through life's challenges and come out on top. And stress is certainly a challenge we all face. Stress can be a problem, but our reaction to the stress is also part of the problem. We get stressed about the stress and then it compounds the experience. If we take away the stressful reaction to stress, we can immediately start to ease a layer of the negative effects caused by the stress.

It may also help to change our perception of the stress. There are, of course, some situations where a certain amount of stress can help keep us alert, motivated, and can play a critical role in protecting us from outside threats. In these situations, we can view stress as something that may be helping us through the situation instead of hurting us. This makes sense when you think about how your body responds to stress surrounding joyful occasions: the adrenaline you get on your wedding day, giving birth to a child, when you find out you passed a huge test you prepared a lot for, or simply when you're trying something new. We almost never think of these rushes of adrenaline as being bad for us, but when our body does the same thing in response to negative events, we typically do.

In a study at Harvard, participants were asked to think of their stress response as helping them by preparing their body to take action. Then they were given an actual stress test. In a typical stress response, our heart rate increases and our blood vessels constrict, but in this study, when participants saw their stress response as energizing them, their heart rates went up, but their blood vessels stayed relaxed, much how they do when we experience positive rushes of adrenaline. Constricted blood vessels are correlated with cardiovascular disease, so keeping those blood vessels relaxed during times of stress can be a real game changer.

So our relationship with stress is part of what determines whether our stress supports us or sinks us. Just remembering that our stress response is there to help us makes stress, well, less stressful! Now this isn't to say that we should stay in circumstances that are chronically stressful. Remember, our stress response is intended to prepare us to take action during times of change or uncertainty. If we recognize that this response is always on while we're at work or in a relationship, it might be a sign that something is not right. Our life balance seems off, and it feels like we can never get out of the hamster wheel. If we can never relax, and it is difficult for our body to activate our parasympathetic nervous system, it makes it harder for our body to maintain homeostasis.

Changing our relationship with stress is one tool that can really help boost our ability to bounce back from life's challenges. We're going to spend the rest of this talk exploring other aspects of stress management so you can give yourself the support you need to move through stress without ignoring why it's there and why you need it.

Let's begin with the concept of de-stressing. When we are stressed, our sympathetic nervous system is activated, so to de-stress, we want to activate our parasympathetic nervous system, or in other words, we want to relax. When we're stressed, it's common to run to a glass of wine or our favorite comfort foods, but there is a much more effective way to relax. It's called the relaxation response. The term *relaxation response* was originally coined by Dr. Herbert Benson of Harvard Medical School. Evoking the relaxation response is characterized by a reduction in the rate of breathing, heart rate, and metabolism. The University of Michigan defines the relaxation response as the "ability to make your body release chemicals and brain signals that make your muscles and organs slow down and [increase] blood flow to the brain."

The relaxation response shifts our body from the fight-or-flight sympathetic nervous system to the rest-and-digest parasympathetic nervous system. Sometimes this shift happens naturally, but we can also train our body to evoke the relaxation response. There are many ways to access the relaxation response, like breathing techniques, qigong, tai chi, progressive muscle relaxation, meditation, prayer, yoga, massage, and even some activities like knitting. In fact, breathing is a tool that everyone can use that actually gives us direct access to our autonomic nervous system. Neuro-Ophthalmologist Mithu Storoni explains how the base of the breathing nerve and the source of stress in the brain are very close to each other, and that this close proximity might be why altering our breathing pattern by taking longer and deeper breaths reduces stress and symptoms of stress in the body. It's as if we were designed with a built-in de-stressing tool. We can even prepare our body to better handle stress by weaving in breathing breaks throughout our day.

Do you remember all of that research I told you about how stress changes the brain? Well, hear this: Initial research on the relaxation response shows that evoking the relaxation response shrinks the amygdala, grows the hippocampus, and gives us more access to our prefrontal cortex, allowing us to stay more focused and rational. A study at Massachusetts General Hospital and Harvard University even found that cortical thickness of meditators between the ages of 40 and 50 was similar to the cortical thickness of non-meditators between the ages of 20 and 30. You heard me right: Meditation can actually keep your brain younger for a longer time, even by as much as a decade! Do you also remember me saying how stress can turn on our stress genes? Well, Herbert Benson's research has started to show that accessing the relaxation response for only 20 minutes a day can turn off, or downregulate, stress genes.

Our stress response gets activated by our emotional brain, and during the stress response, our logical brain, which includes our prefrontal cortex, gets pushed to the back burner. With a stronger logical brain, we have more control over our emotional brain, and therefore, over our stress response. Yoga and meditation are two great tools for strengthening your logical brain. Mithu Storoni explains that yoga can train our stress circuit to increase both relaxation and our ability to use our logical brain during stressful circumstances. She further explains that holding a posture, which often can feel stressful on the body, activates our logical brain, since we have to concentrate on keeping our body steady in the posture, and that when we bend forward, relaxation is activated. So when we're standing in a forward fold, as we'll do during the practice classes, we are simultaneously activating and strengthening our logical brain and our ability to tap into relaxation.

Functional MRIs used in meditation research show that a part of the brain called the anterior cingulate cortex becomes very activated as a result of focused attention that happens during meditation, and that the more experienced someone is at meditation, the more activated this part of the brain becomes. The anterior cingulate cortex has connections to both the emotional and logical brain, and the more it's activated, the more it seems to help people control their emotions, due to the higher activation in our logical brain.

Sometimes mind training doesn't only involve strengthening your logical brain, but it actually requires retraining your thought patterns. As I mentioned earlier, sometimes our belief systems are to blame for contributing to our stress. If we believe that the world is a threatening place, we will likely feel stress most of the time. I've worked with trauma survivors who haven't felt safe in their own bodies, leaving them feeling like there is nowhere to go for them to feel relaxation or safety.

Oftentimes we consume ourselves with our low level problems because we don't really want to tackle the things that scare us the most—the real source of our problems. But when we suffer from chronic stress that stems from these problems, it's imperative that we get to the core of the problem. If we only scratch the surface, the problem will surely arise again. Psychotherapy and tools like iRest can be very effective in changing debilitating thought patterns, creating more access to positive thoughts and emotions, establishing feelings of safety, and accepting circumstances that are beyond our control.

If you've watched my Great Courses series on iRest, I'm sure iRest has come to your mind during this talk. For those of you who aren't familiar with iRest, it's a clinically adapted form of an ancient practice called Yoga Nidra and is the primary tool I use to help both myself and others manage stress. iRest helps with retraining your thought patterns by allowing you to access all of the deeply embedded beliefs that are holding you back and that could be contributing to your stress. In iRest, you learn how to welcome the entirety of what is present in your body and mind, and once you're in a relaxed state, you're invited to bring all of these deeply rooted beliefs to the surface, so that you can safely inquire into their message and how they may be holding you back.

A huge piece of stress management is simply knowing what to take on and when. If you're working on a big project at work, it might be best not to take on an additional big project on top of that. Boundary setting also involves things like making sure we give ourselves time for exercise, healthy food, and sleep, all of which are crucial for resilience. Boundary setting involves recognizing the aspects of our stress that we can control. When you start to feel stressed—and it's not helpful stress—or when you're experiencing second-hand stress from others, try taking a moment to think about what is in your control. So if you start to recognize unhelpful feelings of stress while watching the news on

TV, remember that you can always just turn off the TV. Or if you feel stressed because you and your partner frequently avoid talking about hard topics, try therapy. Instead of letting ourselves be controlled by stress, we can put ourselves in the driver's seat by setting boundaries and making productive choices. This skill becomes much easier once we've practiced mind-training, and our logical brain has more control over our emotional brain during times of stress.

The last component of stress management I want to discuss is social support. I'll devote a whole class to this topic later in the course, but since support is so crucial to navigating stress, I want to take a moment to discuss it here as well. When you think about it, stress is an interpersonal phenomenon. People can contribute to our stress, and we can contribute to theirs. Not only that, but stress can even be "contagious." If someone in your environment is stressed, that person can cause you or others in your environment to feel stressed, too. This is especially the case if you tend to be very in tune with the people around you. But here's the good news: Just as stress can be contagious, so can our ability to de-stress! By actively working on managing our own stress response and changing our own relationship with stress, we are helping those around us in a stressful situation rather than just adding to all of the stress. We're also modeling positive self-care, which can inspire those around us to do the same as they see the benefits in our life.

Stress also manifests differently in different people. I'm sure we've all experienced the feeling of being shocked or surprised at how strongly someone reacted to something that caused them stress, or at how someone didn't react to something that caused you a lot of stress. Everyone has strengths and weaknesses, and because of that, support can be extremely beneficial in helping us bounce back from stress. There is always someone who can help in some form or another.

I'm sure you've heard of oxytocin, also known as the love hormone. But did you know that oxytocin is released in times of stress? This is your body encouraging you to find support during times of need, and stress is certainly a time of need. And the physical benefits of oxytocin, like relaxing your blood vessels, are amplified when we do get support from others. So our oxytocin asks us to find help or to talk to someone about how we're feeling, and when we do, even more oxytocin is released. As you'll learn in the class on community, support is key to resilience, which means that oxytocin is, too! So not only can we thank our stress response for preparing us to take action, but we can also thank it for encouraging us to connect with others.

Stress really provides us with the opportunity to practice what resilience is all about—withstanding difficulties and bouncing back from adversity. The tools in this class teach us how to manage and reframe stress, which shields us from all of stress's many potential harmful consequences. There will always be stress, but stress doesn't always have to be stressful. And once we recognize this, our stress becomes even easier to navigate. This is how we thrive.

Class 5

Mastering Physical Resilience

Physical resilience is the body's ability to bounce back easily from physical stress, illness, or injury, which requires an extra set of skills above and beyond strength training and even physical fitness. This class looks at how you can build these skills. Keep in mind that physical resilience is both what you do and how you do it.

Setting Goals

- Setting physical fitness goals is something many people have done before, only to burn out or let it trickle off. Rather than setting you up for idealistic physical resilience goals that may never be achieved, at which point you will feel like you've failed, this class recommends a different approach.

> The best exercise is the one that you actually do.

- A good starting point is setting out to do something every day. You can pick what it is and how long you do it, but you have to absolutely commit to doing it every day. It could be getting a Fitbit and making sure you walk 10,000 steps a day, or 5,000, or 2,000. It could be doing a half-hour of yoga, taking an aerobics class, or swimming. Pick something and then commit to it.

- Perhaps you want to set a big, audacious goal, like completing a challenging triathlon. Even then, it is still important to create a plan that is made up of many small, obtainable goals along the way that will help you get to your ultimate goal.

- Whatever goal you pick, make sure it is compelling for you. For example, losing 20 pounds is not compelling. The reason you want to lose 20 pounds is compelling.

Willpower

- Many people who set physical fitness goals depend on their willpower alone to make it happen. There are some people who have a tremendous capacity to utilize willpower in achieving their goals, while others are not as capable.

- There are ways to cultivate willpower, and there are also ways to create a backup plan for achieving your physical resilience goals, just in case your willpower fails on a given day. The secret method for boosting your willpower is to create a very strong connection with why you are doing something.

- The stronger your reasons for doing something are connected to your values, the more solid your willpower becomes. The more you reflect upon why you are doing something and feel connected to those reasons, the more likely you are to do it.

- It is also helpful to pick an activity you genuinely love and then do that activity in places where you genuinely enjoy being. Even if it is not fun 100 percent of the time, physical activity should be fun at least a healthy percentage of the time.

- You can also make physical activity a part of your lifestyle. For example, you might walk or bike to your destination instead of getting in the car, or take the stairs instead of an elevator.

- Once you find an activity you like, find ways that you can make it even more fun. For instance, you might do the activity outdoors instead of inside. You can add music, bring friends along, or sign up for a charity race. You will be many times more likely to do something if you enjoy it rather than if it is drudgery.

Choosing Your Exercise

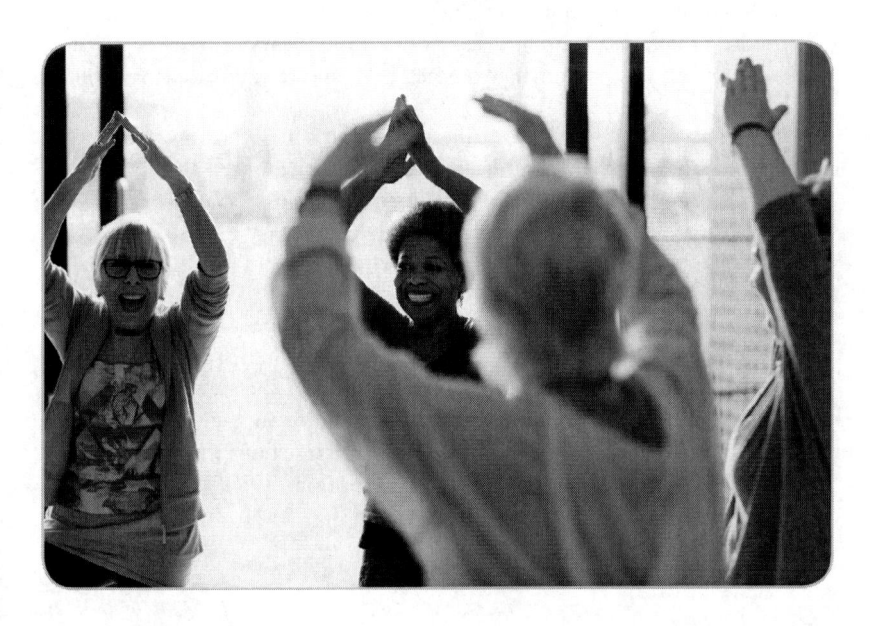

- It is also essential to pick the type of physical exercise that is right for your body. Every human body comes into the world with different needs. People all have different constitutions, ages, tendencies, injuries, and strengths.

- It helps to consult an expert like a doctor, physical therapist, or experienced personal trainer on what activities are best for you. If you haven't worked out in some time or have a history of accidents or injury, go slow and build toward your goals. If you injure yourself the first week, you are far less likely to continue. Keep listening to your body and discovering what it needs.

- When you are selecting the type of training you would like to do, there are several key factors that experts recommend as the pillars of solid physical fitness. These include cardiovascular fitness, strength, flexibility, and balance training.

Measuring Physical Resilience

- People have more ability now to measure physical resilience than ever before. One of the fastest and easiest ways to measure physical resilience is by studying your heart rate and your heart rate variability.

- The heart rate measures the number of times your heart beats per minute. Studying your heart rate both at times of rest and activity can give a good indicator to your level of cardiovascular fitness. Check with your doctor to see what heart rate is optimal for rest and activity, and that honors your age, size, and weight.

- Heart rate variability, on the other hand, measures specific changes in time between your successive heartbeats. Heart rate variability is one of the best ways to measure the state of the autonomic nervous system. This is important because the autonomic nervous system is involved in all of the automatic physical functions that relate to how the body processes stress and recovers from it. This includes blood pressure, cardiovascular disease, blood sugar levels, and other factors.

- Low heart rate variability shows that the heart is under stress while exerting. High heart rate variability is for the most part a good indicator your body is able to tolerate stress or to bounce back quickly when it is stressed. In general, high heart rate variability measured during rest is more favorable to low heart rate variability.

- Measuring heart rate variability easily requires a device. Fortunately, there are many on the market today. They are simple to use and easy to track with a smartphone.

Rest and Sleep

- Another important factor in maintaining physical resilience is to know when to stop and rest. Check in with yourself on a regular basis to make sure what you are doing is still feeling good. Additionally, if you have an injury, give it time to heal to avoid reinjury. Remember to take time to relax after doing any physical activity.

- Sleep is also one of the most important factors in maintaining physical resilience. The average adult needs eight hours of sleep per night. That is the amount of time it takes the body to rest and restore itself. When the body doesn't get enough sleep, the person begins to physically, emotionally, and mentally deteriorate. Committing to healthy sleep patterns is one of the most important things you can do to boost your physical resilience.

Rhythms
Rhythms are important. They teach the body to know naturally when it's time to go to sleep, when it's time to become hungry, and when it's time to wake up. For example, a person will probably be less likely to binge on food if he or she isn't absolutely starving when dinner comes around. He or she will be likely to get a full night's rest by sticking to a regular bedtime and wakeup time.

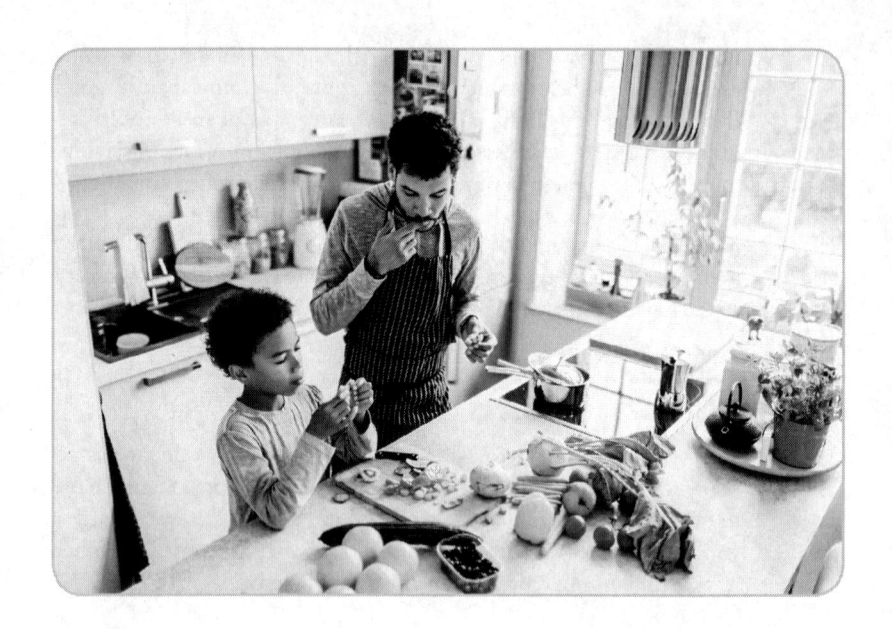

Nutrition

- Nutrition is another essential point for building your physical endurance. The foods you eat can either strengthen your body's resilience or create stress and illness in your body.

- If you want your body to perform well, it needs to be properly nourished, which includes getting the right amount of protein, carbohydrates, fats and oils, vitamins, minerals, and amino acids. Everyone is different; for instance, the optimal diet for a body builder and an elderly person trying to overcome cancer may be quite dissimilar. It's important to stay tuned into what your body needs and always keep listening for what it's asking for, acknowledging how these needs change all the time.

- Integrating food as part of resilience can also include the process of preparing and eating the food. By cooking for yourself and people around you, you can become more aware of what you are putting in your body. It can also be a fun and meaningful way to build connection with people.

- You can also take steps to make obtaining proper nutrition easier on yourself. For example, you are more likely to eat well if there is good food in the fridge than if you have to order takeout every night. If you know you are going to have a busy week, prepare on Sunday by making a couple of dishes that you can heat up throughout the week.

Monitoring Yourself over Time

- As you take the steps to maintain a healthy diet, don't forget that a good doctor can give you a wealth of information about how your body is performing. Blood and urine tests are a great way to see if you are getting all the proper nourishment you need. It is a good idea to get tested at least once a year.

- It is also possible to track certain biochemical markers using metabolic panels for potential disease or imbalances. Nutrition support is often used in cases where there are issues to bring the body back into a healthy state.

- Many people have food allergies that they are unaware of. If you have any physical symptoms of headaches, inflammation, or digestive issues, it's a good idea to get a food allergy test to see if what you are eating may be causing the problem.

- Talk to a doctor, dietician, or health coach to learn more about what diet is best for you. Remember, the way you feel after eating a food is one of the best ways to measure if it is helping you or holding you back.

- Finally, disease prevention and early diagnosis is one of the most important ways to stay physically resilient. If you have not been to the doctor in the past year, call your health-care providers to schedule appointments. Early detection of all diseases and physical injuries is key to bouncing back as quickly and effectively as possible.

Suggested Reading

Van der Kolk, *The Body Keeps the Score*.

Zolli and Healy, *Resilience*.

Activities

- Answer the following questions:
    - » Who do you consider to be a role model for physical resilience?
    - » What do you think makes that person so physically resilient?
    - » What are you doing to build your physical resilience?
    - » How are you measuring it?
- Take some time to really focus on your physical resilience over the next couple of days. What could you do to improve your physical resilience?

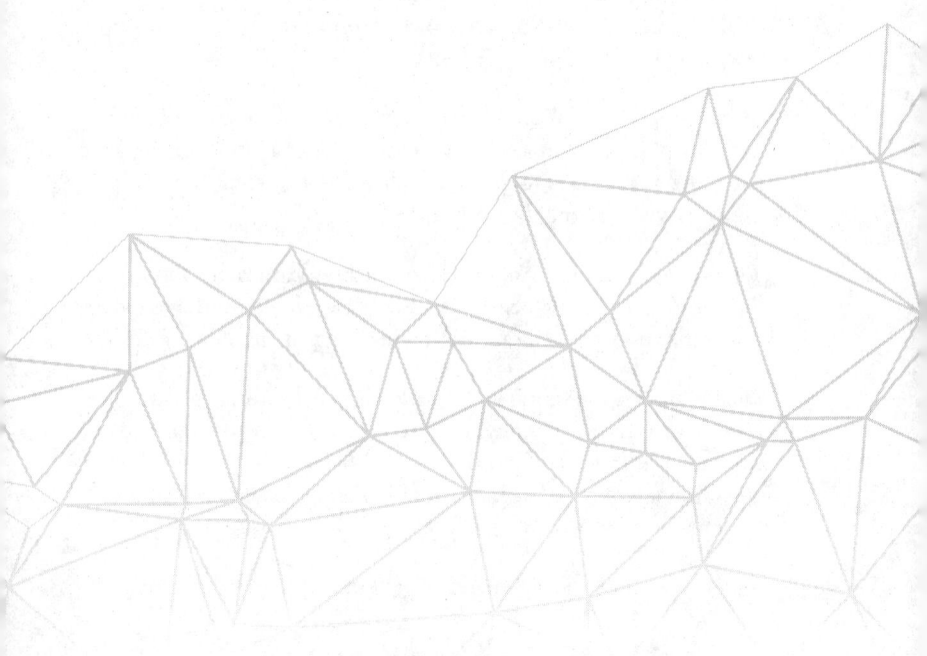

Class 5 Transcript

Mastering Physical Resilience

Take a moment now to close your eyes. Settle into the surface you're seated upon. Take a few deep breaths, and welcome the mind to start to settle. Now envision someone who you perceive as physically resilient. It can be someone you know or someone you've seen on television. What pops to your mind first? What do they look like? What do they do that makes them resilient? How can you tell they are resilient? Now take a few moments to welcome another deep breath as you open your eyes and come back to the class.

It's interesting; I individually asked 20 people to do this practice I just guided you through. 15 of them envisioned an athlete, four envisioned a soldier, and one of them envisioned their mother, who survived cancer and then became a triathlete. Anecdotally, 17 of the people mentioned as physically resilient were male. Serena Williams got two mentions. When I asked them to describe what the person looked like, most of the descriptions were of these Herculean-sounding individuals who were large and physically strong. Even the woman whose mother had cancer described how her mom ended up with bigger muscles than her daughter who played Division 1 college volleyball. When I asked what they did that made them resilient, most spoke about hard work to be the best, exercise, strength training, and maintaining a healthy diet. A few mentioned good genetics. Several mentioned youth as a factor. When I asked how they could tell that they were physically resilient, all but one mentioned they seemed physically strong as one of the factors.

It's always fascinating to see what makes an exceptional person so good at what they do. And certainly it's no mistake that so many people mentioned athletes as their image of physical resilience. Sports are one of the most exciting places to experience the pinnacle of fitness and resilience. The person whose response really stood out to me is a friend and business colleague named Sven Gade, who is also an accomplished triathlete at 60 years old. Sven just finished the Escape from Alcatraz Triathlon, which is a pretty extreme test of physical resilience. When I asked him the question about envisioning a physically resilient individual, he immediately mentioned the tennis champion Roger Federer as his example. For those of you who don't know, Roger has the current record for being the oldest number one singles tennis player in tennis history.

Sven described how Roger's style of play isn't about overpowering the ball, but rather being masterful in his execution of what he does, noting the difference between over-effort and fluidity. There is wisdom in how he plays that comes from his decades of experience. He then mentioned that while, of course, Roger trains hard—unbelievably hard—he also knows when to rest, an essential practice for maintaining physical resilience. Roger knew when he needed to stop, as he did after an injury in 2016. He came back with a vengeance from his break and played better than he had in years. He listened to what his body was asking for, and he took action to give it what it needed.

Sven then spoke about how Roger genuinely loves and enjoys what he does, and that he looks like he is playing—the having fun kind of playing—both when he is in the midst of a match, but also when courtside or between points. He seems like he would be on the court having fun even if no one was there in the stands watching. Between points, he's always playing around with a ball, trying out a crazy shot, or lobbing a shot over to a ball kid. He seems to find joy not just in the big moments but also in the moments between. In the heat of a match, Roger doesn't force it, and he doesn't get distracted. He's relaxed and fully present throughout the flow of his game. Roger is caring for his physical resilience in many ways, and thus, his body is maintaining peak performance far longer than any athlete in tennis history. Sven never mentioned Roger's physical strength.

It is of course important to keep the body strong because being strong does have an impact on physical resilience. However, resilience is really a much larger topic than just strength, just as Sven's description of Roger illustrates. Physical resilience is our body's ability to bounce back easily from physical stress, illness, or injury, which requires an extra set of skills above and beyond strength training and even physical fitness. As you can see from Sven's response, physical resilience is not just what you do, it's also how you do it.

We have a lot to learn from people who have become masters of their physical bodies so that we can become as effective and as efficient as possible in giving our bodies what they need to bounce back from stress, injury, and illness. While most of us will never be a tennis pro on the USTA circuit, the factors Sven mentioned are factors that we can all cultivate. We, more than anyone else, have a deep understanding of what it feels like to be in our bodies and how they operate. We know what feels good and what works, and we know what doesn't. We too have physical activities that we love and have fun doing. We too can take time to rest. We too can cultivate mindfulness while engaging in physical activities.

Somehow this feels like good news to many of us who are living in bodies that are not necessarily in top athletic form. We live in bodies that are aging every moment with a whole history of accidents, illness, and injuries. We also live in bodies that have an incredible capacity to heal and grow stronger. So often when we look at what is wrong with our bodies, when really our bodies are working so hard in this moment to keep us healthy, alive, and strong. Really, even despite whatever might be wrong with our bodies, there are billions of things happening right in this moment to keep us alive.

There's also one factor Sven didn't mention that I believe is one of the most important factors to achieving physical resilience: showing up. To stay physically resilient, we have to show up to do the things that will help our bodies be resilient. What is the best exercise? The one you actually do. Setting physical fitness goals is something many of us have done before, only to burn out or let it trickle off the moment we get a tight hamstring or something else more interesting comes up. As you've probably guessed by now, in this course, I would rather be honest about our humanness, the reality that we as human beings are not perfect. We are not made of just strengths, despite the story our social media profile may tell. We also have weaknesses. Challenges.

So rather than setting you up for idealistic physical resilience goals that may never be achieved, at which point you will feel like you've failed, let's take a different approach. Let's set small realistic goals for ourselves. Let's start by doing something every single day. You get to pick what it is, and you get to pick how long you do it, but you have to absolutely commit to doing it every day. It could be getting a Fitbit and making sure you walk 10,000 steps a day—or 5,00, or 2,000. It could be doing a half hour of yoga, taking an aerobics class, or swimming. Pick something and then commit to it 100%.

For me, it's 20 minutes of yoga a day. Of course, I love doing a long yoga practice, having hours to go into the ocean for a swim, do my breathing exercises, and everything else that I enjoy, but I'm also realistic. I have a kid, I'm involved in my community, I work full time, and I travel a lot. Yet, I always do my 20 minutes of yoga a day. Or, you may want to set a big audacious goal, like Sven wanting to do the Escape from Alcatraz Triathlon in San Francisco. Even so, it's still important to create a plan that is made up of lots of bite-size, obtainable goals along the way that will help you get to your ultimate goal.

Let's talk now about how we're going to achieve this. A lot of times when we talk about starting something new or commit to do an exercise practice, we will depend on our willpower alone to make it happen. I really encourage you to make an honest, and I mean *really* honest, assessment of your own willpower by looking at your track record and then asking the person closest to you if they agree.

Sure, the movies are filled with people who have indomitable will, and it's really exciting and inspiring to watch. There are some people who have a tremendous capacity to utilize willpower in achieving their goals. Others not so much. And let's be realistic here; off the silver screen and back down here on earth, willpower really does not have a great track record. If it did, alarm clocks would not come equipped with snooze buttons, New Year's Resolutions would last past Valentine's Day, and obesity and addiction would not be the leading killers of people who may otherwise be perfectly healthy and strong.

The good news is that there are ways to cultivate willpower, and there are also ways to create a backup plan for achieving your physical resilience goals just in case willpower doesn't show up tomorrow morning when your alarm clock goes off earlier than it usually does for you to start that new meditation and yoga routine. There is an important secret for boosting your willpower, whether you have iron will or can barely keep your exercise regime alive for more than three days. The secret is creating a very strong connection with why you are choosing to do something. The why is the engine that carries you towards your goal. The stronger your why is connected to your values, the more solid it will become. The more you really reflect upon why you are doing something and really feel connected to those reasons, the more likely you are to do it. And that's why so many people who recover from a serious illness like cancer end up committing so fully to their physical resilience. They've had a taste of why their physical health is so important.

Start by taking Sven's advice and pick an activity you genuinely love, and then do that activity in places where you genuinely enjoy being. If you already have a physical fitness regimen, ask yourself if you genuinely like it and why you do it. If you don't, find something that you want to practice all the time because you actually love doing it, something that you think about even when you're not doing it. Physical activity should be fun—perhaps not 100% of the time, but at least a healthy percentage of the time. There are so many types of physical activity. Find one you really love and one that works for your body. If you genuinely enjoy a physical activity, you are far more likely to do it. You can also make a physical activity a part of your lifestyle. Walk or bike to your destination instead of getting in the car. Take the stairs instead of an elevator. Get a dog that needs to be walked every day. You'll soon begin to wonder if you are taking care of the dog, or if the dog is taking care of you.

Once you find an activity you like, find ways that you can make it even more fun. Do the activity outdoors instead of inside. You can add music, bring friends along, or sign up for a charity race. You will be many more times likely to do something if you enjoy doing it, rather than if it's drudgery.

Having a plan for what you want to achieve and supporting it with clear goals can help a lot of people as well. Your goal may not be to do the Escape from Alcatraz Triathlon like Sven; it may be to take your dog for a walk six days per week. When you set your goal, make sure it is *your* goal. You are much more likely to achieve it if you created the goal, if it's meaningful to you, and it reflects the why you want to do something.

When I was recovering from my car accident, I went to a physical therapist. He laid out all these goals for me that had absolutely nothing to do with what was meaningful to me: measurements on a treadmill, weight numbers to meet, distances I could stretch. I didn't even know what half of them meant. One day I got fed up and said, "I couldn't care less about any of these goals! What I really want to do is be able to hike the Inca Trail in the Andes Mountains. That's a goal I want." He looked kind of shocked for a minute, and then he said, "Okay. Let's aim for that." During moments when I wanted to give up, I would picture myself standing on top of Machu Picchu watching the sunrise. That was the magic moment I was aiming for.

Sure enough, one year later, I hiked for ten days and had almost made it to Machu Picchu. I woke up at 3:30 a.m. to hike to a place where I could watch the sunrise. It poured rain the entire way. My flashlight was lost, so I was hiking along muddy paths next to cliffs with no light in the pouring rain. Finally, I got to the spot. I was so disappointed because it was raining so hard that I didn't think I'd get to see the sunrise. But sure enough, the warmth of the sun began to melt away the clouds. And there I was, watching the sun rise as I stood on top of Machu Picchu. I got my magical moment.

Whatever goal you pick, make it really compelling for you. Losing 20 pounds is not compelling at all. The reason why you want to lose 20 pounds is compelling. It's important to remember to also do it for the sake of doing it and not just the goal. Otherwise, once you've achieved the goal, it may seem like there's another endless goal on the horizon. You may also start to feel like you've failed if you don't reach the goal when really lots of benefits may have come from the practice you did. If you're enjoying what you're doing, you'll keep going. It also helps to have people join you along the way.

This brings us to one of the other factors that can increase your physical resilience: community. We have an entire class on community because that is how important community is to resilience. Oftentimes we will do for other people what we won't do for ourselves. It's a great idea to sign up for a series of classes, join a sports team, hire a trainer, or find an exercise buddy. If you enjoy having a goal in mind and that helps you, you can even sign up for a race or plan a dream vacation with friends. Whether it's joining a yoga studio, a rowing crew, a hiking group, or a ski club, nearly every town has group fitness programs that can be a source of community and support. If you don't find one you like, you can start your own.

It is also essential to pick the type of physical exercise that is right for your body. Keep in mind that the type of exercise we did when we were in college might not be what is best for us later in life, and vice versa. Every human body comes into the world with different needs. We all have different constitutions, ages, tendencies, injuries, and strengths. It definitely helps to consult an expert, like a doctor, physical therapist, or experienced personal trainer on what activities are best for you. If you haven't worked out in a while or have a history of accidents or injury, go slow and build towards your goals. If you injure yourself the first week, you are far less likely to continue. Keep listening to your body and discovering what it needs.

When you are selecting the type of training you would like to do, there are several key factors that experts recommend as the pillars of solid physical fitness. These include cardiovascular, strength, flexibility, and balance training. Please keep in mind here that we could do an entire course on each of these aspects of physical fitness. And if you're interested, The Great Courses offers many activities-based series on subjects such as tai chi, fitness, yoga, nutrition, and much more. Please check the resources section of your guidebook for further information on various aspects of healthy living.

As you dive into the resources, here is a reoccurring theme you might notice: We have more ability now to measure our physical resilience than we ever have before. Even companies are seeing the need to measure if their employees are getting everything they need to stay healthy and productive. I personally do a lot of work with companies on developing corporate wellness programs to improve resilience. While hopefully they are approaching this out of a desire to care for their employees, every client I've worked with also reports increases in productivity, teamwork, and overall morale of their staffs.

One of the fastest and easiest ways we can measure our own physical resilience is by studying our heart rate and our heart rate variability. Our heart rate measures the number of times our heart beats per minute. Studying our heart rate both at times of rest and activity can give us a good indicator of our level of cardiovascular fitness. You'll want to check with your doctor to see what heart rate is optimal for both rest and activity and that honors your age, size, and weight.

Heart rate variability, on the other hand, measures specific changes in time between your successive heartbeats. As it turns out, heart rate variability is one of the best ways to measure the state of the autonomic nervous system. This is important because the autonomic nervous system is involved in all of the automatic physical functions that relate to how the body processes stress and recovers from it. This includes things like blood pressure, cardiovascular disease, blood sugar levels, and many more. Low heart rate variability shows that the heart is under stress while exerting. High heart rate variability is, for the most part, a good indicator that your body is able to tolerate stress or to bounce back quickly when it is stressed. In general, high heart rate variability measured during rest is more favorable to low heart rate variability.

Measuring heart rate variability easily requires a device. Fortunately, there are many on the market today. They are simple to use and easy to track with a smartphone. It's been a really useful biofeedback tool that's allowed me to track and measure my body's resilience. Since I started using it, I'm better able to see what activities or thoughts cause me the most stress, as well as what activities and thoughts can help regulate it. It's a great way to raise awareness. Many professional sports teams and the military are using heart rate variability monitors to help people reach peak performance.

Another important factor in maintaining physical resilience is to know when to stop and rest. Just like Roger Federer, we can learn to value *being* as much as doing. We can discover that, sometimes, stopping an activity for a time will give it even more power and strength when we re-engage with it. Check in with yourself on a regular basis to make sure what you're doing is still feeling good. Does pushing yourself a little harder feel like a good idea? Are you feeling like you're ready to lift extra weight or walk for a longer distance? Conversely, if you have an injury, give it time to heal and avoid re-injury. Remember to take time to relax after doing any physical activity.

Sleep is one of the most important factors in maintaining physical resilience. As I'm sure you know, the average adult needs eight hours of sleep per night. That is the amount of time it takes for our body to rest and restore. When the body doesn't get enough sleep, we physically, emotionally, and mentally begin to deteriorate. Committing to healthy sleep patterns is one of the most important things you can do to boost your physical resilience.

A Tibetan Buddhist friend of mine did a three-year, three-month, and three-day silent retreat. When I asked him about what was meaningful in his retreat, one of the things he spoke about was getting in tune with what his body's natural rhythms and needs actually are. He discovered the best time of day to eat and what foods made him feel best at which times of day. He learned how the foods affected his body. He found the connection between the foods he ate and how they made his body feel. He became hyperaware of his cravings and what was at the root of them. He found the best times of day to nap and exactly how long his body needed to nap in order to find that sweet spot between feeling adequately refreshed but not sleepy. Seasons became more apparent to him, as well as what his body needed in each of those seasons. He said he felt so much more healthy and peaceful when his body found its natural rhythms perhaps for the first time in his entire life.

There are so many ways we override this natural system in modern life. We drink caffeine, have homes filled with bright lights, eat at different hours every day, and stare at screens that trick our bodies into thinking that it's always daylight, when in fact it might be time to go to sleep. Rhythms are important. They teach our body to know naturally when it's time to go to sleep, when it's time to get hungry, when it's time to wake up. If we do not give our body predictable patterns, we cause it unnecessary stress. If we don't eat on certain cycles, our bodies will secrete digestive fluids when we aren't necessarily consuming food.

We will be more resilient when our body knows what to expect. We'll be less likely to binge on food if we aren't absolutely starving when we finally go to eat. We'll be more likely to get a full night's rest when we dependably go to bed and wake up at a certain time, and our body will produce melatonin accordingly.

Nutrition is also a really essential point for building your physical endurance. The foods we eat can either strengthen our body's resilience or create stress and illness in the body. If you want your body to perform well and go the distance, it needs to be properly nourished, which includes getting the right amount of protein, carbohydrates, fats and oils, vitamins and minerals, and, of course, amino acids too. Obviously, the optimal diet for a bodybuilder and an elderly person trying to overcome cancer may be quite different. It's important to stay tuned in to what your body needs and always keep listening for what it's asking for, acknowledging how these needs change all the time.

Having food be a part of your resilience can also include the process of preparing and eating the food yourself. By cooking for ourselves and our families, we become more aware of what we're putting in our bodies. It can also be fun and meaningful way to build connection with the people in our lives. And, while you're doing it, make taking care of yourself convenient. You are more likely to eat healthy if there's good food in the fridge than if you have to order takeout every night. If you know you're going to have a busy week, prep cook for yourself on Sunday by making a couple of dishes that you can heat up throughout the week. You can also pre-chop veggies to make it easy to toss them in a salad or stir-fry. Make life easy and you're far more likely to follow through.

As you take the steps to maintain a healthy diet, don't forget that a good doctor can give you a wealth of information about how your body is performing. Blood and urine tests are a great way to see if you're getting all the proper nourishment you need. It is a good idea to get tested at least once a year. It is also possible to track certain biochemical markers using metabolic panels for potential disease or imbalances. Nutrition support is often used in cases where there are issues to bring the body back into a healthy state. Also, many people have food allergies that they are unaware of. If you have any physical symptoms of headaches, inflammation, or digestive issues, it's a good idea to get a food allergy test to see what you're eating that may be causing the problem. Talk to a doctor, dietician, or health coach to learn more about what diet is best for you. Remember, the way you feel after eating a food is one of the best ways to measure if it's helping you or holding you back.

This brings me to my last point of this class. Disease prevention and early diagnosis is one of the most important ways to stay physically resilient. If you have not been to the doctor in the past year, please pick up the phone and call your healthcare providers to schedule appointments. Your chances of surviving most cancers go up by 90% over the next 5–10 years—that's right, 90%—if they are detected early. Early detection of all diseases and physical injuries is key to bouncing back as quickly and effectively as possible. So please take this as a friendly reminder to pick up the phone right now and call for your appointments. As Swami Vishnudevananda used to say, "Health is wealth. Peace of Mind is Happiness." Indeed, it is true. Our health is the most precious asset we have. The more we care for these physical bodies, the better they will serve us in the long run.

Class 6

Improving Emotional Resilience

This class starts by exploring what emotions are and their fundamental purpose. The class then turns to common ways people are socialized to handle emotions and how that socialization may hinder emotional resilience. Next, the class covers the benefits that come from feeling both positive and negative emotions. The class ends with some strategies for building emotional resilience.

Foundations of Emotions

- Scientifically, emotions are neural impulses with a variety of features that prompt us to take some sort of action. A more relatable definition might be that emotions are individual responses to the situations that you experience. Depending on your emotional resilience, your emotions can either support you or hijack you. Either way, they can completely change the way you experience the world.

- Emotions come in primary and secondary varieties. According to neuroscientist and author Antonio Damasio, primary emotions are innate and enable people to act quickly. Think of primary emotions as those that can be observed in an infant. Infants purely react to their environment and have not yet developed the capacity to have a controlled response to their automatic emotions.

- Psychologists Paul Ekman and Wallace Friesen identified six such emotions: sadness, happiness, fear, anger, disgust, and surprise. New research, however, points to there being only four basic emotions: sadness, happiness, fear, and anger. Even further, some researchers and clinicians believe that there are only three basic emotions: sadness, happiness, and fear.

- Anger is often referred to as a secondary emotion. Secondary emotions are what you feel after having your initial reaction to an experience. They come from your ability to have thoughts and opinions about your circumstances and your primary emotions.

- The fundamental purpose of emotions is twofold. The first purpose is to push you to take some sort of action or to learn from your experience, guiding how you choose to respond to similar situations in the future. The second purpose is to help you communicate and interact with others.

Socialization

- Typically, people avoid things they consider to be bad and welcome things they consider to be good. This raises a question: Which emotions are bad? The answer is that there are not any bad emotions. People are socialized to believe that emotions are good and bad, but in reality, they are all good, because they all help people navigate experiences.

- Many cultures seem to value happiness over honoring the full spectrum of life's experiences. For example, you might make an effort to not cry in front of others, and you might smile and say, "I'm fine," even when you're going through something difficult.

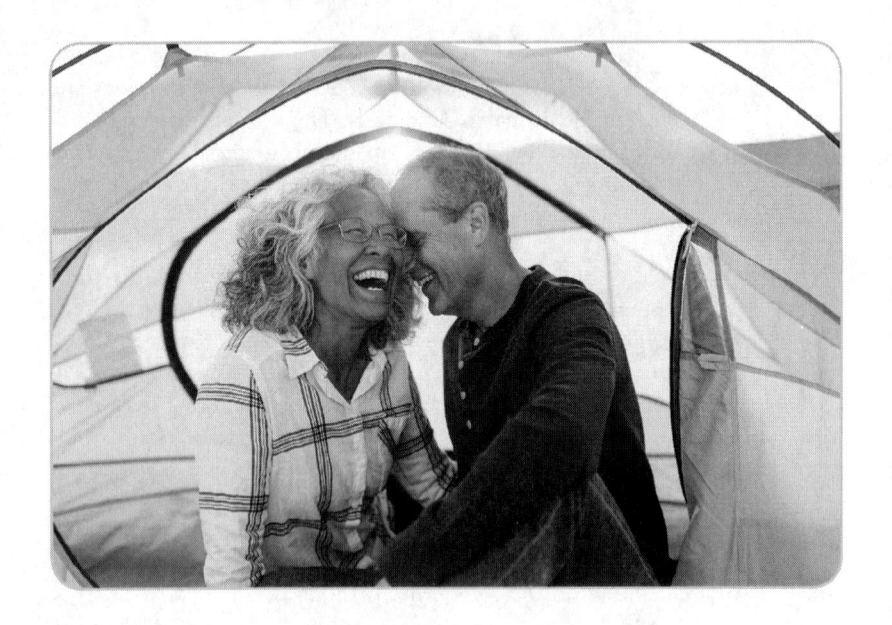

- Two emotions that people tend to have the most difficult time honoring are fear and sadness. For example, when someone says not to cry to a sad person, the goal is usually to make the person feel better. However, this message likely instead sends the message crying is a sign of weakness and makes others uncomfortable. Being told you're OK during times of distress invalidates the emotions you're feeling while distressed.

- Keep in mind that emotional regulation and resilience does not mean you suppress your emotions. Instead, it means listening to the messages they have to give. Try asking yourself questions like these, which can transform the experience:

    » What is present?

» What does that feel like in my body?

» Is there an action this experience is calling me to take in the world?

Positive and Negative Emotions

- When emotions are studied, they are often called positive and negative emotions. Positive emotions are pleasant to feel, like happiness, and negative emotions are unpleasant to feel, like sadness.

- Positive feelings, such as happiness and joy, predict increases in resilience and life satisfaction. According to Barbara Fredrickson's broaden-and-build theory of positive emotions, positive emotions encourage new thoughts and actions that help build internal resources, improve psychological flexibility, and create better relationships.

- However, so-called negative emotions have some positive benefits of their own. Emotions like sadness and fear prepare the body to deal with real or perceived danger by sharpening the memory and helping focus, which can improve one's ability to analyze and act in situations.

- Negative emotions do not interfere with the benefits of positive emotions. Studies on resilience report that all people, no matter how resilient they are, tend to experience negative emotions with similar frequencies. The only difference between the two groups is that more resilient people experience more frequent or higher levels of positive emotions than people who are measurably less resilient. Positive emotions serve as a protection mechanism against the adversities of life, no matter how strong fear, sadness, and other negative emotions become.

- Because positive emotions foster resilience and negative emotions do not detract from it, there is no reason to hide or suppress these emotions. In fact, it is better to address them and learn from their message than it is to keep them pressed down or let them control you.

> **Building Emotional Regulation**
>
> Emotional regulation means you are fully aware and in charge of your emotions. Sometimes being in charge of emotions is defined as not showing emotions, but this is far from the truth. The more you suppress your emotions, the more they're bound to burst out, either as anger or in their original form. The remainder of this class covers three components of emotional regulation that can help you improve your resilience: naming feelings, coping skills, and mindfulness.

Naming Feelings

- In the book *The Whole-Brain Child*, Dan Siegel and Tina Payne Bryson offer brain-based parenting strategies. Many of the strategies for emotional regulation and resilience are geared toward children, but adults can benefit from these exact same skills.

- One of the first ideas in *The Whole-Brain Child* is that in order to control your emotions, you need to know what it is you're trying to control in the first place. The more you practice naming your emotions, both during emotional moments and after, the better you will be able to regulate your emotional experiences.

- There are tools designed to help with this. For instance, the feeling wheel is a tool developed by Dr. Gloria Wilcox to help people name what they are feeling and find the root emotion behind it. You can simply use the wheel to help you name the various emotions you're feeling, or you can use it to trace those emotions back to the center of the circle to help you simplify your emotional experience by bringing it back to a more basic emotion.

- Another way to practice naming feelings is to dig into feelings of anger. Anger is often a secondary emotion that is covering up feelings of sadness or fear. Think about a time you've felt angry in the past or something you are feeling angry about in the present.

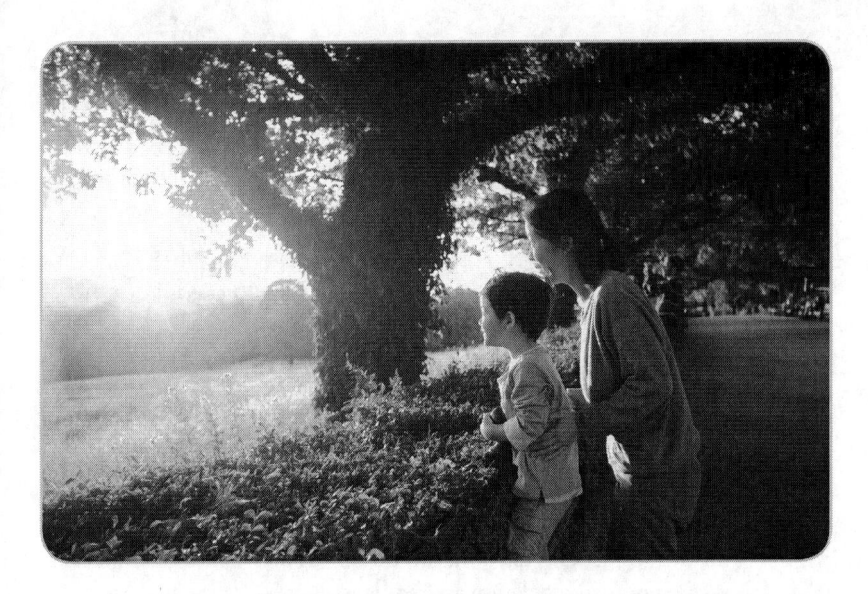

- Look beneath the surface: You might actually be experiencing feelings of sadness or fear that are being masked by anger. For instance, if you yell at your partner for being late, it is possible that your emotion came from a fear that something happened to your partner.

Coping Skills

- When people struggle with emotions, it can lead them to engage in behaviors that harm themselves or others. Managing emotions can be hard, especially when it is a new skill. This is why coping skills are so crucial to developing emotional regulation.

- One simple but very effective coping skill is to normalize the experience of having emotions. No matter what you're feeling, tell yourself, "It's OK that I feel this way." Emotions are always OK; it is the behaviors that follow the emotions that are sometimes a problem.

- Another quick and easy coping skill is to take three deep breaths when you're feeling overwhelmed. Doing this has the potential to quickly lower your heart rate, which will encourage relaxation and feelings of calm.

- Other options for coping skills include going for a walk, taking a yoga class, writing, dancing, cleaning, painting, and so on. These coping mechanisms involve some sort of physical outlet, either through gross motor movements or fine motor movements. Learning to observe where you feel your emotions in your body and giving them an outlet deepens your mind-body connection, which increases your emotional regulation and resilience.

> Make sure your coping skills are healthy, meaning they don't hurt you or someone else.

Practicing Mindfulness

- The ability to be mindful is one and the same with your ability to be emotionally resilient. Mindfulness is the ability to observe and experience emotions in the present moment without judgment.

- Think about how many sensations there are for you to observe around you all the time. There are thousands. Take wherever you are right now: Perhaps you can notice the weight of your shirt on your shoulders or a sensation of coolness on your forehead. There are so many ways to practice mindfulness that Class 10 and Class 21 (a practice class) are dedicated to the concept. These will give you basic strategies for applying mindfulness to your own life.

Suggested Reading

Allione, *Feeding Your Demons.*

Sheehy, *Passages.*

Activities

- Answer the following questions:

    » Which emotions are the most uncomfortable/difficult for you to experience?

    » Do you tend to suppress your emotions? Cling to them? Let them run their course?

    » How were you socialized to deal with emotions?

- Pay attention to the physical experience of emotions in your body. What physical sensations do you notice when you experience different emotions (such as happiness, sadness, fear, anger, disgust, and so on)?

- Try to focus on fostering positive emotions over the next couple of days. Try creating a gratitude list or spending more time on activities that give you a sense of happiness, calm, or peace.

Class 6 Transcript

Improving Emotional Resilience

How many of you remember the marshmallow experiment: the study from the early 1970s at Stanford University, led by Walter Mischel, where researchers measured delayed gratification in preschool-age children. These children were invited into a room and asked to choose whether they wanted one marshmallow now or two marshmallows once the researcher returned to the room, which happened after about 15 minutes. So what happened? Follow-up studies showed that the children who were able to wait for the larger reward had higher SAT scores and overall better educational and social outcomes. This study measured these children's impulse control, which is a component of emotional regulation. One aspect of impulse control is the ability to sit with discomfort—in this case, the discomfort of temptation—in order to gain something more valuable, more important for yourself.

Emotional regulation is a tool that allows us to respond with clarity and a long-term vision in mind to the circumstances in our life, rather than simply react to them. When we respond to our circumstances, we're taking life in stride. When we take life in stride, we're demonstrating resilience. Andrew Shatté, coauthor of *The Resilience Factor,* even goes as far as to say that emotional regulation is the most vital piece of resilience.

So what do you do when you're sitting in front of the proverbial marshmallow in your life? How do you tend to handle uncomfortable or unpleasant emotions? In this class, we'll explore how the more comfortable we are being uncomfortable, the greater our emotional resilience. Being able to sit with the discomfort of temptation prevents us from acting on the temptation. Similarly, being able to sit with the discomfort of feelings like fear and sadness lets us hear the messages behind these emotions rather than suppressing them or feeling ashamed for having them. Learning how to take our emotions in stride improves our relationships, our ability to solve problems, and our overall emotional resilience.

In this class, we're going to start by exploring what emotions are and their fundamental purpose. Then we'll look at common ways we are socialized to handle our emotions and how that socialization may hinder our emotional resilience. Next, we cover the benefits that come from feeling both positive and negative emotions. We will end this class with some strategies for building our emotional resilience.

So before we jump into the pieces of emotional resilience, let's start with the basics. What exactly is an emotion? Well, there is no agreed upon definition. We know that, scientifically, emotions are neural impulses with a variety of features that prompt us to take some sort of action. They also are crucial to our memory and our ability to learn. But I'm going to guess that for most of us, when we experience an emotion, that isn't the definition that comes to mind. A more relatable definition might be that our emotions are our individual responses to the situations that we experience. Depending upon our emotional resilience, our emotions can either support us or hijack us. Either way, they can completely change the way we experience the world.

Even though narrowing down what an emotion actually is has proven to be a difficult task in the science community, for most of us, if someone asks what it feels like to be happy, to be sad, to be scared, we know exactly how it feels. We feel emotions when we interact with each other, when we pet our beloved dog; we can even feel them when we're moved by music or a beautiful sunset. Our emotions depend not only on the situation but also on culture, language, family, and individual differences. Furthermore, what makes one person feel sad could make another person feel a sense of relief, or what makes one person feel happy could make another person feel scared. Clearly, there's a lot of variety—what an emotion is, and who feels what emotion and when.

Some of us tend to ignore or suppress our emotions, which prevents them from doing their job. Others of us feel completely overwhelmed by our emotions, living on a rollercoaster of emotional ups and downs throughout our lives. As you may have guessed, the sweet spot of emotion management lies somewhere between those two. No matter what emotions we feel, our ability to be aware of, express, and apply our emotions is crucial to our emotional resilience.

Let's start by taking a look at our basic, or primary, emotions. According to neuroscientist and author Antonio Damasio, primary emotions are innate and enable us to act quickly. Think of primary emotions as those that can be observed in an infant. Infants are purely reacting to their environment and have not yet developed the capacity to have a controlled response to their emotions.

Just like the definition of the word emotion, there is much debate on how many basic emotions we all possess. Based on their observations for the remote Fore tribe of Papua New Guinea, psychologists Paul Ekman and Wallace Friesen identified six such emotions: sadness, happiness, fear, anger, disgust, and surprise. New research, however, points to there being only four basic emotions—sadness, happiness, fear, and anger—finding that surprise shares the same arousal patterns as fear, and that disgust shares the same as anger. Even further, some researchers and clinicians believe that there are only three basic emotions—sadness, happiness, and fear—explaining that anger is actually what occurs when we have unprocessed fear or sadness.

Anger is oftentimes referred to as a secondary emotion. Secondary emotions are what we feel after having our initial reaction to an experience. They come from our ability to have thoughts or opinions about our circumstances or about our primary emotions themselves. For example, our fear of getting hurt could result in anger, which we could use to protect ourselves, or the alleviation of our anxiety after giving that presentation at work may result in the secondary feeling of relief. Emotional resilience requires a mastery over both the primary and secondary emotions that we experience. Luckily, a few basic emotional regulation skills can be applied to all emotions, no matter whether they happen instantaneously or have been suppressed inside us for many years.

The fundamental purpose of emotions is twofold. The first purpose is to push us to take some sort of action or to learn from our experience, guiding how we choose to respond in similar situations in the future. The second purpose is to help us communicate and interact with others. Our emotional expression is an innate piece of our survival as humans, so why do we put so much effort towards hiding our emotions both from ourselves and others? Well, part of it has to do with the ways we are socialized to deal with our emotions. So let's turn to the next question of socialization. And to do this, let's start with a short activity. It's a writing activity, so go ahead and take a moment to grab some writing materials if you'd like.

Okay. So first, I want you to pause the lecture and take 20 seconds to write down all of the good emotions you can think of. Ready? Go. Okay, now pause the lecture again and take another 20 seconds to write down all of the bad emotions you can think of. Go. Now take a look at how you've divided your lists. My guess is that most of you classified emotions that feel pleasant as good and those that feel unpleasant as bad. Am I right?

But are there really good emotions and bad emotions? There are certainly emotions that are comfortable to feel and uncomfortable to feel, but are the uncomfortable emotions themselves actually bad? How do you tend to handle other things in your life that you consider to be bad—perhaps smoking, harming others, or anything else you consider to be bad? Do you tend to partake in these activities, or do you avoid them? If you partake in them, do you tend to feel guilt or shame about doing so? Typically, we avoid things we consider to be bad and welcome things we consider to be good. So coming back to emotions: Which emotions are bad? The truth is, there aren't any bad emotions. We are socialized to believe that emotions are good and bad, but in reality, they are all good because they all help us navigate our experiences.

Here's how that socialization happens. We live in a culture that often seems to value happiness over honoring the full spectrum of life's experiences. Do you make an effort not to cry in front of others? How many of you smile and say, "I'm fine," even when you're going through something really difficult? We seem to have a chronic problem in this society of shielding our truth for the sake of keeping a happy front—and that is not to say we shouldn't strive to see the positive in life. As we will see in a few minutes, there are many benefits to feeling gratitude and pleasant, or "positive," emotions. The important part here is that we don't want to suppress our actual emotions for the sake of coming across as if everything is fine to those in our lives, but most importantly, to ourselves.

Two emotions that we tend to have the most difficult time honoring are fear and sadness. Have you ever heard the words "Don't cry" after you started crying? Have you ever said those words to someone you care about or tried to stifle their cries because, in some way, you felt uncomfortable or had to do something? When we say things like "Don't cry," our goal is usually to make someone feel better, but what message do these words really send? Probably something along the lines of "Crying is not okay. Crying is a sign of weakness. Your crying makes me uncomfortable."

Let's look at an example through the eyes of a child. When my son Santiago was a toddler, we went to the playground every day. At least once a week, he would get a scraped knee, bump his head, or take a sudden plummet off of the monkey bars that left him not hurt but a little startled. Over time, I watched how my response to his injuries changed the way he experienced them. Most of the time, the "injuries" were little 60-second hurt moments that are a normal part of a young person learning how to maneuver their growing body in the interesting terrain of a playground with lots of different obstacles to navigate. I noticed how, in the beginning, how my previous socialization was to give him a little hug and say things like "You're okay! Shake it off." You know, and this is a very typical response intended to comfort the child and let him know that he will be okay, but when you really break down these words, what message is being shared with the child?

The message is that there is conflict between how he actually feels and how he is being told to feel. Being told you're okay during times of distress invalidates the emotions we're feeling while distressed. It also teaches him to look for how other people respond to the situation to assess how he is feeling. When this message is reinforced to us time and time again through words like "You're okay," "You'll be fine," "Don't cry," "Don't be scared," it makes sense that, over time, we start to either suppress those emotions or to become overwhelmed by them, as though we shouldn't be feeling them in the first place. Also, when we come with parental superhero solutions like "Mommy will fix it," we breed codependency instead of compassionate independence.

Over time, I would always still give him a hug, but instead of saying things like "Shake it off," I would ask questions like "How are you feeling? What did it feel like when you fell? What do you need right now? Can you handle that or is there something I can do to help?" Eventually I would ask, "Does it feel like we need to go home to take care of this, or would you like to play with your friends for a while longer on the playground?" At which point, he all but once went off running back to play some more. What I was trying to share with him was that he had the answers inside of himself. It is a problem-solving paradigm that includes giving him more opportunities to explore how he was feeling and to find the answers of what he needed inside of himself. He knew I was there for backup and love always, but also that his emotions were valid and that he could evaluate the situation and come up with a good solution for himself.

So many of us are walking around with buried emotions we aren't even aware of or feeling overwhelmed by the emotions we're ashamed to have. This results in a lot of unprocessed pain being carried around, and if we're carrying that unprocessed pain around with us, we're not moving through it. Remember, emotional regulation and resilience does not mean we suppress our emotions; it means we accept them and listen to the messages they have to give us. Sometimes just asking ourselves the question "What is present? What does that feel like in my body? Is there an action this experience is calling me to take in the world?"; sometimes just asking these questions can transform an experience.

When emotions are studied, they are often called positive and negative emotions—positive emotions being the ones that are pleasant to feel, like happiness, and negative emotions being those that are unpleasant to feel, like sadness. It probably comes as no surprise that there are benefits to feeling positive emotions. But did you know that there are actual benefits to feeling negative emotions as well? Let's take a closer look at this.

Positive feelings, such as happiness and joy, predict increases in our resilience and life satisfaction. According to Barbara Fredrickson's broaden-and-build theory, positive emotions encourage new thoughts and actions that help us build internal resources, improve our psychological flexibility, and create better relationships. According to this theory, emotions like happiness, interest, and anticipation encourage better health, wellness, and wealth, not because the emotions themselves are pleasurable but because they help create the tools and resources that help us reach our goals.

There is probably no surprise that emotions that inherently feel good have positive benefits, but that doesn't mean that so-called negative emotions don't have some positive benefits of their own. Emotions like sadness and fear prepare the body to deal with real or perceived danger by sharpening our memory and helping us focus, which can improve our ability to analyze and act in situations. Even more interesting is that negative emotions do not interfere with the benefits of positive emotions. Did you get that? Negative emotions do not interfere with the benefits of positive emotions. Studies on resilience report that all people, no matter how resilient they are, tend to experience negative emotions with similar frequencies. The only difference between the two groups is that more resilient people experience more frequent or higher levels of positive emotions than people who are measurably less resilient. Positive emotions serve as a protection mechanism against the adversities of life no matter how strong our fear, sadness, and other negative emotions become. So since positive emotions foster resilience, and negative emotions do not detract from it, we have no reason to hide or suppress these emotions. In fact, it's better to address them and learn from their message than it is to keep them pressed down or to let them control us. Let's take a look at how we can do that.

In his book *The Body Keeps the Score*, Bessel van der Kolk states, "Neuroscience research shows that the only way we can change the way we feel is by becoming aware of our inner experience and learning to befriend what is going on inside ourselves." So how do we do this? How do we befriend our inner experience to improve our resilience? The key to this is normalizing our emotions and our relationship with them, which we can do by practicing emotional regulation. Emotional regulation means we are fully aware and in charge of our emotions. Sometimes being in charge of our emotions is misdefined as not showing our emotions, but this is so far from the truth. The more we suppress our emotions, the more they're bound to burst out either as anger or in their original form. Emotional regulation is like sitting on a boat in the ocean, riding out the waves as they come and go. Today we're going to talk about three components of emotional regulation that can help us improve our resilience: naming feelings, coping skills, and mindfulness.

In the book *The Whole-Brain Child*, Dan Siegel and Tina Payne Bryson offer brain-based parenting strategies. You might notice that a lot of these strategies for emotional regulation and resilience are geared towards children, but even adults can benefit from these exact same skills. Most adults need them too because most of us never learned them as children. How many times have you ever reacted to something emotionally in the moment, only to reflect back on it once you've calmed down and thought, "Oh, I wish I hadn't done that." One of the first strategies in *The Whole-Brain Child* is you need to name it to tame it. In other words, in order to control your emotions, you need to know what it is you're trying to control in the first place. The more we practice naming our emotions both during emotional moments and after, the better we are able to regulate our emotional experiences. There are even tools designed to help us with this. The Feeling Wheel is a tool developed by Dr. Gloria Wilcox to help us name what we're feeling and find the root emotion behind how we're feeling. You can simply use the wheel to help you name the various emotions you're feeling, or you can use it to trace those emotions back to the center of the circle—to help you simplify your emotional experience by bringing it more and more into a basic emotion.

Another way to practice naming feelings is to dig a little bit into feelings of anger. As I mentioned earlier, anger is often a secondary emotion that is covering up feelings of sadness or fear. Think about a time when you felt angry in the past, or maybe you're angry about something right now. Look beneath the surface a little and see whether you're actually experiencing feelings of sadness or fear that are being masked by anger. This trick can work wonders on our communication with others. There is a huge difference between yelling at your partner for being home an hour later than expected and saying, "I was really scared because I thought something might have happened to you" or "I feel sad that you didn't tell me you were going to be late because we've talked about this before."

Let's take an example that many of us can relate to: road rage. Some of us find it gratifying to vent anger on the cars we share the road with, but where does that anger originate from? A fear of being late to a meeting? A fear of being hurt on the road? Or perhaps you're feeling sad about something else in your life, which is then taken out on the car in front of you. Sometimes, we aren't even aware of the emotions that lie underneath our anger because we've been conditioned to think that they're not favorable or even okay to have, but learning how to accept, name, and dig into these emotions is crucial for our emotional resilience.

When we struggle with our emotions, it can lead us to engage in behaviors that harm ourselves or others. Managing our emotions can be hard, especially when it is a new skill that we're working on. This is why coping skills are so crucial to developing emotional regulation. One simple but very effective coping skill is just to normalize the experience of having emotions. No matter what you're feeling, tell yourself, "It's okay that I feel this way." Emotions are always okay; it's the behaviors that follow the emotions that are sometimes not okay. Telling yourself, "It's okay that I feel sad" allows the feeling just to exist. It reminds you that, even though I might not be comfortable, I am allowed to feel the way that I do. Another quick and easy coping skill is to take three deep breaths when you're feeling overwhelmed. Doing this has the potential to quickly lower your heart rate, which will encourage relaxation and feelings of calm. Breathing is so important, we have a whole practice class devoted to it in this course.

There are so many different coping skills, some of which will work better for you than others. Some people like to take a walk or do yoga, write out how they're feeling, dance, clean, take a bath, paint—the list goes on and on. You may have noticed that these coping mechanisms involve some sort of physical outlet, either through gross motor movements or fine motor movements. Learning to observe where you feel your emotions in your body and giving them an outlet deepens your mind-body connection, which increases your emotional regulation and resilience. We all can find what works for us. The important thing is to make sure your coping skills are healthy, meaning they don't hurt you or someone else. It is also important to recognize that these coping mechanisms don't work by distracting us from our emotional experiences. Effective coping mechanisms are actually supporting us in processing these emotions throughout our body and mind. A useful coping mechanism will help you navigate your way through a challenging emotion, helping the emotion tell its tale and share what it has to share.

Recently, over the course of three months, I had three friends get diagnosed with cancer, two of whom are moms with small children. A deep feeling of sadness arose. It was the strongest sense of sadness I had felt in a long time. Then one evening, I went to see the cellist Yo-Yo Ma and the Silk Road Ensemble play in concert. When they began the concert, Yo-Yo Ma shared a story about how there was so much sadness in the world right now, from war to family conflict to damaging the environment. He said that sadness is a universal emotion and the one that can unite us in many ways. He hoped that the concert would help share many different sides of the feeling of sadness being felt individually and collectively. He mentioned that music has a unique ability to bridge cultures and help us find the human qualities we all share.

When I heard that, my first response was disappointment. Part of me was hoping for an inspiring concert to shift me out of the cloud of sadness I'd been feeling. However, as the concert unfolded, it felt like the music gave many unique expressions to the sadness I was experiencing. It helped me feel the full symphony of the experience of sadness. When I left the concert hall, the sadness felt alive, like it had all these different flavors and textures that I wasn't even aware of before the concert. I wasn't just sad about my three friends. Sadness had been building for a long time about a lot of topics. The experience of my friends just brought it to the surface.

I felt like the music helped sadness tell its tale. In the days that followed, I noticed how my sadness had transformed into a deep feeling of connection with others—both the people in my life, as well as the sadness of people I walked past on the street or saw in the news. The sadness was also there helping me see what I valued most in life, as well as how precious this human life really is. Sometimes we don't realize what we value until we're afraid we might lose it. In the days that followed, sadness was still present, but it was there amongst a whole collection of incredible insights and wisdom that was awakened from the deep experience of sadness.

This example also illustrated two of the main points we discover in the practice of mindfulness. There are two main ways that emotions are brought to our attention: The first is that they are so strong we can't help but notice them, and the second way is we use introspection to pay attention to what is going on beneath our surface. Practicing introspection is so important when it comes to resilience because we can't work with the emotions we have if we don't even know what's there in the first place, right?

The ability to be mindful is one and the same with our ability to be emotionally resilient. Mindfulness is the ability to observe and experience emotions in the present moment without judgment. Think about how many sensations there are for us to observe around us all the time. There are thousands! Take wherever you are right now: Perhaps you can notice the weight of the shirt on your shoulders or a sensation of coolness on your forehead. There are so many ways to practice mindfulness that we're going to devote a whole class to this concept, which will give you a basic strategy for applying mindfulness in your own life.

All of these strategies provide a foundation for increasing our emotional regulation, boosting our ability to bounce back from adverse circumstances. Mindfulness strategies are also important in building mental resilience, which you can explore in our class on mindfulness in the practice class. Before that, though, take some time to consider which pieces from this class speak the most to you, and let that guide you as you work to master your emotions and bring your emotional resilience to life.

Class 7

Strengthening Mental Resilience

This class will take you through the components of mental resilience. It starts by looking into thoughts, belief systems, and the role that core values play in mental resilience. Then the class dives into psychological flexibility—the foundation of mental resilience. The class compares rigid and flexible thinking styles, and then it discusses the impact your mindset can have on your psychological flexibility. The class concludes with some practical ways to boost your mental resilience.

Thoughts and Belief Systems

- Like emotions, thoughts are neural impulses that prompt people to take short-term action or work toward long-term goals. The thoughts a person has are a combination of his or her circumstances, life experiences, upbringing, social environment, mood, physical needs, and so on.

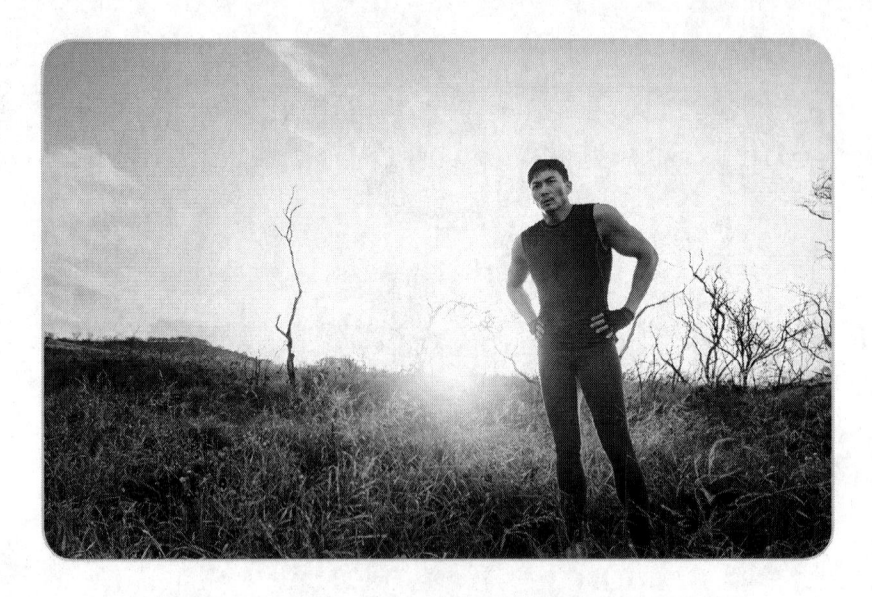

- Your belief system, meanwhile, affects everything that you see, for better or for worse. For example, it can be the difference between feeling sympathy or derision toward a homeless person on the street.

- The brain naturally tries to mold incoming information so that it fits within a person's belief system. Thoughts are the building blocks of your belief system, and the quality of these thoughts can have a huge impact on your resilience. This makes it important to put time toward considering your thinking.

- Keep in mind that trying to stop yourself from thinking simply doesn't work. However, humans have a well-developed prefrontal cortex, which is the part of the brain that helps with complex thinking and decision making. Even though you might not be able to control all of your thoughts, you can use your prefrontal cortex to help control how you react to your thoughts.

Core Values

- The first step in building strong mental resilience is making sure that an internal compass, which directs you toward what you find most meaningful, guides your life. Core values are the building blocks for a life with meaning.

- The most basic level of control you can have over your belief system is uncovering your true core values and living them in your everyday life. If your core values have meaning, it will be much easier to follow them, especially when times get hard.

- Think about your core values. Do you know where they come from? Were they passed down to you, or did you find them on your own? Do any of your core values contradict each other? Do you live your core values in practice? It doesn't matter how you find your core values, so long as they feel right and are meaningful to you.

- Take some time to define your core values, focusing not on what sounds good, but on what is most meaningful to you and why. Everyone grows and changes, and part of resilience is the ability to adapt to changing circumstances, so keep in mind that your core values may adapt with time, too. What you find meaningful might change, but your core values will remain meaningful, no matter what that looks like for you.

Rigid and Flexible Thinking

- A primary cause of problems is when one's expectations don't meet one's reality. When a person's thinking is rigid, he or she can become stuck, holding on tightly to absolute beliefs about themselves, others, and the world, often in spite of evidence pointing against these beliefs. The focus of life shifts from goals and values to the avoidance of discomfort and pain.

- Flexible thinking, on the other hand, can allow you to adapt your thinking so that it fits with changing circumstances, which enables you to continue to move toward your goals in spite of challenges. Psychological flexibility helps people see options in how they look at and respond to circumstances.

- Rigid thinking is not to be confused with discipline and determination. Sticking to goals and core values motivates discipline and determination. Rigid thinking gives a false sense of control over situations that are often out of your control.

- Pay attention to your reaction when your thinking is challenged or questioned by others. If your reaction is to get defensive or indignant, there is a good chance that rigid thinking is at play.

Growth Mindset versus Fixed Mindset

- A large piece of your belief system that also impacts your psychological flexibility is how you view failure, which, according to Stanford professor Carol Dweck, is embedded in your mindset. Dweck distinguishes between two types of mindset: a growth mindset and a fixed mindset.

- When a person has a fixed mindset, the person believes his or her abilities and intelligence are unchanging. A person with a growth mindset believes his or her abilities and intelligence can develop.

- With a fixed mindset, success is determined by an outcome, such as scoring well on a test or securing a coveted job. With a growth mindset, success is determined by the process—for example, the things one learned by studying for a test or the skills acquired in the job search, regardless of the outcome.

- If you're motivated by the process, your determination persists in spite of perceived failure. There is value in the failure. If you're only motivated by the outcome, you may become discouraged by frequent perceived failure and perceive yourself as inherently flawed.

> **Improving Mental Resilience**
>
> The rest of this class discusses two main strategies for improving your mental resilience. The first and most important strategy is learning how to accept your thoughts. Once this has been mastered, it becomes easier to venture into the second strategy: challenging your thoughts.

Accepting Your Thoughts

- You can't always change your circumstances, but you can change your relationship with your circumstances. The key to this is changing your relationship with your thoughts. In order to do this, it's so important to recognize that thoughts are not facts. By recognizing your thoughts as thoughts rather than fact, you can start to detach from them, which increases your psychological flexibility and resilience.

- For example, if someone had the thought, "I am a failure," she could change her relationship to the sentiment by thinking instead, "I had a thought that I am a failure." This small shift changes the perceived truth of this thought from the person being a failure to the person having a thought that they were a failure.

- Recognizing thoughts as thoughts rather than facts makes it easier to welcome every part of your experience. Welcoming thoughts enhances your psychological flexibility, since you are not ignoring or avoiding any part of your experience. Suppressing thoughts or clinging to a thought out of fear of its opposite keeps thinking rigid.

Challenging Your Thoughts

- Once you have mastered welcoming your thoughts, rather than ignoring or avoiding them, it allows you to look at your thoughts more objectively. This makes it easier to transform your thoughts in a way that can better serve you, your values, and your goals.

- Unhelpful thoughts are thoughts that keep thinking rigid and prevent you from being able to work toward your goals. Cognitive Behavioral Therapy, or CBT, is one of the most widely used therapy orientations that focuses on helping people challenge their unhelpful thinking patterns and go-to behaviors.

- One example of an unhelpful thought is worst-case-scenario thinking. This is when your head tends to jump to the worst possible outcome instead of thinking about more likely outcomes.

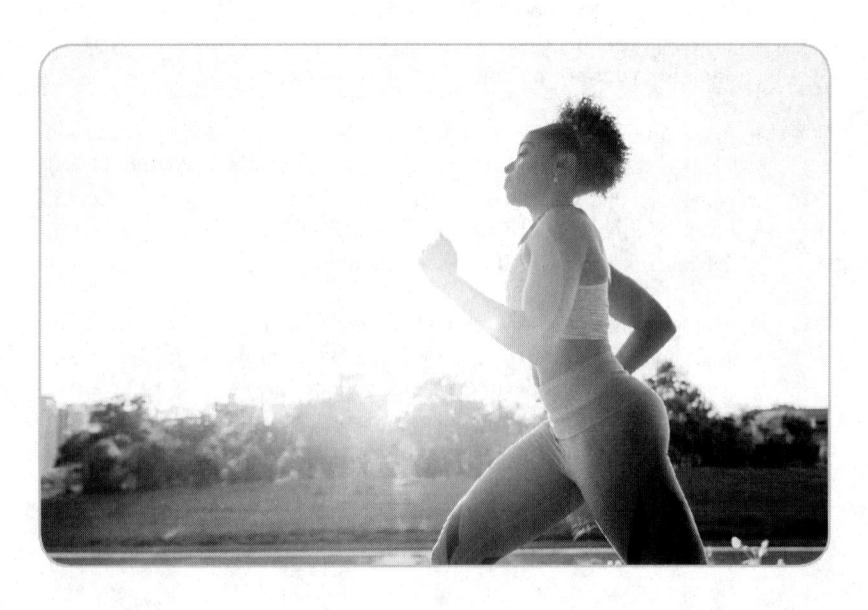

- Another example is the use of the word *should*, as in, "I should've known better." The use of *should* can show judgment of yourself or others, can discourage you, or can show you when you might be holding yourself to outside standards that don't resonate with your truth.

- Here is the same thought without the word *should*: "I want to do better next time." Removing *should* removes judgment and shame, and replaces them with options for the future.

Shifting Your Perspective

- After learning to welcome your thoughts, you can practice shifting your focus and broadening your perspective. If you tend to put most of your energy toward focusing on what could go wrong, try thinking instead of what could go right.

- Shifting your perspective can change how you see the world around you. It can change whether you look at the world as containing good people and bad people or as containing good people who make good and not good choices.

- Making changes to your belief system can change not only how you view others, but how you view yourself, too. For example, think about your self-talk. Do you tend to be nice to yourself or critical of yourself?

- If you notice yourself being self-critical, one thought-shifting exercise you can try is creating a personal gratitude list. Spend time reflecting on everything about yourself that you like and that you're grateful for, such as physical abilities, personality traits, interests, and so on.

- To challenge thoughts, it can also help to shift your perception of thinking as a whole. If you tend to avoid certain thoughts or emotions, try to change your experience of them by generating curiosity about them.

- For example, if you are nervous before a presentation and worry that the nervousness will hurt your performance, try shifting how you see your nervousness. Instead of a detriment, you might view it as a rare life experience that shows how alive and present you are in that moment.

Suggested Reading

Covey, *The 7 Habits of Highly Effective People*.

Farhi, *The Breathing Book*.

Frankl, *Man's Search for Meaning*.

Activities

- Write a list of core values that are most meaningful to you. You can also write down what it is that makes them meaningful.

- Respond to the following prompts:

    » Think of a time your thinking has been flexible.

    » Think of a time your thinking has been rigid.

    » Think of a time you have used a fixed mindset.

    » Think of a time you have used a growth mindset.

- What unhelpful thought patterns do you think you tend to use?

- What can you do to break these patterns?

Class 7 Transcript

Strengthening Mental Resilience

You may have heard the aphorism that is often attributed to the Buddha, "Pain is inevitable. Suffering is optional." The origins of that aphorism root back to a story from one of the Buddha's teachings, *Sallatha Sutra*, where he talks about what is often referred to as the two arrows paradigm. The first arrow is the one that is shot at us. This could represent either physical or emotional pain that happens to us, so to speak, whether it is illness, injury, the death of a loved one, or something else. While the first arrow may cause pain, the suffering is actually caused by the second arrow, which is the arrow we shoot at ourselves.

The worst part of our pain comes not from the first injury but from the way we respond to it. That response to the pain is what holds the key to living a life filled with meaning or a life filled with suffering. When we look at people who have endured the worst pain imaginable, it is their response to the pain that makes all the difference, as we learn when we look at the example of Viktor Frankl. A survivor of the Holocaust, Frankl spent years in concentration camps. His mother, father, brother, and wife all perished at the hands of the Nazis, and Frankl himself had to find a way to persevere through one of the worst horrors mankind has ever known.

While adjusting to life outside of the camps, Frankl depicted his story of survival in a book titled *Man's Search for Meaning*. He said he wrote the book to "convey that life has potential meaning under any conditions, even the most miserable ones. For many, finding meaning is the only path out of suffering." His account is full of examples of mental resilience, which is the ability to harness the power of your mind to recover from adversity. And perhaps no words capture that ability better than when Frankl writes, "Forces beyond your control can take away everything you possess except one thing, your freedom to choose how you will respond to the situation."

According to Frankl, the greatest motivation in life is to find meaning, and this meaning is what enables people to conquer even the worst of suffering. He shares that even the suffering itself is meaningful, reminding us that "What is to give light must endure burning." The ability to find meaning in adversity is central to the ability to bounce back from it. Frankl's message reinforces the truth that perspective is reality. Our perspective of situations is determined by our belief system, or our typical way of interpreting ourselves and the world around us. Our belief system can help or hurt our resilience depending on its quality. If you tend to feel helpless during a challenge, you may give up easily or miss out on opportunities to improve your situation. But if you see challenge and disappointment as opportunities for growth, you are more likely to take advantage of those opportunities, allowing you to endure and even possibly to find meaning and purpose in your challenges. Frankl said, "He who knows the 'why' for his existence will be able to bear almost any hardship."

This class will take you through the components of mental resilience. We'll start by looking more into thoughts, belief systems, and the role that our core values play in our mental resilience. Then we'll dive deep into psychological flexibility, the foundation of mental resilience. We'll compare rigid and flexible thinking styles, and then we'll talk about the impact your mindset can have on your psychological flexibility. We'll end this class with some practical ways to boost your mental resilience, specifically by learning how to welcome and challenge your thoughts.

Like emotions, our thoughts are neural impulses that prompt us to take short term action or work towards a long-term goal. The thoughts we have are a combination of our circumstances, our life experiences, our upbringing, our social environment, our mood, our physical needs, and so on. We can think about our past, our present, and our future; real situations and concepts; or hypothetical and pretend ones. We actually have a lot of control over what we want to think about; all that is required to have a thought is the will to have it. That being said, it is a lot easier to think, "I want to watch that cute puppy video again" and do it than it is to think, "I want to start liking my mother-in-law" and actually do it. That's because our opinions about people and things are deeply rooted in our belief system, which as I mentioned, is our typical way of interpreting ourselves and the world around us.

Think of your belief system as seeing the world through tinted glasses; it affects everything that you see for better or for worse. It's what determines whether we look at a homeless person on the street and think, "That guy really needs to get up off the ground, quit begging, and get a job" or "That guy must've had a really difficult life. I wonder how he ended up where he is and what can be done to help?" Not only that, but our brain naturally tries to mold incoming information so that it fits within our belief system. So if our tinted glasses are green, and we're looking at a blue ocean, we might see it through our glasses as not completely blue but as a shade of green as well. Our thoughts are the building blocks of our belief system, and the quality of these thoughts can have a huge impact on our resilience. This makes it so important to put time towards thinking about your thinking.

While we have control over what we actively think about, such as where we want to eat or deciding we really need to focus on a work project, it can feel like we have less control when we want to change our thoughts or when we don't want to think about something. Trying to stop yourself from thinking something just simply doesn't work. Part of this is because, in trying to stop our brain from thinking about something, we have to remember that we don't want to think about it, which, ironically, keeps us thinking about it. Lucky for us, as humans, we have a well-developed prefrontal cortex, which is the part of the brain that helps us with complex thinking and decision making. Even though we might not be able to control all of our thoughts, we can use our prefrontal cortex to help us control how we react to our thoughts, which, as we'll explore during the second half of this class, can help you change your belief system over time.

As Frankl said, meaning gives us purpose. It gives us a will to live. So the first step in building strong mental resilience is making sure that our lives are guided by an internal compass directing us towards what we find most meaningful.

Core values are the building blocks for a life with meaning. If someone asked us what our core values are, all of us could most likely rattle off a few: dependability, honesty, and compassion, for example. But if someone were to ask you why your core values are meaningful to you, could you do that? It's easy to acknowledge that core values matter, but it's harder to put thought into what makes them such an important piece of your life.

The most basic level of control we have over our belief system is uncovering our true values—those that give us real meaning—and then living them in our everyday lives. If your core values have meaning, it will be much easier to follow them, especially when times get hard. Think about your core values. Do you know where they come from? Were they passed down to you, or did you find them on your own? Do any of your core values contradict each other? Do you live your core values in practice? It doesn't matter how you find your core values so long as they feel right and are meaningful to you. So if you haven't done it before or haven't done so in a while, take some time to define your core values, focusing not on what sounds good, but on what is most meaningful to you and why. We all grow and change, and part of resilience is the ability to adapt to changing circumstances, so keep in mind that your core values may adapt with time, too. What you find meaningful might change, but what shouldn't change is that your core values *are* meaningful, no matter what that looks like for you.

Even once we have our core values that are meaningful to us, we are bound to find some areas of life in which we aren't living them completely. This is often due to passively assumed belief systems, or parts of our belief system that have been influenced by outside sources but that we haven't put much critical thought into. Parenting styles is a common one; without intervention or a conscious effort to change, parents will typically parent in the same way they were parented. Making sure we are living our meaningful core values in every facet of life requires the ability to make changes to these more rote aspects of our belief system.

How well we are able to make changes to our belief system depends largely on our psychological flexibility, or our ability to be adaptable in our thoughts and behavior. A primary cause of our problems is when our expectations don't meet our reality. When our thinking is rigid, we can become stuck, holding on tightly to our absolute beliefs about ourselves, about others, and about the world, oftentimes in spite of evidence pointing against these beliefs. When this happens, our long-term goals and core values are inadvertently put on the back burner. The focus of life shifts from our goals and values to the avoidance of discomfort and pain. Flexible thinking, on the other hand, allows us to adapt our thinking so that it fits with changing circumstances, which enables us to continue to move towards our goals in spite of challenges. Psychological flexibility helps us see that we have options in how we look at and respond to our circumstances. It tells us that even if we don't have an answer or explanation for a problem quite yet, we know that an alternative answer or explanation is out there.

Rigid thinking is not to be confused with discipline and determination. Discipline and determination are motivated by sticking to goals and core values. Rigid thinking gives us a false sense of control over situations that are often out of our control. Determination is thinking, "I will reach my goals," whereas rigid thinking is thinking that "The only way I can reach my goals is this." *Only* is a common word in the land of rigid thinking. "This is the only way someone should behave." "He's a bad person. That is the only explanation." "My income and job title are the only ways to define my success."

Both rigid thinking and determination involve sticking to what you think. There is a solidity to each of them, but the solidity is very different. Rigid thinking is like glass; it's easily shattered when it's dropped or hit too hard. Determination is like steel; it's more durable and able to weather the same rough and tumble that glass cannot. Pay attention to your reaction when your thinking is challenged or questioned by others. If your reaction is to get defensive or indignant, there's a good chance that rigid thinking is at play. Determination has life. It has a humanity to it. When we cannot possibly see the other side, when it seems unfathomable why someone else may think the way they do, when you assert that there is no other option—these are sure signs of rigidity.

A large piece of your belief system that also impacts your psychological flexibility is how you view failure, which, according to Stanford professor Carol Dweck, is embedded in your mindset. Dweck distinguishes between two types of mindset: a growth mindset and a fixed mindset. When we have a fixed mindset, we believe that our abilities and intelligence are unchanging. When we have a growth mindset, we believe that our abilities and intelligence can develop. Think of the implications that this has on failure and success. With a fixed mindset, success is determined by an outcome, such as scoring well on a test or securing a job we wanted. With a growth mindset, success is determined by the process; for example, the things we've learned by studying for a test or the skills we've acquired in our job search, regardless of the outcome. If we're motivated by the process, our determination persists in spite of perceived failure because there's value in the failure. If we're only motivated by the outcome, we may get discouraged by frequent perceived failure and see ourselves as inherently flawed.

Dr. Dweck makes an interesting observation that people who succeed don't believe that failure is a permanent condition. The way we explain our failures determines whether we give up or push through, which, as you may remember from our class on the science of resilience, is a key piece of grit. The more and more we repeat our thought patterns, such as how we see failure, the more they become a part of our belief system. By not believing that failure is a permanent condition, you are setting yourself up for positive change in the future. Taken more broadly, when we can't change our circumstances, we improve our resilience by changing our relationship with our circumstances. This is the essence of psychological flexibility.

Think of your belief system like an iceberg. We are actually only aware of a small portion of our belief system—the tip of the iceberg. Most of our belief system is shaped by our early experiences and socialization, which determine how we view our place in the world and our beliefs about how the world should work. It's important to look below the surface when addressing our belief system because otherwise we are limiting our perspective to what is in our conscious awareness, which leads to an incomplete assessment of our circumstances. And with less information, we have fewer options, which reduces our ability to be resilient.

We're going to discuss two main strategies for improving your mental resilience. The first and most important strategy is learning how to accept your thoughts.

Once this has been mastered, it becomes easier to venture into the second strategy—challenging your thoughts. Both of these strategies will help you dive below the surface to see the whole iceberg and uncover what might benefit from change. These practices will help you harness the power of psychological flexibility, and if you use that flexibility to make practical changes in your belief system, you're just about guaranteed to notice an increase in your mental resilience.

As I mentioned before, we can't always change our circumstances, but we can change our relationship with our circumstances. The key to changing our relationship with our circumstances is changing our relationship with our thoughts. In order to do this, it's so important to recognize that thoughts are not facts. Just like our emotions, our thoughts are transient, but it can be easy to forget this in the moment. Remembering that our thoughts are not facts helps us change our relationship with them because we remember that they are just that—thoughts. When we recognize our thoughts as thoughts rather than facts, we can start to detach from them, which increases our psychological flexibility and resilience. So let's take a look at the thought "I am a failure" as an example. If someone had the thought "I am a failure," they could change their relationship to the sentiment by thinking instead, "I had a thought that I am a failure." This might seem like an insignificant change, but the implications are huge. This small shift changes the perceived truth of this thought from the person being a failure to the person having a thought that they were a failure.

Recognizing thoughts as thoughts rather than facts makes it easier to welcome every part of our experience. Welcoming thoughts enhances our psychological flexibility since we're not ignoring or avoiding any part of our experience. Suppressing thoughts or clinging to a thought out of fear of its opposite keeps our thinking rigid. It limits our options, and, as we've seen, it keeps our focus on the avoidance of discomfort rather than our values and long-term goals. Not only that, but welcoming your thoughts can actually help you uncover the core values that are truest to you. Welcoming your experience allows you to look truthfully at why you have the values you do. Do you think you should act or feel a certain way? Does someone else want you to live a certain way? Is living in this way meaningful to you? By digging into what your values are and where they come from, and welcoming everything that comes up in this process, you can come out the other side feeling secure and content with values that are right and meaningful for you.

Welcoming and acceptance are the opposite of avoidance. Acceptance is the process of being aware of your experience without trying to change what it looks or feels like. If we're not afraid of our thoughts, we are more open to them. If we're not busy suppressing or avoiding our thoughts or the emotions associated with them, we can work through the information they're trying to give us. Resilience increases when we feel we have options. Let me repeat that because it's really crucial: Resilience increases when we feel we have options. When our thinking is more open, we become more aware of all the options that lay before us. This doesn't mean we can't act in response to a situation or to take actions to try to change it. It just means our happiness is not dependent upon it. We accept and welcome the fact that pain is present while knowing it doesn't have to disturb our peace. Then we are operating from a more clear-headed mindset about how to respond. It's just like the double arrow paradigm we shared at the beginning of class. The first arrow causes the pain, but the suffering arises—or not—from our response to the pain.

As discussed in the class on emotional resilience, mindfulness is the ability to practice acceptance by observing our experience in the present moment without judgment. The ability to practice this with our thoughts is just as important as the ability to practice it with our feelings and emotions. Luckily, the tools you need to do it are the same. When using mindfulness with thoughts, you learn how to observe and describe your thoughts rather than use them to judge people and situations or to make predictions about the future. Check out the practice classes on mindfulness and guided meditation to get firsthand experience on what it's like to practice mindfulness in real time.

Once you have mastered welcoming your thoughts rather than ignoring or avoiding them, it allows you to look at your thoughts more objectively, which then makes it easier to transform your thoughts in a way that can better serve you, your values, and your goals. Unhelpful thoughts are thoughts that keep our thinking rigid and keep us from being able to work towards our goals. Cognitive behavioral therapy, or CBT, is one of the most widely used therapy orientations that focuses on helping people challenge their unhelpful thinking patterns and go-to behaviors. The Great Courses offers a whole course on cognitive behavioral therapy if you're interested in a thorough explanation of this therapy orientation.

For our purposes, let me just give you a couple of examples of unhelpful thoughts, and I invite you to keep track of whether you tend to find in your own thinking habits. The first example is worst-case scenario thinking. This is when your head tends to jump to the worst possible outcome instead of thinking about more likely outcomes. Another example of unhelpful thoughts is our use of the word *should*. "I should've known better." "He should really go back to school." Our use of *should* can show judgment of others or ourselves, can discourage us, or can show us when we might be holding ourselves to outside standards that don't resonate with our truth. Watch what happens when we remove the word *should* from our vocabulary. "I should've known better" becomes "I want to do better next time." "He should really go back to school" becomes "Has he thought about going back to school?" Removing *should* from our vocabulary removes judgment and shame and replaces them with options for the future.

These examples of unhelpful thoughts are certainly not exhaustive, but it gives you a taste of the types of thoughts that could hold us back and could benefit from being changed. So what can we do about these thoughts? The first thing we can do after learning how to welcome all of our thoughts is to practice shifting our focus and broadening our perspective. If you tend to put most of your energy towards focusing on what could go wrong, try instead thinking of what could go right—or, as I learned from my friend Suzi Landolphi, who you'll hear from in another class, "It's not what's wrong; it's what happened." This is what Suzi and other guides remind the veterans who participate in their Progressive and Alternative Training for Healing Heroes, or PATHH, program at Boulder Crest Retreat. It's a valuable piece of wisdom that helps these warriors reframe their tragic life experiences.

Shifting your perspective can literally change how you see the world around you. It can change whether you look at the world as containing good and bad people or as containing good people who make good choices and not so good choices. There is a quote I love by Yogi Bhajan that very well captures the peace that comes from shifting our perspective on our interactions with the people in our lives: "If you are willing to look at another person's behavior toward you as a reflection of the state of their relationship with themselves rather than a statement about your value as a person, then you will, over a period of time, cease to react at all." Making changes, such as those on how you choose to see another person and their behavior, can, over time, change your belief system in ways that will allow you to bounce back from hardship with more ease.

Making changes to your belief system can change not only how you view others but how you view yourself, too. We'll talk about more about the impact that our self-worth has on our resilience in the next class, but what's important to recognize in this class is how our automatic thoughts often reflect our underlying feelings of self-worth. And since this is the case, we can actually make changes to our sense of self-worth by shifting some of our thoughts. For example, think about your self-talk. Do you tend to be nice to yourself or critical of yourself? If you notice yourself being self-critical, one thought-shifting exercise you can try is creating a personal gratitude list. Spend time reflecting on everything about yourself that you like and that you're grateful for, such as your physical abilities, personality traits, interests, and so on. It's amazing the power that our relationship with ourselves can have on our relationship with the world around us.

To challenge our thoughts, it also helps to shift our perspective on the experience of thinking as a whole. If you tend to avoid certain thoughts or emotions, try to change your experience of them by generating curiosity about them instead of judging yourself for having a certain thought. Try thinking "Oh, that was an interesting thought—I wonder where it came from." Or if you get nervous before a presentation and worry that your nervousness will hurt your performance, try shifting how you see your nervousness from a detriment to a rare life experience that shows you how fully alive and present you are in that moment. These small shifts are very powerful when it comes to your ability to generate more positive emotions, as well. As you might recall from the last class, resilience is correlated with the frequency and intensity of our positive emotions and is not affected by the presence of what science would call negative emotions.

The examples I've offered, such as being intentionally nice to yourself and altering your views on others' behavior, are ways of shifting your experience of the world in a way that can foster more positive emotions. While hardship may temporarily deplete our energy, enthusiasm, and other resources, our underlying beliefs remain, and when these beliefs are helpful and flexible, they improve our ability to bounce back from difficult circumstances. Our mind is the gatekeeper to our perception of our lived experience, and it has the power to make or break our ability to recover from adversity. In our next class, we'll take a closer look at a fundamental piece of our belief system—ourselves. Join me for a class all about self-care, where we'll explore how the way we think about, feel about, and care for ourselves affects our resilience.

Class 8

The Practice of Self-Care

Not taking care of yourself can result in problems with sleep, difficulties with concentration, damage to your mood, and other problems, so self-care is essential. This class starts by looking at basic principles of self-care. It also looks at the impact that self-worth has on self-care. The class ends with some tools you can use to create a self-care plan.

Basic Principles of Self-Care

- The concept of self-care is not new, but for many people, actually putting it into practice is new. A good self-care routine is like a good set of armor, allowing you to endure the challenges of life with greater ease.

- The first core principle is balance, which is not an end state. It is an ongoing, constantly changing process. Balance is making sure that, day by day, aspects of your life aren't being neglected. For example, if you find yourself having fits of anger, it's a message that something is out of balance. Perhaps your emotional needs aren't being met.

- The second core principle of a self-care plan involves setting boundaries. The foundation of setting boundaries is knowing when to say no to other people and to yourself. Boundaries often come into play in careers: A person who constantly works 60-hour weeks, checks email around the clock, and puts everyone's needs above her own may need to set better boundaries.

- The third principle is that a good self-care plan should keep your energy reserves full. A lack of balance and boundaries can drain your energy reserves, so looking at self-care in terms of energy reserves is the simplest way to make sure you are giving yourself the care you deserve.

Self-Worth and Self-Efficacy

- A huge piece of self-care and your ability to be resilient is simply being nice to yourself, valuing yourself, and believing in your importance to the world. Your self-worth can be seen in your behaviors, self-talk, and interactions with others.

- The only way to accurately uncover your sense of self-worth is through deep, honest, self-reflection. Think about how you talk to yourself. Are you harsh and self-critical? Would you ever talk to a friend the way you talk to yourself? Do you build yourself up by tearing others down? These can speak to a lack of self-worth.

- The companion to self-worth is self-efficacy, or your belief that you can accomplish something. It is very common for self-worth to affect self-efficacy. If you don't think highly of yourself, you might not be confident in your abilities. It is possible, though, to have a high sense of self-efficacy while also having low self-worth.

- Research on both self-worth and self-efficacy shows that these qualities improve one's ability to cope with and bounce back from difficult circumstances. This can be seen in action by looking at the concept of codependency: If your sense of self-worth is dependent on something external, it goes down or away when that person or object is absent or disengaged from you.

- For instance, if a dating prospect decides they do not want to be with you, you might internalize that as a belief that you are not good enough. However, if you recognize your self-worth, you can understand that someone not wanting a life with you does not take away from your value as a person. This in turn can improve your self-efficacy—the belief that you can navigate your personal life successfully, in spite of challenges.

Self-Compassion and Self-Worth

- Cultivating self-compassion can help work through deep feelings of shame that may seep through in actions that hurt yourself and others. Self-compassion fuels self-worth, and when you recognize your worth, you will naturally be more inclined to take care of yourself.

- Keep in mind that building self-compassion is a process: Creating habits and rewiring thought patterns doesn't happen overnight. Even if your reaction is to be frustrated that it is hard to show yourself compassion, try to have compassion for that.

> Sometimes working through shame and building your sense of self-worth is best accomplished by a professional trained in helping people work through these emotions.

Self-Care Tool: The Wheel of Life

- The Wheel of Life is a helpful tool that will allow you to evaluate how well you take care of yourself. The purpose of the wheel is to measure and map out how you feel you are doing in each category of life. You can use the wheel included on the next page or create your own by following these steps:

  1. Draw a circle and create spokes on the wheel. You can make as many spokes on the wheel as you find helpful.

  2. Divide the wheel into different categories of life. It is recommended that you pick between 6 and 12 categories. Each category has its own spoke of the wheel. You can use these example of categories, choose your own, or both:

  - » Family Life
  - » Career
  - » Social Life
  - » Personal Development
  - » Health
  - » Finances
  - » Free Time
  - » Romantic Relationships
  - » Life Purpose
  - » Religion/Spirituality
  - » General Housekeeping
  - » Giving Back

  3. Each spoke starts at 0 at the center of the wheel and ends at 10 at the outermost part of the wheel. To complete the wheel, place a dot on each section of the wheel somewhere on the line between 0 and 10. A score of 0 in a category means you have a lot of room for improvement in that category, whereas a score of 10 means you are already living at your fullest in that category.

The Wheel of Life

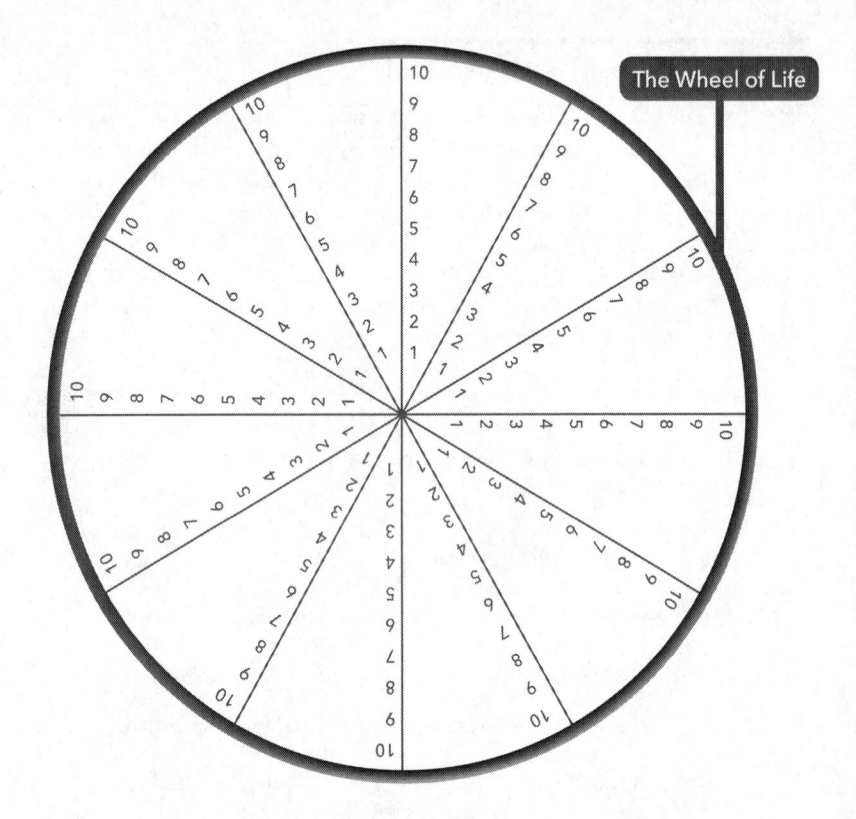

- As you add dots to your wheel, you'll start to see that you're thriving in some aspects of your life, whereas you feel more constricted in other aspects. Once you're done placing a dot in each category, connect the dots. Ideally, you'll see a round wheel, but it is more likely that your wheel will look somewhat bumpy.

- A bumpy wheel lets you know that your life is asking for more balance. Often, the key to that balance is in your self-care practice.

- The end goal isn't a round wheel that is all 10s. Rather, it is to simply have a round wheel, hopefully in the higher range of numbers. For instance, if your career is a 10 but your family life is a 5, you might realize that boosting your family score requires pulling back from your career score. A good goal might be striving for an 8 in both categories.

Self-Care Tool: The Needs Wheel

- Another tool you can use is a wheel divided not by category of life but by category of need. You can use the blank Needs Wheel below or create your own. To create your own, draw a circle, just as you did for the Wheel of Life. Then, create 5 to 10 spokes on your wheel.

- Feel free to label the spokes with whatever needs are pertinent to you. For example, the sample Needs Wheel below covers physical needs,

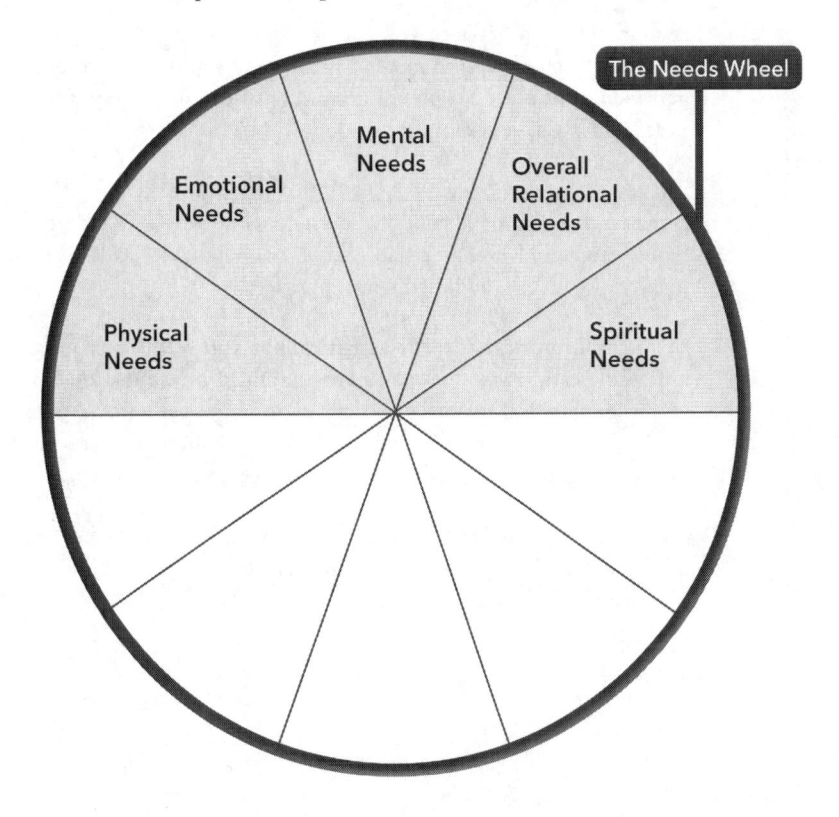

The Needs Wheel

- Mental Needs
- Emotional Needs
- Overall Relational Needs
- Physical Needs
- Spiritual Needs

emotional needs, mental needs, overall relational needs, and spiritual needs. It also has five blank spokes for any other needs you want to add.

- Keep in mind that if you feel an obligation to do something, it loses some of its value in nourishing you. If exercising, attending a service, meditating, or conducting volunteer work is seen as a line item on a checklist, it is unlikely that it is actually meeting your need for purpose or meaning. Find something that truly serves you when you look to fulfill your needs.

Self-Care Tool: Journal

- A journal is another tool you can use to evaluate how well you're doing with self-care. One method is to create a grid in a spreadsheet and then print out 52 copies of it on the first day of the year. On the next page is a blank example:

- To create your own, down the left side of the grid, write the different activities that you spend your time doing, including working, sleeping, family time, and exercise. The grid can also include fields like the quality of your diet and meditation practice.

- In the column next to your activities, put your ideal goal in each applicable category so that you have a point to measure against. For example, one ideal might be to sleep eight hours per night. Another might be a certain number of minutes of meditation. Place seven blank rows for each day of the week next to each ideal.

- From here, you can track how you do each week. For more examples of activities and measures with which to track them, refer to the audio or video class.

Self-Care Journal

Activity										
Ideal										
Monday										
Tuesday										
Wednesday										
Thursday										
Friday										
Saturday										
Sunday										

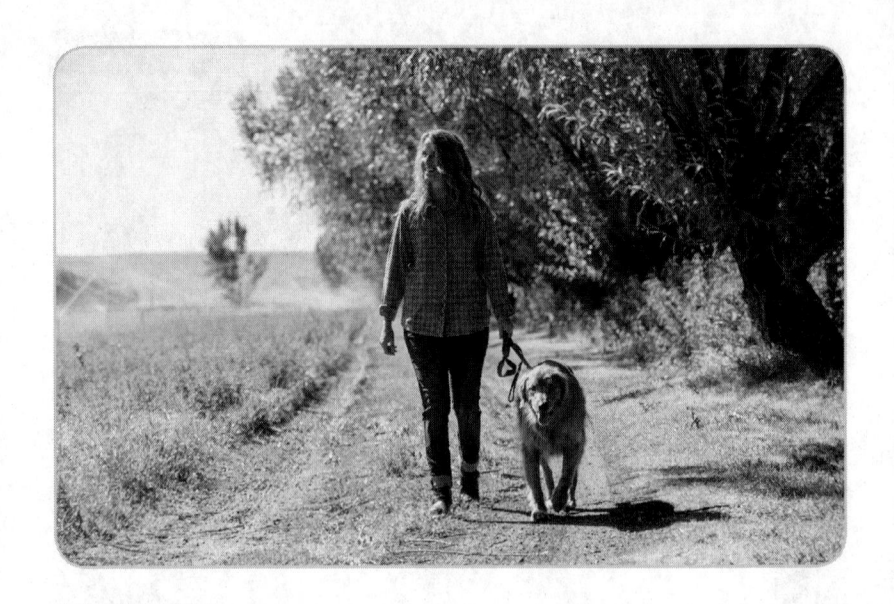

Conclusion

- Every person's self-care plan will look different. Your plan may include daily activities, such as time for deep breathing and self-reflection. It may also include weekly or monthly activities, such as a massage or a retreat in nature. It could also include reminders to simply let yourself feel your feelings or to set time aside each day to write three kind things about yourself.

- Self-care creates the foundation for your resilience by keeping your tank full and ready to go. Tracking and reflecting on self-care can bring your attention to a few simple changes that can bring more balance and freedom to your life, improving your overall resilience.

Suggested Reading

Gawande, *The Checklist Manifesto*.

Tiwari, *The Path of Practice*.

Activities

- Complete at least one self-care Wheel of Life. If desired, also complete the Needs Wheel.

- Answer the following:

    » Is your life balanced? How so or how not?

    » Do you set appropriate boundaries? How so or how not?

    » Are you able to keep your energy reserves full? If not, what would help you supplement your energy?

- Create a self-care journal.

- Complete Practice Class 4 (Class 20), titled "Relaxing Yoga for Self-Care."

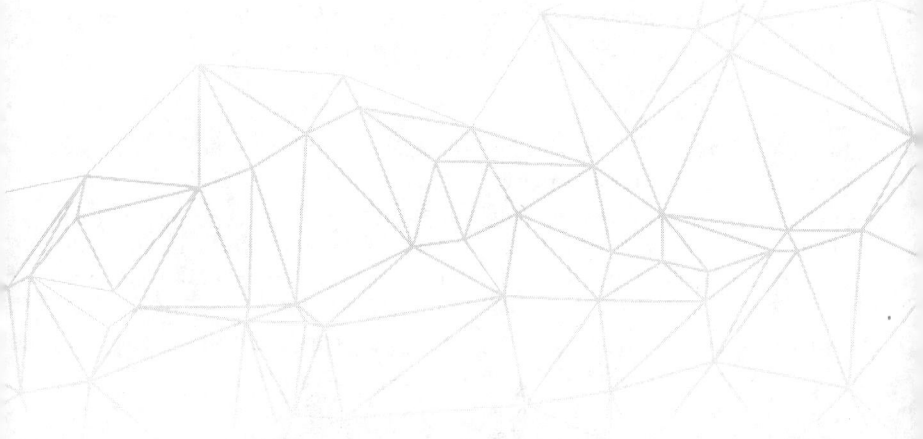

Class 8 Transcript

The Practice of Self-Care

Think of the last time that you were on an airplane. Everyone has been seated, and you're asked to pay attention to a brief safety presentation. What do the airline attendants always say when describing how to use the oxygen masks? That's right! Put on your own mask before assisting others. Even though I, fortunately, have never had to follow these words in a literal sense, I know them to be true in my life.

If we truly want to help others to the best of our ability, we need to make sure that we're taking care of our own basic needs first. Taking care of our needs is not only important in our ability to help others, it's also incredibly important to support our own resilience as well. When we properly nourish ourselves, we keep our energy reserves full. And with full energy reserves, we're more prepared to move through the challenging circumstances that arise in our lives. Not taking care of ourselves can result in problems with sleep, difficulties with concentration, distractibility, detachment, low mood, anger, isolation, anxiousness, and so on. Many of us are also modeling self-care for others in our lives, whether it's children, employees, students, friends, or others. It's important to make sure we are modeling healthy self-care strategies to the people who look up to and relate to us as well.

In this class, we're going to start by looking at a tool that can help us evaluate how well we take care of ourselves. It's called the Wheel of Life. Then we're going to spell out the basic principles of self-care and look at the impact that our self-worth has on our ability to take care of ourselves. We'll end this class with some more tools that you can use to create a self-care plan of your own.

Having your own self-care plan will ensure you're keeping your energy reserves full, leaving you ready to take on and bounce back from life's challenges.

The Wheel of Life is a really helpful tool that will allow you to evaluate how well you take care of yourself by giving you a bird's-eye view of your life. I'm going to describe how to do this now, and then you can come back to create your Wheel of Life after class. We've included an example in the guidebook. It's really quite simple to make your own. Draw a circle and create spokes on the wheel. You can make as many spokes on the wheel as you find helpful. The wheel is divided into different categories of life, such as family life, career, social life, personal development, health, finances, free time, and relationships. Each category has its own spoke of the wheel. We use the wheel to measure and map out how we feel we are doing in each category of life.

Each spoke starts at zero at the center of the wheel and ends at ten on the outermost part of the wheel. To complete the wheel, you place a dot on each section of the wheel somewhere on the line between zero and ten. Giving yourself a zero in a category means you have a lot of room for improvement in that category, whereas a score of ten means you are already living at your fullest potential in that category. As you add dots to your wheel, you'll start to see that you're thriving in some aspects of your life, where in other aspects, you feel more constricted. Once you're done placing a dot in each category, connect the dots around the circle. Ideally, you'll see a nice round wheel, but it's more likely that your wheel will look a little bumpy.

Just as you can't drive a car with a flat tire, a bumpy wheel of life lets us know that our lives are asking for more balance, and oftentimes, the key to that balance is in our self-care practice. Balance is a process, not a destination. There likely will not be a day when everything is a ten. Remember, the end goal isn't a round wheel that's all tens—it's just to have a round wheel, hopefully in the higher range of numbers. This could mean that you may need to pull back from some categories to find balance. If your career is a 10, but your family life is a five, you might realize that boosting your family score requires pulling back from your career score, perhaps striving for an eight in both categories.

The concept of self-care is not new, but for many of us, actually putting it into practice is new. A good self-care routine is like a good set of armor, allowing you to endure the challenges of life with greater ease. So much of our life can be out of our control, but one thing we can control is how we care for ourselves. Now, there's no such thing as a one-size-fits-all self-care routine. But any good self-care plan will be built around three core principles. First, it should give your life balance; second, it should give your life boundaries; and third, it should keep your energy reserves full.

The first topic already came up with the Wheel of Life—balance. Balance is a funny word. Many people look at finding balance as an end state or a final destination—a place we will finally reach when all our bills are paid, when we spend lots of quality time with our family, and when we have a healthy body. The truth is, balance is not an end state. It is an ongoing, constantly changing process. Balance is making sure that, day by day, aspects of your life aren't being neglected. If you find yourself blowing your top in fits of anger, it's a message that something is out of balance; perhaps your emotional needs aren't being met. And if you're finding yourself chronically exhausted, maybe it has to do with the fact that you're working 15-hour days and aren't looking out for your physical needs.

The second core principle of a self-care plan involves setting boundaries. We need boundaries to keep our lives balanced. Boundaries look different for everyone, but their purpose is the same, which is to set limits in aspects of our lives that tend to get too much of our attention or that bring us down. If someone is a negative force in your life, are you able to walk away from the relationship or say, "No, I'm not going to be treated that way," or do you tend to be passive about this? The foundation of setting boundaries is knowing when to say no to other people but also to yourself.

Our careers are a common area where it's important to consider setting boundaries. Do you regularly work 60 or more hours per week? Do you take every call that comes in? Do you check your email around the clock? Do any of these have an impact on other parts of your life? On you as a person? Do you put everyone's needs above your own? Asking yourself these questions can help you see where your life could be supported by better boundaries. Studies on clinicians and other high-stress helping professions have shown that professionals with higher hours of contact with clients have lower concentration, reduced memories, lower work satisfaction, and increased stress and irritability. A lack of boundary-setting hurts not only ourselves, but it can also hurt the people we're trying to help in the first place. Boundaries help support us and the people in our lives, and they ensure that our lives don't fall out of balance.

Which brings us to the third key principle of a good self-care plan: It should keep your energy reserves full. During 2017, I traveled across the country interviewing brilliant and inspiring women for my Women's Empowerment Initiative course, which is offered through Yoga International. One woman I interviewed is Dianne Bondy, a celebrated yoga teacher and leading voice in the Yoga For All movement. Dianne spoke on self-care for the Women's Empowerment Initiative, and one of her lines from that talk really stuck with me: "You have to support people from the overflow of energy, and not from your depths, because once you start pulling from your depths, you burn out very quickly." Dianne really captures the essence of self-care in this quote. Self-care is all about keeping your energy reserves so full that they don't become depleted when we live out all the responsibilities we have in our lives. A lack of balance and boundaries can drain our energy reserves, so looking at self-care in terms of energy reserves is the simplest way to make sure you're giving yourself the care you deserve.

Now that we have the basic principles of a self-care plan in place, let me tell you a little secret: A huge piece of self-care and our ability to be resilient is simply being nice to yourself. Valuing yourself. Believing in your importance in the world. How nice we are to ourselves usually can trace back to our own sense of self-worth. Our self-worth is the value we see ourselves as having. It is a combination of how we think about, feel about, and treat ourselves. Our self-worth is how we truly feel about ourselves deep down, all the way at our core. Our self-worth can be seen in our behaviors, in our self-talk, and in our interactions with others. It often is affected by our early experiences and how we've been socialized to see ourselves and our role in the world.

Sometimes someone's lack of self-worth is apparent to us, whereas other times it is less evident; sometimes insecurity and a lack of self-worth are masked by an outward appearance of over-the-top confidence, arrogance, or even narcissism. The only way to accurately uncover your own sense of self-worth is through deep, honest self-reflection. Think about how you talk to yourself. Are you harsh and self-critical? Would you ever talk to a friend the way you talk to yourself? Or on the flipside, do you build yourself up by tearing others down? Both of these can speak a lot to a lack of self-worth. A lot of times, our self-worth is reflected in our lack of self-care routine. But when we put our self-care routine back on the back burner, we're also putting our self-worth there, too.

The sister to self-worth is self-efficacy, or our belief that we can accomplish something. It is very common for our self-worth to affect our self-efficacy. If we don't think highly of ourselves, we might not have a very strong belief in our abilities. It is possible, though, to have a high sense of self-efficacy, while also having low self-worth. We might be really good at completing tasks and knowing we'll complete them well, but due to low self-worth, we may not think that we deserve the benefits of our hard work.

Research on both self-worth and self-efficacy shows that these qualities improve our ability to cope with and bounce back from circumstances. Let's see this in action by looking at the concept of codependency. When we are codependent, we find our self-worth through something or someone else—a husband or wife, a child, a pet, a title, or a career. If our sense of self-worth is dependent on something external, it goes down, or goes away completely, when the person or object is absent or disengaged from us. So, for example, if a dating prospect or current partner decides they don't want to be with us, we might internalize it as we're not "good enough." This thought implies that if only we were better or had more value, then we would have been the "good enough person." This thought ultimately comes from a lack of self-worth. When we fully recognize our worth, our feelings of not being good enough transform into an understanding that just because someone doesn't see their life with us, it doesn't take away from our inherent value as a person. This belief in turn can improve our self-efficacy, or our belief that we can navigate our personal life successfully in spite of challenges.

Everyone has unconditional worth just because they exist. No one is perfect, and it is possible for good people to make not good decisions. Cultivating self-compassion can help us work through deep feelings of shame that may seep through in actions that hurt ourselves and others. Self-compassion fuels our self-worth, and when you recognize your worth, you will naturally be more inclined to take care of yourself. We make time for what is most important to us. If you believe you're of value, you will find the time to take care of yourself.

Keep in mind that building self-compassion is a process; creating habits and rewiring thought patterns doesn't happen overnight. Even if your reaction is to be frustrated that it's hard to show yourself compassion, try to have compassion for that! Try to give yourself the same support that you might give to a baby learning how to walk; they make progress, they stumble or fall, and then they try again. And they're encouraged and supported by the people around them while they learn. Sometimes working through shame and building your sense of self-worth is best accomplished by a trained professional in helping people work through these emotions. Ultimately, the higher our sense of self-worth, the higher our resilience.

At the beginning of this class, we showed you how to use the Wheel of Life to rate yourself in different areas of life. Another way you can use this tool is to divide your wheel not by category of life but by category of need. Draw a circle, just as you did for the wheel of life, then create eight or 10 spokes on your wheel. There are many different ways you can label the spokes of the wheel, and you can, of course, feel free to label the spokes with whatever needs are pertinent to you. For the Needs Wheel that is included in your guidebook, we use physical needs, psychological (or emotional) needs, mental needs, overall relational needs, and spiritual needs. You can then add additional spokes for particular areas of focus. For instance, if you haven't gone to the doctor in a while, you may want to add a spoke for healthcare needs. Another example is to include needs in different relationships, such as your partnership, kids, etc. For spiritual needs, I have a category that includes things like going on an annual yoga and meditation retreat, as well as a daily meditation practice. Those are important and essential for me, but they might not be for you.

You'll notice that many of these needs are covered in other classes in this course. Some of you might be surprised to hear me list spirituality as a need, but it might not be what you think. While religion might be a piece of spiritual needs for some, what our spiritual needs really embody is our need for meaning, purpose, and connection with that which is greater than us as individuals. These needs can be met through meaningful work, frequent time for introspection and self-reflection, meditation or prayer, volunteer work, and time spent in nature.

No matter what you do to meet all types of your needs, it's important to ask if you're really being served by the way you're spending your time. Are you doing what supports the life you really want to lead, or are you living your life through habit, custom, obligation, or because someone told you to do it a certain way. When we feel an obligation to do something, it loses some of its value in nourishing us. If exercising, attending a service, meditating, or conducting volunteer work is seen as an item on a checklist, it is unlikely that it is actually meeting your need for purpose or meaning. Find something that truly serves you when you look to fulfill your needs.

Self-care is a huge piece of my life, but that hasn't always been the case. In fact, I didn't even go looking for self-care; self-care found me. Sometimes we don't care for ourselves until we get a wake-up call where we have no choice but to change. After my taxicab accident, I needed to heal, not only physically but emotionally, mentally, and spiritually. It was immediately apparent that my old regimen of running two to five miles a day on a treadmill, working 80 or 90 hours a week as an investment banking analyst, unwinding by drinking a glass or two of wine at night, and eating takeout on the run was entirely unsustainable. During this time, someone introduced me to the concept of keeping a self-care journal to track how I spend my time.

I went to the store, and I bought a little pocket-sized notebook. For one week, I wrote down all the activities I did and how long I spent doing them. This was nearly two decades ago, and there are now lots of phone tracking apps that can organize your time and track how you spend your time if you prefer a tech solution. Some apps even allow you to track how you spend time on your phone. Anyway, tracking my time was a really illuminating experience.

Overwork. Eating terribly. Not sleeping. Not exercising in a way that supported my healing body.

I then created my ideal Self-Care Journal that chronicled how I wanted to spend my time. Personally, I create a grid on a spreadsheet and then print out 52 copies on the first day of each year. There's an example in your guidebook. Down the left side of the grid, I write down all the different activities that I spend my time doing, including working, sleeping, family time, exercise, quality of my diet, meditation practice, and several more. Then in the column next to my activities, I put my ideal in each category where it's applicable so I have a point to measure against. For example, my goal is to sleep eight hours per night. Then I place seven blank rows for each day of the week next to my ideal.

I'll be honest. I tried for years keeping my spreadsheet online, and I found that it works better if I actually print out my daily practice log and just leave it next to my bed in a three-ring binder so I don't forget or get distracted late at night or on the computer. I have a ritual. On January 1st, I re-evaluate the way I'm spending my time, make any changes to the log that need to be made, and then I print out 52 copies, one for each week of the year. I then put them in a three-ring binder and place it next to my bed. Every night before I go to sleep, I spend 60 seconds recording what I did that day.

Now I'll go through the rows on the spreadsheet so you can get a better idea about how to work through it. These categories include what I do to take care of myself. The things you do may be completely different than what I'm sharing here. As always, feel free to make this practice your own. Let's dive in:

The first item is simple: wake up time. Just jot down what time you wake up.

The next is hours of sleep. Write down how many hours sleep you got the previous evening. If you don't sleep well, I would suggest adding an additional line item for quality of sleep.

The next is state of being. You can also call this row health. I put one or two words here to give a brief, instinctual glimpse of how I feel that day, such as strong, energized, clear, or exhausted. They don't have to mean anything to anyone but you.

After that comes quality of diet. Write down a couple of simple words that capture how you ate that day; for instance, if you ate really healthy that day, you can write, "fresh and light," or if you went out for burgers, you can write, "overate junk food."

The next row on my personal list is contemplation. Again, this may or may not resonate with you. For me personally, this usually takes the form of my personal mantra—a prayer I have for the day or something that I'm contemplating. For instance, yesterday, I prayed for a friend of mine and his family who just lost their beloved mother. Some people like to choose a prayer from their particular religion, like the Hail Mary if you're a Christian or the Three Daily Prayers if you're Jewish. If you like a more secular approach, you can also write down a personal affirmation, such as "I am healthy, whole, and complete just as I am."

Next is one of my favorites: silent meditation. Personally, I like doing my silent meditation practice in the morning because my mind is more still. Here, I enter the number of minutes I spend in meditation.

Then I like doing the next category, Yoga Nidra, which is a guided form of meditation, at night. We'll practice together in a future class. Right after I finish filling out my activity log, I put on my Yoga Nidra CD. It really feels like a filing system for the mind. Typically, I fall asleep within a few minutes and that's fine. There is some clinical research out that shows it has an effect on the subconscious mind even if you're in the deep sleep states. Again, I'll record the number of minutes I practice, even if I'm practicing while asleep.

Next comes the physical practice of yoga. I do a minimum 20 minutes every day. Then two or three times per week, I do an hour-and-a-half or a two-hour class, typically in a yoga studio, which is a great way to feel the support of a teacher and also to connect with a community.

After that is breathing. While you could of course put down 24 hours for the breathing practice every day, this section is devoted to time spent consciously breathing. I do my breathing exercise every morning right when I get out of bed and sit down on my meditation cushion. It's a great way to wake up the mind and bring some fresh air into your system after a long night's rest.

Next comes physical exercise. You can capture both your cardiovascular and your strength training here or break them into two separate categories—whatever is best for you. I swim or bike three to five times per week and do free weights a couple days per week, so I record that here.

Reading: Typically, I may, of course, be reading other things for work, but this space is reserved for my spiritual or inspirational readings. Typically, I list the title of what I'm reading here, and it's interesting because I oftentimes will see that becoming the focus of other aspects of my life as well.

Which brings us to our next category, which is the hours we spend with our family or those most important to us. It's interesting that many people say that family is the most important thing to them, and yet unless you are a stay-at-home parent with young children, the amount of time we spend with family can be one of the smallest numbers. You may want to set goals in relation to how this interacts with the next category, hours of work. If you are retired, you are welcome to pick whatever time focus feels most important for you.

You can also make a category for hours of social or fun. This includes things you do for fun: game night with the family, going for tea with a friend, dancing with your kids after finishing washing the dishes—whatever you do to play and enjoy life. It can also be interesting to include a separate category for screentime. There are some great apps that can help you track this.

The next category is selfless service. My personal definition for selfless service is something you do for someone or something else with no personal gain for yourself. I also try not to tell people what I do for my selfless service practice so that my ego doesn't get ahold of it. This can include simple things like calling someone you know is having a hard time or dropping dinner off for an elderly neighbor. It can also include bigger volunteer commitments to causes that are important to you.

After this, I keep a category for virtue focus. Each month, my son and I pick a virtue we want to cultivate more of in our lives. This month, our virtue focus is compassion. Each day, I write down a quick note about some way that I lived that virtue even if it was just an internal experience and not an external one.

Our next category is one of the most important on the list, which is the number of lies told. Sounds like a funny one, but it's really important. I try to count the number of times I tell a lie throughout the day. And if you say you never lie, add one to that number. Psychologists have shown that everyone lies sometimes, even if it's an exaggeration or an underplaying of something. While hopefully most of us don't walk around telling big whopper lies all day long or trying to knowingly deceive people, how many times does someone ask, "How are you?" and you say, "fine" or "great" when it's really not true? It's a really powerful practice because I start noticing the places where I lie, exaggerate, or downplay are the places where I feel vulnerable or weak. We also tell lies to ourselves mentally as well. It's really powerful to become more aware of when and how we do this.

Self-care is my next category. This can be doing something like getting a massage, taking a warm bath, having some downtime with a good book, or whatever you consider really nurturing for you. Any intentional time that focuses on your physical, emotional, mental, social, or spiritual needs is perfect to include here as well.

Gratitude is my second to last category and the perfect way to end the day. Here I record something that I was particularly grateful for that day.

And finally, you can record your time of sleep. This should be the last thing you write down before you turn out the lights and close your eyes.

And that's it! Typically, it takes me about 60 seconds to complete my self-care journal each day. I'm going to give you a non-money back guarantee that if you actually do this every day, you will learn a tremendous amount about yourself. You will begin to notice that when you don't take care of yourself, your health and mental state start to decline. When you do take care of yourself, everything starts to change. You also have to be accountable to the page every day, and personally, I feel this adds a layer of mindfulness to my life. It's really important to be accountable to ourselves, just as we would be accountable to our boss, partner, or child.

For about a decade, I had a friend who I would share my log with once a month. We would talk about what was working for us and what was not. It was a great point of reference, and it helped me stay accountable to know she was going to be seeing it. Again, health and resilience should not be an accident. When I started doing this practice, I very quickly realized that my self-care routine wasn't only helping me recover from the physical and emotional trauma from my accident, but it was also helping me heal from years and years of not really caring for myself. As I focused on self-care, I noticed that my ability to bounce back from the adversities of life skyrocketed, too.

Every single one of our self-care plans will look different, just how each of us have different needs. Your plan may include daily activities, such as time for deep breathing and self-reflection, and it may also include weekly or monthly activities, such as a massage or a retreat in nature. It could also include reminders to simply let yourself feel your feelings or to set aside time each day to write three things that you like about yourself.

Many of us live very full lives, and it can be easy to see self-care as an extra item on our to-do list, but self-care is so much more than that. Self-care really creates the foundation for our resilience by keeping our tank full and ready to go. Tracking and reflecting on self-care can bring your attention to a few simple changes that can bring more balance and freedom to your life, improving your overall resilience. Hopefully throughout this class, you've been thinking about your own life and ways to boost your own self-care. Now take those thoughts with you and put them into action. Enjoy giving yourself the nourishment that you deserve.

Class 9

The Rewards of Sleep

Having healthy sleep patterns can transform your life. There is significant evidence that sleeping can help you live longer, improve your memory, decrease anxiety and depression, improve physical and mental health, and promote safety. All of these can help boost your resilience. This class looks at what happens to the body during sleep and ways you can improve your sleep.

The Body during Sleep

- When you sleep, you move through several distinct sleep stages. Stage 1 is the process of beginning to fall asleep where your muscles start to relax, your eyes may have a difficult time staying open, and the world around you starts to disappear. Stage 2 is a light, dreamless sleep where the body is settling into rest. You may still be able to wake up easily from this stage of sleep.

- Stages 3 and 4 are when slow-wave sleep starts to kick in and the body gets to rest. Brain and muscle activity significantly decreases. These are the stages where you truly replenish your physical and mental energy reserves.

- Rapid eye movement (REM) sleep is another stage that occurs throughout the night. The REM phase is the one most closely associated with dreaming. The mind becomes extremely active, but the muscles and body are in a state of paralysis. Some describe REM sleep as a "rinse" of the brain, where it clears away toxins and byproducts that have accumulated throughout the day.

- People move through these stages four or five times throughout the course of a healthy night's rest. If you do not receive seven to eight hours of sleep, the body doesn't have the opportunity to move through these cycles several times. Additionally, sleep interruptions inhibit the ability to move cleanly through these sleep cycles.

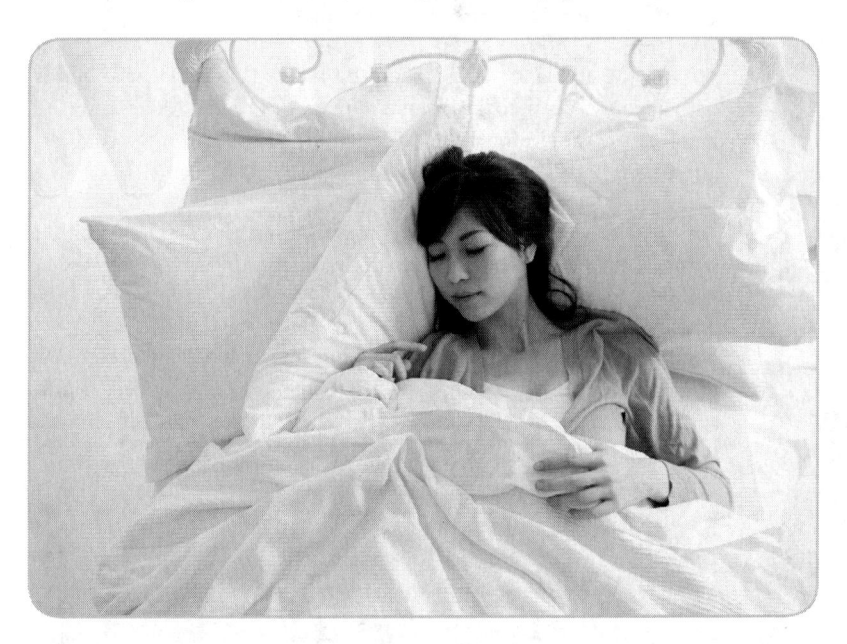

> **Preparing for Sleep**
>
> Just as you prepare yourself for a workout, you can also prepare yourself for sleep so that you get the most out of it. The following are several tips for sleep preparation.

Creating the Right Bedroom

- Take a look at your bedroom and ask yourself if everything in there helps you feel peaceful, nurtured, comfortable, and at ease. If not, remove it. Try to make sure that everything in the room is something uplifting and that it's free from clutter.

- Instead of the stack of books next to your bed, just keep the one you are reading. Instead of piling your clothes on a chair in the corner, try putting them in the laundry or hanging them up. Choose soft lighting or candles before sleep rather than bright overhead lights.

- Prepare the ambiance of the room by making sure you have blinds or blackout shades to keep light out of the room. Make sure the temperature is right for sleep: The room being too hot or too cold can affect your body's ability to relax throughout the night.

- You may also want to invest in a new mattress. It's crucial to find a mattress that it is right for your body. Then, top it off with sheets, blankets, and pillows that make you feel comfortable.

- Some people who have trouble sleeping find that weighted blankets are helpful to them. It can help the body feel more protected and secure, much like swaddling a baby. It's also important to keep animals off the bed if they disturb your sleep.

Televisions and Phones

- Many people have televisions in their bedrooms; however, televisions are highly stimulating to the brain, which can disturb it before sleep. If you watch television, try to do it earlier in the day or evening and set limits on it. Nearly every television comes with a timer. Set limits for yourself and try to stick to them.

- It is also a good idea to put your cell phone in another room of your house while you sleep and to put the phone on silent mode, so as to not be disturbed by notifications. Taking the phone into your bedroom also can rob you of extra sleep, as many people end up reading the news, surfing social media, or playing games.

- Instead of using the alarm clock on your phone, buy an old-fashioned alarm and use that to wake you up instead of your phone. If you want to use your smartphone for something useful related to sleep, most smartphones come with sleep timers that will remind you when to go to sleep.

Exercise, Water, Caffeine, and Alcohol

- If you find that you have trouble sleeping, you may want to increase the amount of exercise you do during the day. It's important to get some sort of physical movement or exercise every day.

- If you have trouble sleeping, also look at how much caffeine, sugar, or other stimulants you are consuming. For example, caffeine is a double-edged sword: People turn to it when they don't feel rested, and then it perpetuates the cycle of their bodies not being able to rest. Try not to drink any caffeinated beverages after 12:00 pm if you have trouble sleeping at night.

- Be sure to drink plenty of water during the day. People often feel fatigued when their bodies are dehydrated. Many people turn to caffeine during these moments, when they may instead need water.

However, try not to drink too many liquids after dinner, as these can lead to having to go to the bathroom frequently throughout the night.

- Many people turn to alcohol to help them fall asleep. The problem is that alcohol also causes the body to wake up in the middle of the night. It both disrupts sleep and diminishes sleep quality. Additionally, it is a diuretic, which can wake you up for multiple trips to the bathroom when you should be sleeping.

Preparing the Body and Mind for Sleep

- It is much better for the body to use natural ways to fall and stay asleep, and there are ways you can prepare your body for sleep. If you are someone who tends to harbor tension in your body, you may want to start by doing some gentle stretches, tension and relaxation exercises, or breathing exercises that evoke the relaxation response.

- Just as it is a good idea to avoid looking at television or checking the news before bed, it is also a good idea to calm down the mind before sleep. Read something relaxing or inspiring instead of something that can disturb the mind. Additionally, try to have uplifting conversations or interactions instead of going into a sticky emotional issue that may cause agitation before sleep.

- Avoid checking work email or messages before sleep, which can get the wheels of the mind turning. You'll be more effective at whatever you have to do the next day when your body and mind have had enough time to rest and restore.

- Another practice that can help calm down the mind before bed is to do a day's review. Every night before going to sleep, mentally go through your day and think about what went well. Think about why those actions felt so good to you and how perhaps you helped other people or made a positive difference.

- If there are memories from the day that you don't feel good about, bring those to mind. Think about how you would do them differently next time or something good that may come from those actions eventually. This will help create positive thought patterns and can help to clean up any lingering issues in the brain.

> **Yoga Nidra**
> Yoga Nidra guided meditation may be able to help you sleep more deeply. It is also an excellent tool for napping. Some initial research has found that 20 minutes of Yoga Nidra is equal to approximately two hours of sleep in terms of how the brain restores itself.

- Taking a bath before bedtime can be yet another nurturing way to calm down the body and mind before bedtime. The hot water elevates the body temperature, but when you get out, the flash of cooler air causes the body to naturally start producing melatonin. Adding Epsom salts to your bath can amp up the healing properties.

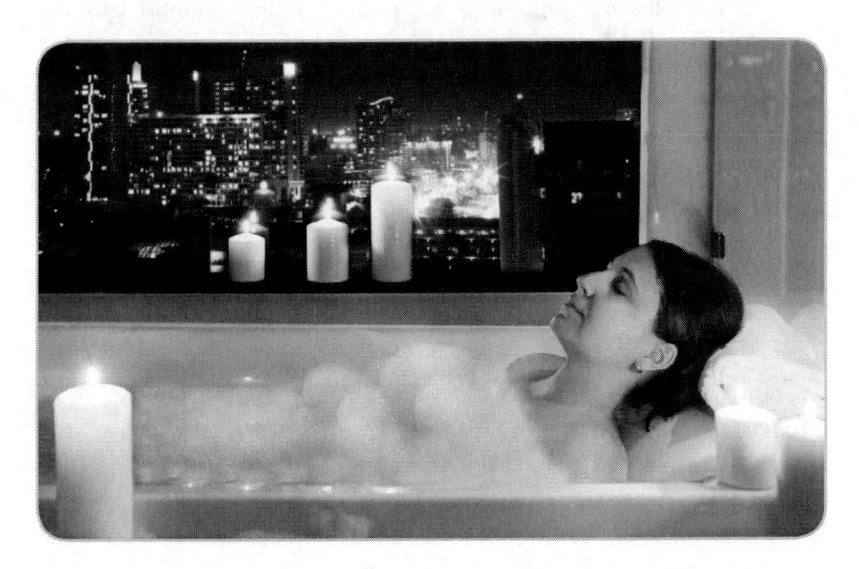

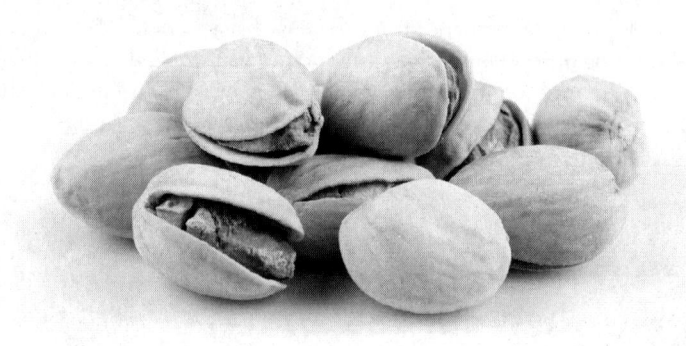

- It is best to avoid eating two hours before going to sleep to give your body a chance to properly digest. If you are going to snack pre-bedtime, choose foods that are high in B vitamins, magnesium, and protein. Try to avoid high-calorie foods at this time.

- Reliability is an important trait to have when cultivating a sleep routine. The human body loves rhythms and patterns. If you promise yourself you are going to get eight hours of sleep, follow through every night. If you have a late event, plan to start your morning later the next day so that you can get a full eight hours.

- The best practice is to set a time that you are going to go to sleep every night so that your body naturally starts producing melatonin and serotonin. Find your body's natural biorhythm—that is, when your body prefers to fall asleep and then to wake up when it is fully rested. You will know you have succeeded at this when you no longer need an alarm clock. Invest in finding the pattern that is right for you. Your body and mind will thank you.

Suggested Reading

Huffington, *The Sleep Revolution*.

Mednick, *Take a Nap!*

Activities

- Transform your bedroom into a sleep sanctuary.

- Over the next couple of days, complete a day's review before going to sleep.

- Answer the following:

    » In what ways do you have good sleep hygiene?

    » In what ways do you have bad sleep hygiene?

- Complete Practice Class 3 (Class 19), titled "Promoting Sleep."

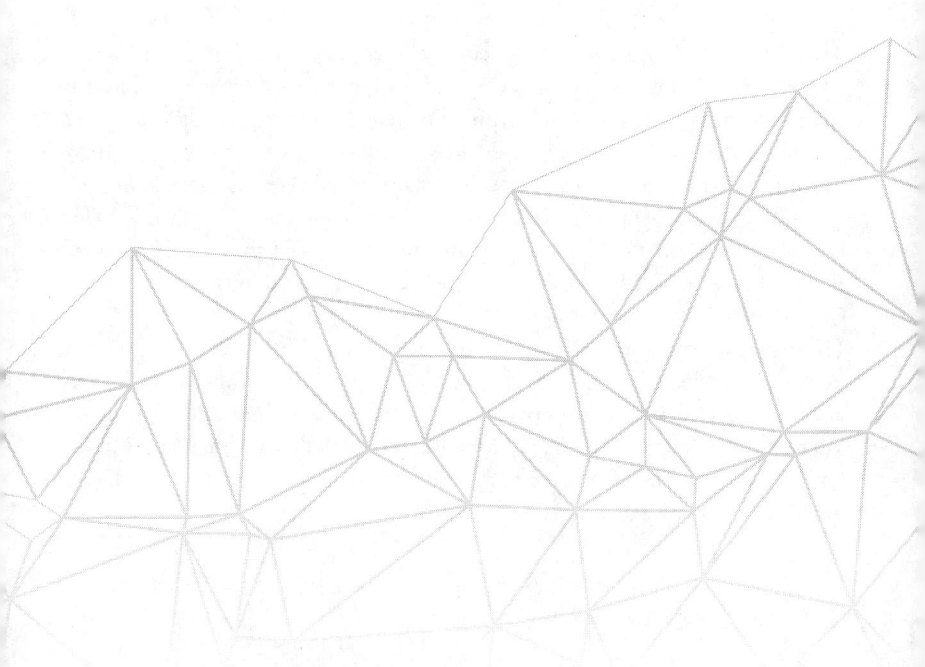

Class 9 Transcript

The Rewards of Sleep

Oh, I am so excited about this class. I love to sleep. I love teaching people how to sleep. I love learning how and why the body loves sleep so much. And I'm so excited about everything I have to share here with you because it has the potential to transform how your body sleeps, your health, and quite honestly, the quality of your entire life. I did not come at this information in an easy way. I earned this knowledge the hard way after my car accident through navigating years and years of insomnia, using a whole lot of trial and error. If you suffer from sleep issues, I feel your pain, and I sincerely hope this class will help you.

This class is also based on my experience helping trauma survivors learn to sleep. My car accident was nothing compared to the experiences of veterans and human trafficking survivors I've worked with who were awoken repeatedly throughout the night, some for years or even decades, during what can only be considered living nightmares. I will tell you sincerely that I've had veterans come to me who claim they haven't slept more than two consecutive hours since the Vietnam War, but when they apply these principles, they're able to sleep six and eight hours a night. These practices can work when diligently applied and followed.

Having healthy sleep patterns can transform your life. There is significant evidence that sleeping can help you live longer, improve your memory, decrease anxiety and depression, improve physical and mental health, and promote safety. Sleep affects how we learn, connect, think, work, eat, react, and interact with each other. Nearly every aspect of life can be improved by improving the quality and quantity of sleep.

The damage you can do to your body through not sleeping can manifest in the blink of an eye in situations like a car crash, or it can occur over time, as is the case with the long, long list of chronic health conditions that can result from lack of sleep, including heart disease, diabetes, high blood pressure, kidney disease, obesity, stroke, and many more. Sleep affects our hormones, including ghrelin, which makes us feel hungry, and leptin, which makes us feel full. If we don't sleep enough, our ghrelin levels increase, and our leptin levels decrease, causing us to feel hungrier than when we are well-rested and the opposite occurs. Sleep also affects how our body reacts to insulin, such that sleep deprivation can lead to high blood glucose levels. Long-term sleep deficiency can also change the way our immune system responds, increasing our likelihood for both minor and major illnesses.

That's just our physical body. If we turn to look at the brain, sleep affects decision-making, concentration, memory, productivity, reactivity, and our ability to regulate emotions and access higher-level thought functions. Sleep deprivation can even change the function and shape of our brains. Memory, problem-solving, and decision-making are affected due to decreased activity in the frontal and parietal lobes of the brain. A 2017 study found that sleep deprivation can cause our brain cells to eat portions of the brain's synapses. In short bouts of sleep deprivation, this may affect our short-term memory and recall abilities. Sounds like a good reason not to stay up all night cramming for a test. In the long term, this type of activity is seen in brain disorders like dementia and Alzheimer's.

Yet, another study found that the amygdala in the brain of a sleep-deprived person was 60% more reactive than the amygdala in the brain of someone who gets healthy sleep. This increase in reactivity means that sleep-deprived brains apply more emotional weight than necessary in many situations, which is why it's never a good idea to start a difficult discussion when you're sleep deprived! Sleep is important to our entire society. Drowsy drivers contribute to about 100,000 car accidents in the US every year, which result in more than 1,500 deaths. There are some horrific stories about how even just one person not sleeping can lead to catastrophe, including nuclear reactor meltdowns, aviation accidents, and even the Exxon Valdez oil spill.

Many people don't even realize that they're sleep deprived. In many ways, it's become a way of life. Something called microsleep happens for many people every day. This is when the body is essentially awake, but the brain goes into brief episodes of sleep. Perhaps there are moments of your morning commute that you don't remember by the time you get to work. There may be moments during a meeting when you just blank out or can't remember what was shared, or times that you glaze over while staring at the computer screen and can't remember what you were doing. You may forget something your partner or child tells you during dinner. If these experiences sound familiar, you may be microsleeping, which is itself a sign of sleep deprivation. Certainly, if you are nodding off throughout the day, this is a very clear sign that your body is begging for rest!

Our society in many ways values doing above all else. Sleep gets left on the back burner far too often. We sleep when we fall over from exhaustion. And unfortunately, falling over from exhaustion is oftentimes what it takes to get people to really value the importance of sleep in their lives. By not sleeping, we are robbing ourselves of one of our body's most essential natural instincts. There are billion-dollar industries built around how to avoid sleep through stimulants, and there are also billion-dollar industries built around getting people to sleep, whether through pharmaceuticals, devices, or natural remedies. Really, it doesn't have to be that complex. Our bodies know how to sleep. They want to sleep desperately. We just need to give our bodies the conditions for sleep to naturally unfold and find solutions for whatever may be standing in the way.

So what actually happens to the body when we sleep? When we sleep, we move through several distinct sleep stages. Stage one is the process of beginning to fall asleep where our muscles start to relax, our eyes may have a difficult time staying open, and the world around us starts to disappear. Stage two is a light, dreamless sleep where the body is settling into rest. We may still be able to wake up easily from this stage of sleep. Stages three and four are what we call slow-wave sleep. It starts to kick in, and the body then gets to rest. Brain and muscle activity significantly decrease. These are the stages where we really replenish our physical and mental energy reserves.

Rapid eye movement, or REM sleep for short, is another stage that occurs throughout the night. The REM phase is the one most closely associated with dreaming, when the mind becomes extremely active, but the muscles and the body are in a state of paralysis. Some describe REM sleep as a rinse of the brain, where it clears away toxins and byproducts that have accumulated throughout the day. It makes sense, too, from a psychological perspective, given many times dreams seem like they are trying to process the events of our conscious and subconscious minds.

We move through these stages of sleep four and five times throughout the course of a healthy night's rest. You can see that if you don't get seven to eight hours of sleep, the body doesn't have the opportunity to move through these cycles several times. Also, when we suffer from interrupted sleep due to a crying baby, a snoring spouse, a phone dinging all night long, or due to alcohol or caffeine consumption, we inhibit our ability to move cleanly through these sleep cycles.

Many people take sleep for granted. They think if they put their head down on the pillow, they should be magically granted eight long hours of deeply restorative sleep. For some, this naturally happens. For billions more, this is just not the case. In reality, healthy sleep is not an accident. Just as you prepare yourself for a workout, you can also prepare yourself for sleep so that you're getting the most out of the time with your eyes closed. We're going to go through some things you can do now before you even get into bed. You might think of these as tips for transforming your bedroom into a sleep sanctuary.

First, I encourage you to take a look at your bedroom and ask yourself if everything in there helps you feel peaceful, nurtured, comfortable, and at ease. If not, remove it. Ideally, our bedrooms are for two things: Sleep and sex. Try to make sure that everything in the room is something uplifting and that it's free from clutter. Instead of the stack of books next to your bed, just keep the one you're reading. Instead of piling your clothes on a chair in the corner, try putting them in the laundry or hanging them up. Choose soft lighting or candles before sleep rather than bright overhead lights. Someone told me once that the state of your bedroom reflects the state of your mind. I've watched that over time, and I've found it to be almost alarmingly true.

You will want to prepare the ambiance of the room by making sure you have blinds or blackout shades to keep light out of the room. You'll also want to make sure the temperature is right for sleep. Too hot or too cold can affect your body's ability to relax throughout the night. Some say that having a cold sleep space increases the production of melatonin, which is a natural hormone that plays a role in sleep. For some people, however, a cold sleep space can make it hard to relax.

Once you've uncluttered your bedroom, made adjustments to keep the light out, and found the ambient temperature that's right for you, you may want to invest in a new mattress. It's crucial to find a mattress that it is right for your body. Then top it off with sheets, blankets, and pillows that make you feel perfectly snuggly and cozy. Think about if the sheets and comforter you're using are right for your body. This may change with the seasons. Some people who have trouble sleeping find that weighted blankets are helpful for them. It can help the body feel more protected and secure, much like swaddling a baby. It's also important to keep animals off the bed if they disturb your sleep.

This brings me to a really important topic: television in the bedroom. Even if you love having your television in your bedroom, please try to listen open-mindedly to what I'm about to share. A television is one of the most stimulating things in your household, if not the most stimulating. Just take a moment to reflect on what TV does to the brain. When we watch anything that is stimulating, from news to drama or action shows, we're engaging circuits of arousal and emotion in the brain. Clinical studies have shown that watching television causes increased aggressiveness, mood disorders, and a thickening of the hypothalamus, which is characteristic of patients with borderline personality disorder. Another study found that for each additional hour of television watched per day in childhood, the odds of developing symptoms of depression increase by 8%, and the odds of developing type 2 diabetes increase by 20%. If you do watch television, try to do it earlier in the day or evening and set limits on it. Nearly every television comes with a timer. Set limits for yourself and really try to stick to them.

Above and beyond how the content of the television may be disturbing your brain before sleep, the light emitted by the television stimulates a nerve pathway that runs from the eyes to the places in your brain that control hormones, body temperature, and other functions that control whether we feel wide-awake or ready for a long night's rest. Many studies show that the light emitted from devices like phones, tablets, and televisions can prevent someone from falling asleep by tricking the brain into thinking that it is still light outside and therefore time to be awake. It is recommended to stop looking at screens two hours before bedtime, but if that is impossible for you, try at least 30 minutes.

It is also a good idea to put your cell phone in another room of your house while you sleep and to also put the phone on silent so as to not be disturbed by notifications. A shocking survey by Huffington Post and YouGov found that 63% of smartphone users between the ages of 18 and 29 actually keep their cell phones in their bed when they sleep. Listen people, you can't use your cell phone while you're asleep, and you are much more likely to check your phone in the middle of the night if it's lying in your bed, which can really disturb your sleep patterns.

Taking the phone into your bedroom can also distract from intimacy and can rob you of extra sleep, as many people end up reading the news, surfing social media, or playing games much farther into the night than they would if they simply left the phone somewhere else when they headed for the bedroom. Instead of using the alarm clock on your phone, buy an actual alarm clock—the old fashioned kind—and use that to wake you up instead of your phone.

If you want to use your smart phone for something useful related to sleep, most smartphones come with sleep timers that will remind you when to go to bed. You can also download an app like Moment that tracks your cell phone usage throughout the day and also reminds you of when you're going over the limit you set for yourself. The app also tracks which applications on your phone you spend the most time on, which can be a very shocking experience. When people say they don't have enough time to get eight hours of sleep or exercise, I invite them to download Moment and then report back to me in a week how much time they spent on their phone doing all sorts of things. Through awareness, we can become more conscious of our actions and make better choices about how we spend our time.

Now that you've prepared your bedroom sanctuary for sleep, how can you prepare your body and mind? First of all, the things that you can do during your day set you up for a good night's rest. If you find you have trouble sleeping, you may want to increase the amount of exercise you do during the day. Many people use their minds a lot during the day, but their bodies are sitting at a desk. While you may be mentally exhausted, your body might not have moved at all. It's important to get some sort of physical movement or exercise every day. For those of you who have ever had a small child, you know this is true. On the days when they get a ton of exercise, they pass out at night. When they don't, it can be a total disaster trying to get them to slow down or to go to bed! As adults, we are very much the same. Make sure you're taking time to get all of your energy out.

If you have trouble sleeping, you will also want to look at how much caffeine, sugar, or other stimulants you're consuming. When I was teaching at the Miami Department of Veterans Affairs, I would frequently have veterans coming to my 4:00 p.m. meditation class, sipping on an energy drink or a cup of coffee, telling me they can't go to sleep at night. Caffeine is really a double-edged sword because people turn to it when they don't feel rested, and then it perpetuates the cycle of their bodies not being able to rest. Try not to drink any caffeinated beverage after 12:00 p.m. if you have trouble sleeping at night. Also, be sure to drink plenty of water during the day. Oftentimes, we feel fatigued when our bodies are dehydrated. Many people turn to caffeine during these moments, which only dehydrates the body more. What they really may need is a big, fresh glass of water with some lemon in it. Try not to drink too many liquids after dinner, as these can lead to having to go to the bathroom frequently throughout the night.

Now let's take a look at alcohol consumption and sleep. It turns out that alcohol is the most common sleep aid with 20% of people turning to it to help them fall asleep at night. In truth, alcohol can help the body fall asleep. The problem is that alcohol also causes the body to wake up in the middle of the night. It both disrupts sleep and also diminishes sleep quality. If that wasn't enough, it is a diuretic, which can wake you up for multiple trips to the bathroom when you should be sleeping. Also, when alcohol is used frequently to fall asleep, it can cause insomnia when you don't have it.

It is much better for the body to use natural ways to fall and stay asleep. So how can we prepare our bodies for sleep? If you're someone who tends to harbor tension in your body, you may want to start by doing some gentle stretches, tension and relaxation exercises, or breathing exercises that evoke the relaxation response. We have a whole practice class devoted to exercises that evoke the relaxation response, a practice class devoted to breathing exercises, and another devoted to sleep, so you will definitely want to check those out for directions and suggestions.

Just as it's a good idea to avoid looking at television or checking the news before bed, it's also a good idea to calm down the mind before sleep. Read something relaxing or inspiring instead of something that can disturb the mind. Also, have uplifting conversations or interactions instead of going into a sticky emotional issue that may cause an argument or for the mind to get agitated before sleep. My grandmother once told me, "If you're ready to pick a fight before you go to bed, give it 24 hours and a good night's sleep." I have to say that at least 75% of the time, the issue resolves itself.

It's also important not to check work email or messages before sleep, which can really get the wheels of the mind turning. You'll be more effective at whatever you do the next day when your body and mind have had enough time to rest and restore. Do everything you can to give your mind the opportunity to be calm when you put your head down on the pillow.

Another practice that can really help calm down the mind before bed is to do what's called a day's review. Every night before going to sleep, mentally go through your day and think about what went really well: the things that you felt really good about. Think about why those actions felt so good to you and how perhaps you helped other people or made a positive difference. If there are memories from the day that don't feel good, bring those to mind and think about how you would do them differently next time or perhaps something good that may come from it eventually. This will help you create positive thought patterns and can help to clean up any lingering issues in the brain.

Oftentimes the things that keep us awake at night are places in our life where we don't feel safe. This may include being safe in a relationship or work setting, or it could include feeling safe just being alone with ourselves. In our class on the importance of safety, we'll learn about a tool called the inner resource, which can also be very valuable for sleep. An inner resource is an internal place of safety and wellbeing. It may be a place in nature that, when you imagine it, helps you feel calm and relaxed, or an inner resource might involve thinking about people or spiritual figures who help you feel peaceful and at ease. But whatever your inner resource might be, I encourage you to spend time knowing that when you snuggle up into bed, you are safe, healthy, and whole just as you are.

The next practice is probably my favorite in my own personal sleep routine. That's Yoga Nidra guided meditation. The Sanskrit phrase *Yoga Nidra* is often translated as "the yoga of sleep" because it is the one form of meditation that can intentionally put you to sleep while you're practicing it. I like to think of it like a filing system for my mind that gently takes me by the hand and guides me through a journey of witnessing my body, breath, feelings, emotions, beliefs, and down into a deep state of awareness where rest and relaxation naturally unfold. I fall asleep every night doing a Yoga Nidra. I find that I sleep more deeply, and also that the emotions or challenges from the day naturally process themselves. Yoga nidra is also an excellent tool for napping. Some initial research has found that 20 minutes of Yoga Nidra is equal to approximately two hours of sleep in terms of how the brain restores itself. Sometimes I do a short practice in the middle of the afternoon when I may otherwise be tempted to reach for a caffeinated beverage. Yoga nidra leaves me feeling refreshed and relaxed instead of wired and scattered.

This is one of the reasons that the military has adopted the use of Yoga Nidra. We're also finding it can be highly effective for insomnia. It's so easy to practice: You simply play a recorded guided meditation either from a CD or on your phone. If you use your phone, please make sure to put it on airplane mode. It's also good to make a playlist with only one Yoga Nidra session on it so that the next one doesn't start immediately after the first one finishes, which can happen if you play a whole CD or album. If you happen to wake up in the middle of the night, try putting on a short version recording of Yoga Nidra as a tool to guide you gently back to sleep. I have several recordings devoted to sleep which do not bring you back to wakefulness at the end, including the Yoga Nidra practice class included with this course. I am an iRest Yoga Nidra Teacher Trainer and I actually teach an entire Great Courses program on iRest Yoga Nidra. So if you are interested, you will definitely want to check that out.

Taking a bath before bedtime can be yet another really nurturing way to calm down the body and mind before bedtime. The hot water elevates the body temperature, but then when you get out, that flash of cooler air causes the body to naturally start producing melatonin. Adding Epsom salts to your bath can amp up the healing properties. Some people find that salt baths can help relax muscles, reduce inflammation, lessen joint pain, and even lower blood pressure. One study found that taking a hot bath can even burn calories! Just be sure not to fall asleep in the tub.

It is best to avoid eating two hours before going to sleep to give your body a chance to properly digest. If you're going to snack pre-bedtime, choose foods that are high in B vitamins, magnesium, and protein, including pistachios or dates, which can help produce the hormone melatonin. Almonds contain tryptophan, the amino acid also found in turkey that everybody talks about making us sleepy after Thanksgiving dinner. Cherries, oats, and nuts are also natural sources of melatonin that can help your body relax. Just don't eat too much. Foods that are high in calories can keep you awake. Of course, the old chamomile tea or ginger tea remedy can calm your nerves pre-bedtime as well.

Reliability is a really important trait to have when cultivating a sleep routine. Our bodies love rhythms and patterns. If you promise yourself you're going to get eight hours of sleep, follow through every night. If for some reason you have a late dinner or event, plan to start your morning later the next day so that you can get a full eight hours. The best practice is to set a time that you are going to go to sleep every night so that your body naturally starts producing melatonin and serotonin. Find your body's natural biorhythm—when your body prefers to fall asleep and then to wake up when it's fully rested. You will know when you have succeeded at this when you no longer need an alarm clock to wake up. Invest in finding the pattern that's right for you. Your body and mind will thank you.

Keep in mind that you may have been cultivating negative sleep patterns your entire life, so it may take a little while before your body adjusts to using these new techniques. Be patient and give it your best effort to do all the things you've learned in this class. In time, a healthier sleep life will follow. And with that in place, you're on your way to building a more resilient mind and body.

Sweet dreams!

Class 10

Finding Equanimity with Mindfulness

This class explores how mindfulness and meditation can contribute to your physical and emotional resilience. All forms of mindfulness and meditation are designed to help you have a direct experience of stillness so that you can live from a place of peacefulness. There are many pathways to the same destination, and this class covers several of them.

Meditation as a Tool

- Meditation is a practical and simple tool that you can use to train your mind to be more focused, healthier, and happier. Meditation is scientifically validated now by thousands of clinical studies.

- However, meditation is not about escaping your reality. It is about being present with what is so that you can move through it effectively.

> Although many religions do use meditation as a part of their practice, meditation is not a religious practice. Meditation can be an entirely secular activity.

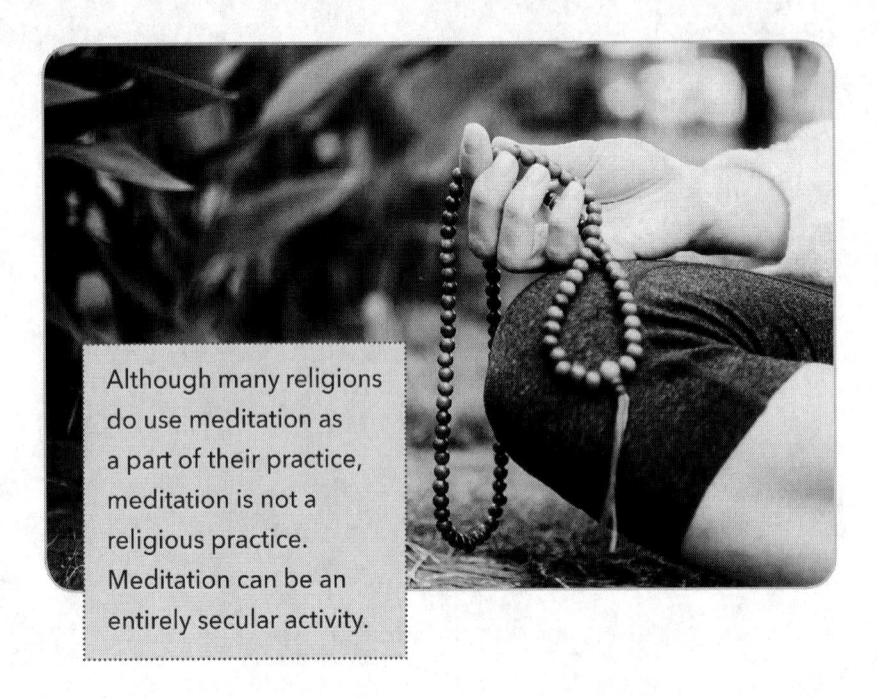

You do not have to make your thoughts stop to meditate, and you do not have to spend hours a day meditating.

Concentration-Based Meditation

- There are many forms of meditation, but they mostly fall into two main categories: concentration-based meditation and mindfulness meditation. Concentration-based meditation involves sitting quietly and picking a point of focus for the mind to rest upon.

- Typically in the Eastern traditions, a mantra or syllable was used to help focus the mind. You can also pick a point of focus like a flower, stone, or sound. Once the mind becomes focused on the mantra or object, the thoughts begin to slow down, and the mind is then able to settle into deeper states of stillness. During practice, you may find that your mind is particularly distracted in the beginning, but then it starts to calm down as you repeat the word or mantra.

- Concentration-based practices root back to the Hindu and Buddhist traditions that use mantras, such as *om*, *om namah shivaya*, and *om mani padme h m*, as a point of focus during the meditation. You can use these traditional mantras, or you can use a phrase or affirmation that will help your mind to focus. One example is the phrase, "I am happy, healthy, and peaceful, just as I am." You can also pick a word such as *love* or *courage* to repeat to yourself. If you have a particular religious prayer or mantra that works for you from your religious tradition, you can use this as well.

- If you are deeply connected to nature, you can choose to focus on a flower, stone, or tree. Some people enjoy focusing on the flame of a candle. As the mind begins to calm down, you can release the mantra and just let the mind rest in stillness. If the mind begins to get distracted again by various thoughts, you can begin again with the mantra.

Mindfulness Meditation

- The second type of meditation is mindfulness meditation. At its core, mindfulness is the ability to pay attention on purpose. It involves observing your experience in the present moment without judgment, and it can be practiced at any moment in your life. The more it is practiced, the more it becomes a natural way of life. The more natural it becomes, the more helpful mindfulness can be in building your resilience.

A Brief History of Mindfulness

One of the pioneers in introducing mindfulness to the medical field is Jon Kabat-Zinn, who developed a treatment program known as mindfulness-based stress reduction, or MBSR. In 1992, researchers Zindel Segal, Mark Williams, and John Teasdale sought to create a group that utilized dialectical behavior therapy, acceptance therapy, and commitment therapy, but during the development process, they participated in an MBSR session. They were amazed by the experience.

Instead of their original idea, the trio created mindfulness-based cognitive therapy, which became one of the first integrations of mindfulness and traditional cognitive therapy to be used in the mental health field. Some other common and well-known mental health treatment orientations that use the power of mindfulness are dialectical behavior therapy and acceptance commitment therapy.

Another application is Integrative Restoration, or iRest Yoga Nidra, which uses mindfulness to promote healing, relaxation, and resilience. Richard Miller, a clinical psychologist, author, researcher, and yogic scholar, adapted traditional Yoga Nidra, which has been around for over 2,000 years, into the secular practice of iRest.

- Mindfulness practices are not about fixing what you are experiencing. You witness it, observe it, and allow it to tell its story. The moment you begin trying to fix and change yourself, tension and stress begin to arise.

- This is the essence of resilience. It is essential to learn to keep your peace amidst whatever happens in life rather than letting it be dependent on outward conditions. That does not, however, mean that you don't work to affect change in your life. It just means that your peace of mind is not dependent upon it.

How to Be Mindful

- When you're awake, most of your time is spent doing things, such as work and caring for your family. When doing a task, you might not be fully present in what you are doing. For instance, you might be thinking of something else while completing the task at hand.

- The first piece of mindfulness is reminding yourself that people are not called human *doings*; they are human *beings*. The word *being* implies being present in the moment. But when people are overtly attached to the end goal, they often lose the ability to be fully present in the moment.

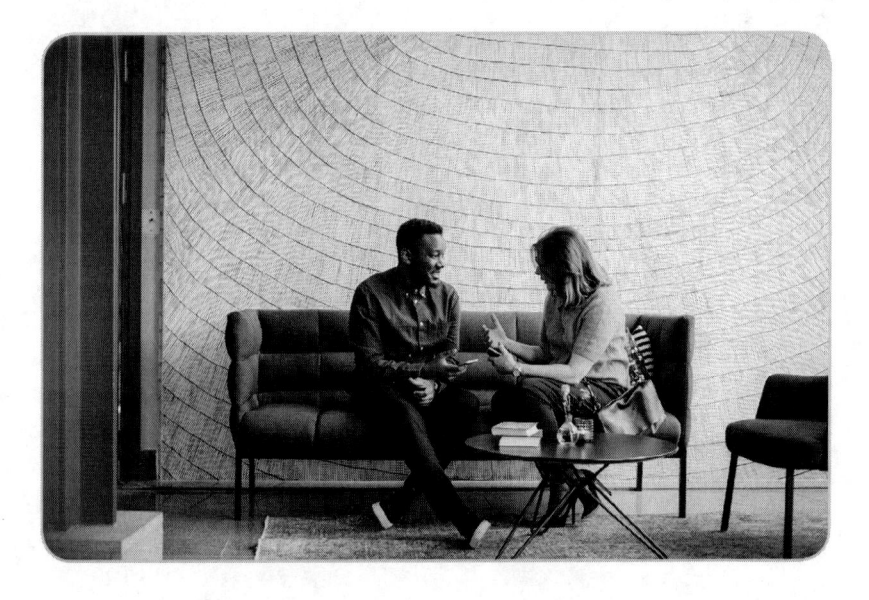

- Instead, people form attachments to some point on the horizon that may or may not ever come. It is important to value how you do things just as much as the end state of what you are doing. Ideally, if you are fully present in the moment as you are doing something, you will be even more efficient and effective in achieving your goals. Additionally, you will arrive there with a present and peaceful state of mind rather than a stressed-out sense of urgency.

- It is likely that your attention is constantly being grabbed by different stimuli, such as someone calling your name, a loud noise outside, or a notification on your phone. To practice mindfulness, try bringing your attention to things that aren't screaming for your attention.

- Orient yourself to your entire surrounding, and try using all of your senses. Pay attention to the sensation of your clothes on your body or note every sound in your surroundings. You might also try pointing out five things that are a certain color around you, four tactile sensations you have, three things you can hear, two things you can smell, and one thing you can taste.

Connecting to Your Body

- Once passively observing your surroundings becomes easier, it will become easier to learn how to passively observe uncomfortable emotions and thoughts as well. Much of your ability to do this comes from your ability to connect with your physical body.

- Your body constantly gives you information about how you're feeling and what you're doing. For example, you might hold stress in your shoulders. Such sensations are messages that you need to listen to. Mind-body practices like yoga and qigong can help you improve your connection to your own body so that you can learn to feel and interpret these messages.

- Co-meditation is another tool that can be used to practice connecting with what is happening in your body while, at the same time, being present for another person as well. It is a partner practice that is easy to do and takes a surprisingly short amount of time to bring you fully into the present moment.

- Sit with a trusted friend, family member, or your partner and take turns sharing what sensations you each feel in your body. Both participants can either keep their eyes opened or closed, whichever is most comfortable for them.

- Set a timer for two minutes. For the first two minutes, one person shares and the other person listens. Once the timer goes off, you switch, and the other person shares for two minutes while the person who shared first listens. Each two minutes, switch from person to person.

- During the successive two-minute increments, participants share answers to these questions without being asked: What is present? Where do I feel what is present in my body? For instance, one person might share, "I feel tension in my stomach and an sense of uneasiness about a conversation I had this morning."

- Parts of the practice may be done in silence as the person feels into what is present. The person sharing may speak for the entire two minutes about one thing that is present. Alternatively, the person may spend some portions of the time in silence observing what is present, and then sharing the same experience or a new one.

- You can alternate back and forth as many times as you would like in two-minute increments. Keep in mind that you don't have to comment on what the other person shares. It may naturally become a part of your experience, but it isn't a conversation. It is a practice of deep listening.

Practicing Mindfulness in Everyday Life

- Mindfulness can truly be practiced anytime and anywhere. Even taking a five-second break to take some deep breaths and check in with your body sensations, emotions, and thoughts can give you the resilience-building benefits of mindfulness.

- Some of the best times to practice being mindful come during your rote daily tasks, like your morning routine or washing dishes. During rote tasks, it is common to find the mind wandering.

- The next time you're in the midst of a task that seems mindless, try to be fully present in that moment. For example, when you're brushing your teeth, pay close attention to the way the bristles feel against your teeth and gums. Pay attention to taste changes, to the way the brush feels in your hand, and to the sounds caused by the bristles hitting your teeth.

- Some people like taking mindful walks, where they fully pay attention to their surroundings and sensations: the sense of their feet hitting the ground, the chirping birds, the warmth of the sun on their forehead. Take some time to think about your own routines and consider where it might be best for you to add in some mindfulness to your everyday life.

- Additionally, both the concentration and the mindfulness forms of meditation can help you experience the peace that is always present in every moment. Experiment with different types of meditation at different times of day. You may want to weave a couple of shorter practices into your daily life. If you find yourself getting stressed, try even a five-minute silent mantra meditation or a brief guided mindfulness practice.

Suggested Reading

Hanson and Mendius, *Buddha's Brain*.

Kabat-Zinn, *Meditation Is Not What You Think*.

Miller, *Yoga Nidra*.

Activities

- Try to meditate for at least seven minutes every day for one week (or more if you like it). You can try either concentration-based or mindfulness meditation.

- Try at least once to practice mindfulness during your whole morning routine.

- Complete Practice Class 5 (Class 21), titled "Practicing Mindfulness."

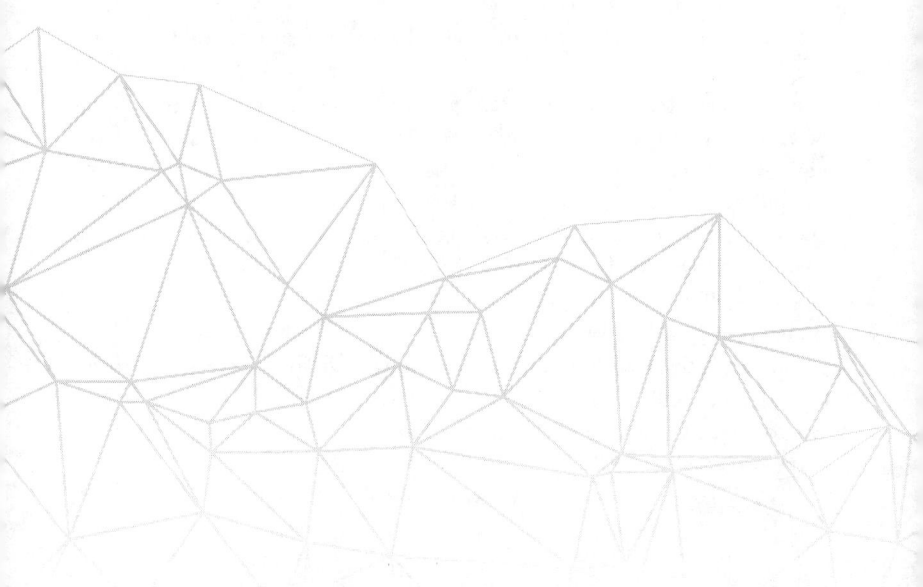

Class 10 Transcript

Finding Equanimity with Mindfulness

Welcome. Today we're going to explore how meditation can contribute to your physical and emotional resilience. This is a topic that's had a huge impact on my life, and I hope that by the end of the class, you'll be motivated to start weaving meditation and mindfulness practices into your daily routines. But to set the stage for all the information I want you to absorb, let's begin in a very practical way. Let's take a few moments to do a brief mindfulness practice.

Start by closing your eyes and feeling the surface that your body is seated upon—the chair or the floor. Feel all the places your body is supported. Notice where in your body you're applying effort to support yourself. See if you can really give your body to that surface you are resting upon so very little effort is involved. Feel as if your body is truly being held by the surface and by the air.

Open up the five senses and notice any sounds, smells, tastes, feelings, or images that arise. Tune in to your surroundings. Feel the physical sensation of your body now. Noticing your head, face, arms, hands, chest and upper back, lower back and abdomen, hips and pelvis, legs, and feet. If only your body were present, what are you feeling? What parts of your body are obvious? Now notice which parts of your body you don't feel at all.

Observe your breath, noticing the natural flow of your breath. Now take a few long, deep breaths, breathing deep down into your abdomen then up in to your chest, breathing all the way up to your clavicle. Then exhale, emptying the lungs completely. Take a few more deep breaths.

Now observe the mind, noticing any feelings, emotions, or images that are present. As you notice a feeling, emotion, or image, observe: Where in your body do you feel it? Notice how every emotion has an associated physical sensation as well. Now, ask yourself the question, who is the observer of your body? Who is the observer of your breath? Who is the observer of your feelings, emotions, thoughts, and beliefs? There is a part of you that is unchanging amidst all of these changing sensations of life. Feel into that state of stillness that is always present, always here, healthy, whole, and complete just as you are.

Watch for a moment, noticing the changing sensations that are occurring, all on a backdrop of unchanging stillness. This stillness has been here every moment of life. It is always present, awake, aware, and peaceful. Now rub the palms of your hands together until you create heat between your hands, and place the palms of your hands over your eyes and rest here for a moment. Then slowly open your eyes.

The process I just guided you through is a quick and easy way to practice mindfulness. You can do the practice anytime, anywhere. It is extremely simple, and you may notice that even a couple of minutes, just like we just did, can leave you feeling more relaxed and present. All forms of mindfulness and meditation are designed to help us have a direct experience of stillness so that we can live from a place of peacefulness. There are many pathways to the same destination, and we'll talk about several of these during the class today.

In daily life, we notice the obvious activity in our life that grabs our attention. But have you noticed that something is aware of this? In actuality, we rarely notice that we are observing these experiences that occur in daily life. Ask yourself now, who is aware of this moment? Who is aware of the body, the breath, the mind, feelings, emotions, and beliefs that may be occurring right now? Who is aware of what the five senses are experiencing? When we step back and really observe what is occurring in daily life, we suddenly become more attuned to our experience.

When we become mindful of the moment, we are more open to fully experience what is occurring. We listen, feel, connect, and experience more deeply and completely. We really taste the food we are eating instead of just chowing down. We hear the sound of birds singing as we make our way to the office. We actually listen more fully to what someone is trying to share with us. We start to sense the way someone is feeling in our bodies even if they don't tell us. We also become more aware of the stillness that is present, every moment of every day. Meditation is our conscious, direct experience of the stillness that is present every single moment of our lives. The stillness has always been here, and it will always be here; we just may not be directly perceiving it because we spend so much of our lives paying attention to what is present outside of ourselves—the world around us that is constantly calling out for our attention. Meditation and mindfulness are invitations to uncover the stillness that is always present both during the formal practice of meditation and also in our daily lives.

Does that match your understanding of meditation? Take a moment right now and think about the word *meditation,* as well as what it means to you. What is your definition of mindfulness? You may already have a very specific definition. Your answer may also be influenced by preconceived notions about how you've experienced the practice in the past. Well here are a few definitions of meditation that I've found particularly helpful. Many ancient scriptures describe meditation as the practice of stilling the waves of the thinking mind so we can experience stillness and peace. The Free Dictionary says, "Meditation is a practice of concentrated focus upon a sound, object, visualization, the breath, movement, or attention itself in order to increase awareness of the present moment, reduce stress, promote relaxation, and enhance personal and spiritual growth." And to define mindfulness meditation, Jon Kabat-Zinn says, "Mindfulness is not about getting anywhere else—it's about being where you are and knowing it."

Each of these descriptions has elements that we'll be unpacking together today. I also want to point out here what meditation is and is not. Meditation is a really practical and simple tool that you can use to train your mind to be more focused, healthier, and happier. Meditation is scientifically validated now by thousands of clinical studies. It's a tool that can help enhance nearly every aspect of your life, from your productivity at work to the quality of time you spend with the people in your life. Meditation is a practice that can help you respond to life on life's terms instead of reacting impulsively to it.

Meditation is not about escaping your reality. It is about being present with what is so that you can move through it effectively. You do not have to make your thoughts stop to meditate. You do not have to spend hours a day meditating. Meditation does not mean that you will eventually have to become a monk and move to a monastery in the Himalayas. Meditation is not about getting to a certain place, but instead about learning to experience the peace that is already present amidst the changing experiences of our daily life. Meditation is also not a religious practice, although many religions do use meditation as a part of their practice. Meditation can be an entirely secular practice. I have taught a very secular form of meditation to the military and other communities for more than a decade.

There are many forms of meditation, but mostly they fall into two main categories: concentration-based meditation and mindfulness meditation. Although they employ different methods, both of these broad types ultimately have the same end goal, which is to experience peace in the present moment. It's important to point out that you don't have to pick one type or the other type. Personally, I practice both every day and find that they serve different aspects of my life. I've also found that, over time, these two types of meditation enhance each other.

Let's look at concentration-based meditation first. This form of meditation involves sitting quietly and picking a point of focus for the mind to rest upon. Typically in Eastern traditions, a mantra or syllable was used to help focus the mind. You can also pick a point of focus, like a flower, stone, or sound. Once the mind becomes one-pointed through focusing on the mantra or object, the thoughts naturally begin to slow down, and the mind is then able to settle into deeper states of stillness. The mantra or object serves as a little perch for the mind to rest upon so that it doesn't wander all over the place. During practice, you may find your mind is particularly distracted in the beginning, but then it starts to calm down as you repeat the word or the mantra. Personally, I like practicing this form of meditation in the morning when I first wake up because the mind is more predisposed to being calm and attentive after a good night's rest. If you're tired when you practice, you may tend to fall asleep instead of meditating.

Concentration-based practices root back to the Hindu and Buddhist traditions that use mantras such as *om, om namah Shivaya,* and *om mani padme hum* as a point of focus during the meditation. You are welcome to use these traditional mantras, or you can use a phrase or affirmation that will help you focus, such as, "I am happy, healthy, and peaceful just as I am." You can also pick a word, such as "love" or "courage," to repeat to yourself. If you have a particular religious prayer or mantra that works for you from your religious tradition, you can, of course, use this as well. Nearly every religious tradition uses some form of prayer beads to aid as a tool in keeping the mind focused. In Eastern traditions, they use mala beads. Christian traditions use a rosary. Similar prayer beads are used in other faiths including the Sikh tradition and Islam. If you are deeply connected to nature, you can choose to focus on a flower, stone, or tree. Some people enjoy focusing on the flame of a candle. As the mind begins to calm down, you can release the mantra and just let the mind rest in stillness. If the mind begins to get distracted again by various thoughts, you can begin again with the mantra.

The second type of meditation we will discuss today is mindfulness. You've heard the term *mindfulness* multiple times during this course, and there is a good chance you may have heard it at some other point in your life as well. The meditation we did at the beginning of class today is a form of mindfulness. In fact, mindfulness is quickly becoming a buzzword in modern society—and with good reason, because it's got a strong ability to promote growth, healing, and resilience. In fact, many studies show that resilience can be taught specifically through mindfulness-based interventions. At its core, mindfulness is our ability to pay attention on purpose. It involves observing our experience in the present moment without judgment, and it can be practiced at any moment of our lives. The more it is practiced, the more it becomes a natural way of life. And the more natural it becomes, the more helpful mindfulness can be in building your resilience. So let's dive a bit deeper into the story of how mindfulness is changing people's lives for the better.

The concept of mindfulness is not new. In fact, it has been practiced in Eastern traditions for thousands of years. But Western society is quickly starting to see its benefits thanks to both yogic scholars, such as Swami Vivekananda, bringing yoga practices to the West, and scientists applying mindfulness practices to mental health treatment. One of the pioneers in introducing mindfulness to the medical field is Jon Kabat-Zinn, who developed a treatment program known as mindfulness-based stress reduction, or MBSR. Started at the University of Massachusetts' Medical School in 1979, MBSR draws from Buddhist traditions but teaches them in a secular way. It uses mindfulness techniques to help alleviate stress, pain, and other illnesses. While typical cognitive therapy focuses on changing thoughts to fix a problem, MBSR invites practitioners to welcome so-called negative emotions and thoughts as a part of their experience. UMass has a whole Center for Mindfulness created by Kabat-Zinn, which conducts mindfulness research and trains practitioners in mindfulness-based interventions.

In 1992, researchers Zindel Segal, Mark Williams, and John Teasdale sought to create a group that utilized dialectical behavior therapy, acceptance therapy, and commitment therapy, but during the development process, they participated in an MBSR session. They were amazed that "the simple act of recognizing your thoughts as thoughts can free you from the distorted reality they often create and allow for more clear-sightedness and a greater sense of manageability in your life." So instead of their original idea, the trio created mindfulness-based cognitive therapy, which became one of the first integrations of mindfulness and traditional cognitive therapy to be used in the mental health field. Some other common and well-known mental health treatment orientations that use the power of mindfulness are dialectical behavior therapy and acceptance commitment therapy. The fact that so many different mindfulness-based therapy orientations have been created shows just how much the mental health world has caught on to the healing and resilience-building powers of mindfulness.

And for those of you who have watched my Great Courses series on Integrative Restoration, or iRest Yoga Nidra, you probably already know that iRest is another intervention that uses mindfulness to promote healing, relaxation, and resilience. Richard Miller, a clinical psychologist, author, researcher, and yogic scholar, adapted traditional Yoga Nidra, which has been around for over

2,000 years, into a secular practice called iRest. The basic premise of iRest is that peace is our true nature. It is present every moment of every day. And the potential to experience this peace is already here. iRest is a 10-step guided meditation protocol that takes you through the various layers of consciousness. I like to think of it like a filing system for my mind that helps me observe what is present in any given moment or on any given day. Similar to the mindfulness interventions I've just mentioned, iRest invites practitioners to welcome their sensations, emotions, and thoughts rather than try to fix or change them.

And this is a key principle. Mindfulness practices like iRest aren't about trying to fix what we are experiencing. We are witnessing it, observing it, and allowing it to tell its story. The moment we begin trying to fix and change ourselves, tension and stress begin to arise. iRest is really about learning to find our peace in the midst of daily life no matter what is occurring. This is really the essence of resilience. We need to learn to keep our peace amidst whatever happens in life rather than letting it be dependent on outward conditions. That does not, however, mean that you don't work to affect change in your life. It just means that your peace of mind is not dependent upon it. I have been teaching iRest Yoga Nidra for over a decade, and to this day, it is my go-to tool for both myself and the people I work with. There is a Yoga Nidra practice later in this course if you'd like to try it for yourself.

Let's talk now a little bit more about how to be mindful amidst your life. Earlier I described mindfulness as the ability to observe our experience in the present moment without judgment. So let's break that down some more. When we're awake, most of our time is spent doing things: doing our work, caring for our families, scrolling through pictures and articles on our phones, thinking about what we have to do, and even looking for things to do when we're bored! And oftentimes, when we're doing a task, we aren't fully present in what it is that we're doing. We're either doing something with the intention of finishing it, or we're thinking about something else while completing the task at hand. The word *auto-pilot* might come to mind.

The first piece of mindfulness is reminding ourselves that we are not called human doings—we are called human beings. *Being* implies being present in the moment. But when we're overtly attached to the end goal, we often lose our ability to be fully present in the moment. Instead, we are attached to some point on the horizon that may or may not ever come. We want to value how we do things just as much as the end state of what we're doing. Ideally if we're fully present in the moment as we're doing something, we will be even more efficient and effective in achieving our goals. And, we will get there with a present and peaceful state of mind rather than a stressed-out sense of urgency.

Our attention is constantly being grabbed by different stimuli: a loud noise outside, a pop-up on our phone, or someone calling our name, just to name a few. Our attention is often grabbed rather than placed on what is around us. In reality, there are thousands of sights and sensations to explore in any moment, most of which go unnoticed or is drowned out by stronger external and internal stimuli. Just how our attention can be automatically grabbed, we often have automatic thoughts, opinions, and judgments about the things we experience, too. When we don't question these automatic responses, they can result in the biases that reinforce our belief system. When we're mindful, we notice thoughts and sensations without making judgments about them. Being mindful is being able to passively observe your thoughts, emotions, and sensations in the same way you might watch clouds float by above you. The cloud floats in, you see it, and it floats away. Being mindful is viewing your experience in this exact same way. A thought, emotion, or sensation comes, you experience and observe it, and it goes away.

To practice mindfulness, try bringing your attention to things that aren't screaming for your attention. Orient yourself to your entire surrounding and try using all of your senses. Pay attention to the sensation of your clothes on your body or note every sound in your surroundings. Try pointing out five things that are yellow around you, four tactile sensations you have, three things you can hear, two things you can smell, and one thing you can taste. Once passively observing your surroundings becomes easier, it will become easier to to passively observe uncomfortable emotions and thoughts as well. Much of our ability to do this comes from our ability to connect with our physical bodies. Our bodies are constantly giving us information about how we're feeling and what we're experiencing. We might hold stress in our shoulders, we might feel heaviness in our chest when we're sad, and we might feel butterflies in our stomach or a rush of energy down our arms when we're happy or excited. These sensations in our body are messages that we need to listen to. Mind-body practices like yoga and qigong can help you improve your connection to your own body so that you can learn to feel and interpret these messages. During the mindfulness and Yoga Nidra classes, I lead you through a body scan, which is a tool you can use anytime and anywhere to strengthen your mind-body connection.

Co-meditation is another tool that can be used to practice connecting with what is happening in your body while, at the same time, being present for another person as well. It is a partner practice that is easy to do and takes a surprisingly short amount of time to bring you fully into the present moment. Sit with a trusted friend, family member, or your partner and take turns sharing what sensations you each feel in your body. Both participants can either keep their eyes open or closed—whatever is most comfortable for them. I like to use a timer on my phone and set the timer for two minutes.

For the first two minutes, one person shares and the other person listens. Once the timer goes off, you switch, and the other person shares for two minutes while the person who just shared listens. Each two minutes, switch from person to person. During the successive two-minute increments, participants share without being asked: What is present? Where do I feel what is present in my body? I can also describe the sensations and experience I'm having of what is present. For instance, if it was my turn to share, I could say, "I feel tension in my stomach and a sense of uneasiness about a conversation I had this morning." Or perhaps, "I feel warmth in my heart and a lot of love for my son, who I just talked to on my lunch break." Parts of the practice may be done in silence as the person feels into what is present. The person sharing may speak for the entire two minutes about one thing that is present, or they may spend some portions of time in silence observing what is present and then sharing the same experience or a new one.

You can alternate back and forth as many times as you would like in two-minute increments. Keep in mind that you don't have to comment on what the other person shares. It may naturally become a part of your experience, but this is not a conversation. It is a practice of deep listening together with another person. It's a beautiful way to be fully present with yourself and another person and a powerful way to cultivate connection. As the other person is speaking, notice how what the other person shares is reflected in your body and breath. This can be a powerful way to cultivate deep connection between two people. It's highly effective in helping both people feel seen and heard, especially in relationships where one person is typically more dominant.

We do not live in isolation. The experiences of other people are constantly being reflected in our own experience. Co-meditation is a great way to experience that. As you practice, you will most likely find that you're able to be more present with people in your daily life as you learn to really listen to them. Being really present for another person is one of the greatest gifts we can give someone. Being present for ourselves is a state of mind we may have been waiting our whole lives to experience.

Mindfulness can truly be practiced anytime, anywhere. Even taking a five-second break to take some deep breaths, check in with your body sensations, emotions, and thoughts can give you the resilience-building benefits of mindfulness. Some of the best times to practice being mindful is during our otherwise mindless daily tasks—those tasks that become rote, like our morning routine or washing dishes. In rote tasks, it is common to find our minds wandering or thinking about something other than what we're actually doing. So the next time you're in the midst of a task that seems mindless, try to be fully present in that moment. When you're brushing your teeth, really pay attention to the way the bristles feel against your teeth and gums; it may even feel like a mini massage! Pay attention to taste changes, to the way your brush feels in your hand, to the sounds caused by the bristles hitting your teeth. You can apply this to your whole life. When you're washing dishes, pay attention to the different sensations you feel from the changing water temperatures on your skin. Actively pay attention to how the soap smells and the sound of the bubbles popping. Some people like taking mindful walks where they fully pay attention to their surroundings and sensations—the felt sense of their feet hitting the ground, the chirping birds, the warmth of the sun on their forehead. Take some time to think about your own routines and consider where it might be best for you to add in some mindfulness to your everyday life. Personally, I like practicing before I go to bed every evening and typically fall asleep while listening to an iRest Yoga Nidra practice.

Both the concentration and the mindfulness forms of meditation can help you experience the peace that is always present in every moment. Experiment with different types of meditations and at different times of day. You may want to weave a couple of shorter practices into your daily life, for instance, around 3:00 p.m. when you may typically go for that extra cup of coffee that could end up keeping you awake at night. If you find yourself getting stressed, try even a five-minute silent mantra meditation or a brief guided mindfulness practice.

The more we can weave meditation throughout our lives, the more we will find ourselves abiding in a peaceful state of mind no matter what we face in daily life. Living connected to a deep feeling of peacefulness that is not dependent on outside conditions is one of the best things you can do to live a truly resilient life. Next time you're feeling stressed, try mentally just dropping back into the peace that is always present. It's right here. You don't have to find it. You just have to turn your attention upon it and draw it up into the present moment.

Class 11

Understanding Trauma

Trauma changes brains, bodies, and the way people experience life. This class explores what trauma is. It also looks at what is occurring in the body and brain as a result of trauma, and at how to respond to trauma in a healthy way.

Defining Trauma

- A traumatic event is an experience that is extremely distressing and often life-threatening. Trauma can happen as a result of a single event, such as a natural disaster, a car accident, or an assault. It can also be complex trauma, which is trauma that has occurred over a prolonged period of time, such as being in an abusive relationship, living in a war-torn country, living in poverty, or experiencing childhood abuse or neglect. It can also be traumatic to hear about the trauma that someone else has experienced, particularly if it's someone you're close to.

- When you are in danger or perceived danger, the body and brain respond in a way designed to keep you safe. Common responses include the fight-or-flight reflex, but there are also other ways that the body responds to danger, too. Sometimes people freeze, just like a deer attempting not to be seen. Sometimes people scream or cry for help.

- When all else fails, sometimes people submit. When you submit, the brain goes into a state of hypo-arousal. The purpose of this response is to shut down the experience of thought and emotion so that you aren't as present for the trauma.

- The stress, panic, anxiety, and terror that happen as a result of a trauma are all normal, and they typically last for a few weeks following the traumatic event. However, if a person is experiencing complex trauma or their fight-or-flight reflex doesn't successfully help escape the danger, the person is more likely to develop symptoms of post-traumatic stress disorder (PTSD), which can last for a lifetime if left untreated.

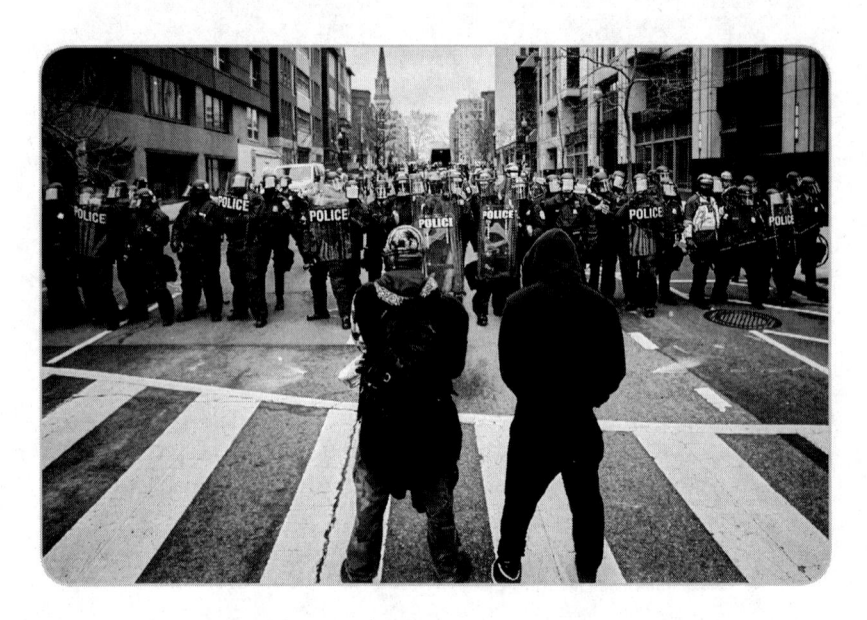

> **Post-Traumatic Stress Disorder**
>
> The rates of PTSD following two national disasters—the 9/11 attacks on the World Trade Center and Hurricane Katrina—are illuminating. While statistics vary, there are some significant statistics showing that 5 percent of 9/11 survivors experienced symptoms of post-traumatic stress disorder. However, 33 percent of Hurricane Katrina survivors developed symptoms of PTSD.
>
> Some experts, including trauma experts, noticed that many survivors of 9/11 were able to escape the trauma by walking back to homes that were safe. Compare this to survivors of Hurricane Katrina, many of whom were stuck on their rooftops with nowhere to run. Survivors of Hurricane Katrina were sent to other cities, and many of them completely lost the safety and security of having a home and a community. Since many of the survivors of Hurricane Katrina were also low income, many of them had less access to mental health services following the disaster, especially since most of the relief funding was spent on relocation and housing issues.

Trauma and the Brain

- When a person experiences a trauma that is too big for the brain to process, it becomes stuck in the brain as a current problem rather than being stored as a processed memory of a past event. In this condition, people often avoid anything that brings reminders of the trauma, including thoughts and feelings associated with it. It is also common to be hypervigilant, making the person almost always tense and alert.

- When someone has post-traumatic stress, their amygdala is extremely reactive, which creates almost a constant flood of stress hormones in the brain. Like stress, trauma also causes the hippocampus to shrink. The hippocampus is largely responsible for the ability to form memories, and when it shrinks, it becomes harder to process events and form memories. When the hippocampus is unable to process a memory, all it can do is hold on to the fragmented pieces of unprocessed information, which makes it feel like the trauma is still a current problem.

- Trauma also inhibits the functioning of the prefrontal cortex, which makes it difficult to plan, problem solve, and control emotions. One part of the prefrontal cortex that is specifically affected by trauma is Broca's area, which controls speech production. This, combined with fragmented memories, can make putting trauma into words extremely difficult.

> **The Intergenerational Transmission of Trauma**
>
> There are multiple ways that trauma can be passed down from parents to their children. Sometimes, people simply have a genetic makeup that makes them more vulnerable to stress and trauma, and these genotypes are passed to later generations. Trauma can also be passed down to children via the environment they're raised in. However, just as trauma can be transmitted from one generation to the next, research is showing that resilience patterns can be transmitted from one generation to the next, too.

Traumatic Memories

- Denial and minimization are two common defense mechanisms that people unconsciously use to avoid having to deal with the reality of a traumatic experience. These mechanisms are also normal, and they do serve a purpose, as they can prevent a person from feeling overwhelmed immediately following a trauma or loss. However, a person can only suppress experiences for so long before the underlying trauma wreaks havoc on the body and mind.

- Sometimes people don't recognize or fully experience symptoms of post-traumatic stress until months or even years after the trauma. Additionally, most people don't have any conscious memories until the age of three, which means it is possible for the body to respond to trauma from birth or early childhood that the person doesn't even remember.

- New research is even showing that sometimes the brain stores traumatic memories that can only be accessed when the brain is in the same state it was in when the original trauma occurred. This state-dependent learning explains why people can't access some traumatic memories from a normal state of consciousness; they are only accessible when the brain is in the state it was in when the trauma occurred. It also explains how environmental triggers that bring the brain back to the state it was in when trauma occurred can result in fragmented memories of the pain endured.

Effects of Trauma

- It is often the small details that affect trauma survivors the most. Smells, sounds, images, and particular thoughts or fears in the moment can alter the way one thinks and acts in the wake of a traumatic event. This is the way trauma can become insidious and can affect entire lives.

- Trauma often disrupts feelings of safety and trust. People can be left feeling as though the world is unsafe, and no one can be trusted. They can feel unsafe in their environments and sometimes even within their bodies. Feeling safe allows people to welcome and respond to what happens in their daily lives; however, feeling unsafe can leave people stuck in a constant state of looking for threats, making it difficult to move on and heal from trauma.

- Another common side effect of trauma is dissociation. Dissociation leads to feelings of detachment and disbelief, as though the experience was not real. A person might feel numb or separate from his or her body. Suppressing thoughts and emotions, which can be done consciously or subconsciously, is another way a person might try to detach from an experience.

- Suppression will only work for so long. Suppressed emotions are likely to become triggered and express themselves as anger, rage, or other reckless behavior. In order to heal traumatic memories, it is necessary to allow thoughts, emotions, and experiences to be expressed and acknowledged.

- If suppression is one possible effect of trauma, fusion is another. In fusion, a person fuses with his or her experience. In fusion, people define themselves by their trauma, or they feel like their lives and identities have been entirely taken over by it. The trick is to find the sweet spot—that is, to be curious about thoughts and emotions without actually identifying with them.

- Shame is another feeling that commonly comes after trauma, especially interpersonal trauma. Shame is the foundation of so many problems: Addiction, violence, and codependency all have roots in shame. It is common to interpret internal distress as though something is wrong, but this is far from the case. Distress is uncomfortable, but it is normal and even purposeful.

A Healthy Conceptualization of Trauma

- Responding to trauma can be difficult, but keep in mind that it is normal. If you go through trauma, keep in mind that your responses don't mean you are broken. You are reacting to a distressing event.

- When you aren't afraid of your response, it becomes easier to plan for how you will handle it if and when it comes up again. An important piece of this is to choose people who are willing to be there when you are reminded of your trauma. Find at least one person—a family member, friend, or professional—who won't tell you to "just get over it."

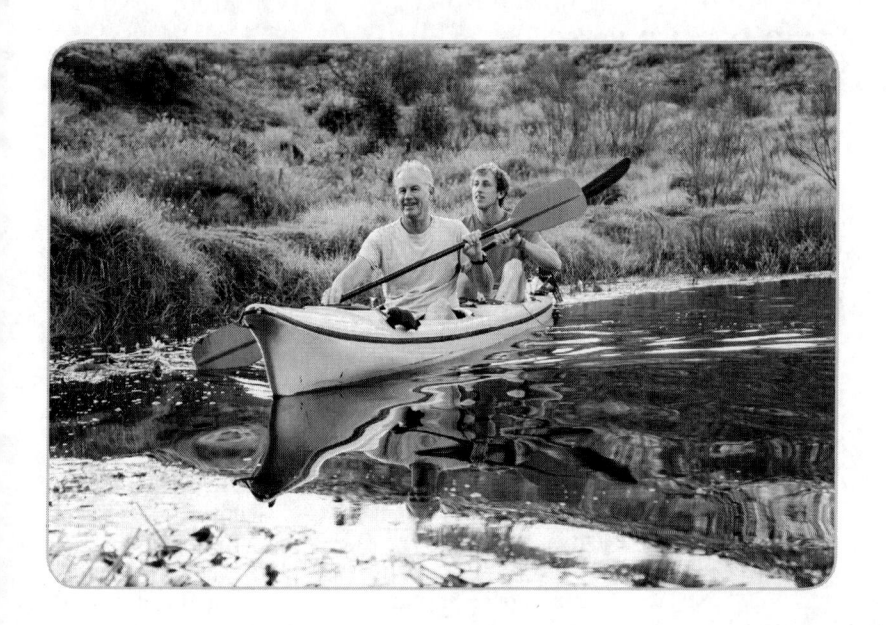

- Survivors often feel as though they have to choose between being vulnerable or being strong, but the truth is that being vulnerable is being strong. Avoidance can keep you stuck, but being vulnerable opens you up to your whole experience. Acknowledging trauma can certainly be uncomfortable, but this, too, is normal. When you acknowledge the sensations, emotions, thoughts, and memories that are associated with your trauma, you are able to recognize them as little pieces of information that each have a message to share.

- You start to see that you are not your trauma; rather, you just went through a traumatic experience. When you start to pay attention to how your experience has affected you, you are able to find the part of you that is unaffected, too—the part of you that is always healthy and whole, and that is completely untouched by your traumatic experience.

Suggested Reading

Brown, *I Thought It Was Just Me.*

Levine, *In An Unspoken Voice.*

———, *Waking the Tiger.*

Activities

Note: Answer these questions only if you feel safe while doing so—that is, only if they will not be triggering for you. If these questions are triggering for you, you may want to talk to your doctor or a therapist.

- Answer the following:

    » Have you experienced trauma? Do you know someone who has experienced trauma?

    » Which aspects of trauma and/or trauma response did you (or they) experience?

    » What was the most helpful way to work through the trauma (for you or someone else)?

    » How have you experienced shame?

- Complete Practice Class 6 (Class 22), titled "Evoking the Relaxation Response."

Class 11 Transcript

Understanding Trauma

For the past 10 years as a trauma educator and yoga and meditation instructor, I've worked with survivors of some of the most horrific traumas, which include terrorist attacks, human trafficking, war-related trauma, and much more. On February 14th, 2018, one of these horrific traumas struck my own community. I live in Fort Lauderdale, Florida, just down the road from Parkland, Florida, which is home to Marjory Stoneman Douglas High School, the scene of the school shooting that left 17 people dead.

The week after the shooting, I began leading classes for a group of teachers who had classrooms in the building where the shooting occurred. While the whole school had mental health resources available, the teachers in the building with the shooting experienced something uniquely different than the others: They saw their students and one of their fellow teachers killed before their eyes. Their classrooms became crime scenes, and they weren't allowed to touch or remove anything from them, even their own purse in some situations. They were pulled between having to cope with their own extreme traumatic experiences while also having to support students, families, and other teachers. We had to plan our first and second sessions between the funerals of those who were killed. Sometimes there were even two, and even three, and one day four funerals in the same day. In the midst of this, the teachers were interviewed by the FBI and launched into a national debate about gun control. Two weeks after the shooting, they all had to return to school with no supplies and no classrooms to finish out the school year. They had to push carts around to different classrooms.

Trauma affects us at every level. For the teachers at Marjory Stoneman Douglas, the first level was obviously their sense of physical safety, something that had been completely shattered that day. While of course it was important to account for why they weren't safe that day and to trace through everyone's experience of what happened, they also needed to know that proper security measures were being taken so that it never happened again. Their minds raced through all the things that made them safe or not safe that day—everything from whose classroom came first, closest to the main door, to what kind of furniture proved to be the most effective to hide behind. Creating a full picture of the narrative was important to them. Unknowns felt dangerous.

They also needed to understand what was happening to their brains and bodies after the trauma. They weren't going crazy; they were having a normal psychological response to a traumatic event. Once they were able to understand what was happening in the body and in the brain, they needed tools and support to help them calm down the effects of the trauma—practices like breathing and mindfulness. The creation of boundaries was essential for them as they were mobbed with requests for interviews. For weeks and even months, they had to navigate their way past reporters and news trucks to get into the school. They needed to give themselves permission to only do what they felt comfortable and inspired to do. In addition, they needed tools to support them with their interactions with students, as well as an understanding of what steps to take if someone else had a flashback or abreaction in the classroom. The teachers needed trusted community and a multi-level support system to shepherd them through the healing process. They also needed moments of joy where they didn't have to think about any of it—time to splash in a pool or dance to a favorite song. Together, these essential factors became the framework for how they began their lives again.

Much of the content of this course you're taking draws on what we've been using to help the teachers of Marjory Stoneman Douglas heal and build their resilience as they continue going to work every day and educating these amazing kids who are simultaneously going through their own healing process. Some people are born amidst a traumatic experience, a violent home, a war-torn country; others, like police officers and active military members, immerse themselves in situations that can induce trauma. And for some, like the teachers and students at Marjory Stoneman Douglas, trauma comes unannounced and changes their lives in the blink of an eye.

Trauma changes our brains, bodies, and the way we experience life. Fully understanding trauma and how it affects you can make you more resilient. When you realize that you're not crazy and that your body is simply having a normal response to a traumatic experience, it improves your ability to withstand and learn from your body's reactions to the trauma. Trauma can keep us feeling stuck when it's unprocessed, but trauma does not have to take over your life. In this class, we're going to thoroughly explore what trauma is, and what is occurring in the body and brain as a result of the trauma. There are many tools in this course that can be helpful in the process of healing after a traumatic experience, but please remember that this course does not substitute as a treatment by a medical professional. If you have experienced trauma, it is very important to have a system of support, and there are many resources, like talk therapy, that can support you in your healing process. We've listed some resources in the course guidebook, which you can use as a starting point if you're looking for additional assistance.

A traumatic event is something we experience that is extremely distressing and often life-threatening. Trauma can happen as a result of a single event, such as a natural disaster, a car accident, or an assault, or it can be what is known as complex trauma, or trauma that has occurred over a prolonged period of time, such as being in a domestic violence relationship, living in a war-torn country, living in poverty, or experiencing child abuse or neglect. It can also be traumatic to hear about the trauma that someone else has experienced, particularly if it's a loved one or someone we're close to.

When you are in danger or perceived danger, the body and brain respond in a way designed to keep you safe. The two responses that we most normally think of are fight and flight, but there are also other ways that our body responds to danger, too. Sometimes we freeze, like a deer who is attempting to not be seen. Sometimes we cry or scream for help. And when all else fails, sometimes we submit. When we submit, our brain goes into a state of hypoarousal. The purpose of this response is to shut down our experience of thought and emotion so that we aren't as present for the trauma we are about to endure.

The stress, panic, anxiety, and terror that happen as a result of a trauma are all normal and typically last for a few weeks following the traumatic event. But if we're experiencing extreme trauma, complex trauma, or if our fight-or-flight response doesn't successfully help us to escape the danger, we're far more likely to develop symptoms of post-traumatic stress, which can last for a lifetime if untreated. The rates of post-traumatic stress disorder following two national disasters, the 9/11 attacks on the World Trade Center and Hurricane Katrina, depict these differences. While statistics vary based upon when the study was conducted and the group that was measured, there are some significant statistics showing that 5% of 9/11 survivors experienced symptoms of post-traumatic stress disorder, or PTSD. Guess what percentage of Hurricane Katrina survivors developed symptoms of PTSD: 33%.

So why did a third of Hurricane Katrina survivors experience symptoms of PTSD compared to only 5% of survivors in the attack on the World Trade Center? Some experts, including trauma expert Bessel van der Kalk, noticed that many survivors of 9/11 were able to escape the trauma by walking to homes that were safe. Compare this to survivors of Hurricane Katrina, many of whom were stuck on their rooftops with nowhere to run, on top of their homes that were in the process of being destroyed. Survivors of Hurricane Katrina were sent to other cities, and many of them completely lost the safety and security of having a home and a community. Since many of the survivors of Hurricane Katrina were also low income, many of them had less access to mental health services following the disaster, especially since most of the relief funding was spent on relocation and housing issues.

When we experience a trauma that is too big for our brain to process, it becomes stuck in our brain as a current problem rather than being stored as a processed memory of a past event. We still live our traumatic experience as if it's happening in the present. Because our brain hasn't yet processed it as a memory from the past, we relive the traumatic experience through nightmares, flashbacks, intrusive memories, and by experiencing physical and emotional distress when we're reminded of the trauma. To prevent this re-experiencing, we often avoid anything that might remind us of the trauma, including thoughts and feelings associated with it. It is also common to be hypervigilant, making us almost always tense and alert so that we feel more prepared to face any potential future trauma. So much subconscious focus on staying prepared for trauma can make it difficult to sleep or concentrate on anything else. We might also find ourselves overcome with negative thoughts about ourselves and the world, irritability, aggression, feelings of isolation, and difficulty experiencing positive emotions.

As I mentioned in the class about stress, chronic stress causes our amygdala, or our brain's fear center, to grow. When someone has post-traumatic stress, their amygdala is extremely reactive, which creates almost a constant flood of stress hormones in the brain. Studies have shown that when people are reminded of their trauma through images, sounds, and words, their amygdala becomes incredibly activated, preparing their body for danger again. Like stress, trauma also causes the hippocampus to shrink. Our hippocampus is largely responsible for our ability to form memories, and when it shrinks, it becomes harder for us to process events and form memories. When our hippocampus is unable to process a memory, all it can do is hold on to the fragmented pieces of unprocessed information, which makes it feel like the trauma is still a current problem. Trauma also inhibits our functioning of our prefrontal cortex, which makes it difficult to plan, problem solve, and control our emotions. Part of our prefrontal cortex that is specifically affected by trauma is Broca's area, which controls our speech production. In Dr. van der Kolk's studies, he notes that Broca's area goes offline when a trauma survivor experiences a flashback. Imagine the difficulty that comes with trying to explain your experience when your speech center isn't fully functioning.

When we put all of these pieces together, we can see a trauma response in action. As we know, trauma survivors tend to be hypervigilant, meaning they're on the lookout for potential threats. When a potential threat that reminds the survivor of their trauma is noticed, it triggers the hippocampus to recall a piece of the unprocessed traumatic memory. The amygdala then reacts to this, which can result in the survivor re-experiencing the trauma. Unprocessed emotional and physical memories of the trauma come up to the surface, and the body thinks this means that the trauma is happening in this moment. The amygdala activates the survivor's stress response, which puts our mental energy towards more primitive survival mechanisms, causing the prefrontal cortex to go offline. This prevents the survivor from recognizing that they are not currently in danger. A lack of activation in Broca's area combined with the fragmented memories makes it nearly impossible for the survivor to put this whole experience into words. Because these thoughts and feelings can be extremely distressing, we tend to avoid them, which keeps the memory from being integrated and continues the cycle.

Now that we've covered some of the physiological aspects of trauma and post-traumatic stress, let's turn to an important phenomenon that's often ignored: the passing of trauma from one generation to the next. Have you ever been told that you look like a parent or that you have the same mannerisms or smile? Do you have any similar interests? Do you follow the same holiday traditions that you did as a child? It comes as no surprise that traits, quirks, interests, and traditions can be passed down from older generations. So should it really surprise us that trauma can be passed down from older generations, too?

There are multiple ways that trauma can be passed down from parents to their children. Sometimes, people simply have a genetic makeup that makes them more vulnerable to stress and trauma, and these genotypes are passed down to later generations. Trauma can also be passed down to children via the environment they're raised in. Studies have shown that survivors of traumatic interpersonal violence are more likely to use authoritarian parenting strategies, such as corporal punishment, verbal hostility, and less nurturance, all of which can result in a child's own trauma. Then there's the effect of modeling and imitation. According to social learning theory, children copy behaviors that are modeled by their parents and react to their environments in the same way they observe their parents reacting to their environment. Keep that in mind the next time you see a kid being a bully. There is a good chance that kid is just behaving in a way that has been modeled to him or her elsewhere. That kid very well could have experienced his or her own trauma and actually might be in need of help rather than punishment.

Most recently, science has uncovered another intriguing way in which trauma can be passed down from parents to their offspring. One study uses the phrase "intergenerational transmission of trauma" to describe trauma that is passed down to offspring as a result of experiences that have altered the parent's biology. Science is finding that trauma can alter men's sperm and women's eggs and gestational uterine environments, which, in turn, can alter offspring biology. Everyone has a genotype and a phenotype. Your genotype is the set of genes given to you by your parents. Your phenotype is your actual observed characteristics, or essentially the interplay between your genetics and your environment. Phenotype is why identical twins, who share the exact same DNA, aren't completely identical in looks, preferences, or behavior. The study of this is called epigenetics. According to epigenetics, genes can be made active or inactive due to changes in our phenotype without any changes being made to our genotype. So trauma and stress can change our phenotype, which can basically turn on or off certain genes. And these epigenetic changes in the biological systems of adults can be passed down to their children.

Here is some good news: As I mentioned, our phenotype is essentially a combination of our genetics and our environment, so even if these trauma-induced changes are passed down from parents to children, we can prevent unfavorable gene expression from continuing so long as parents and children are given enough genuine support and intervention. And some more good news: Just as trauma can be transmitted from one generation to the next, research is showing that resilience patterns can be transmitted from one generation to the next, too.

We can never be 100% sure which experiences will be traumatic to us and which experiences will result in us having post-traumatic stress. For some people, hearing trauma stories can be traumatic, a phenomenon known as vicarious trauma. Extreme, chronic stress can also be traumatic. In fact, many of us have experienced trauma without even realizing it.

Denial and minimization are two common defense mechanisms that we unconsciously use to avoid having to deal with the reality of our experience. These mechanisms are also normal, and they do serve a purpose, as they can prevent us from feeling overwhelmed immediately following a trauma or loss. But we can only suppress our experiences for so long before the underlying trauma wreaks havoc on our body and mind. Sometimes we don't fully recognize or experience symptoms of post-traumatic stress until months or even years after the trauma. And sometimes our brains don't even have a conscious awareness of the trauma we're reacting to. We've already seen that children can unknowingly inherit trauma from their parents. What's more is that most people don't have any conscious memories until age three, which means it's possible for our bodies to be responding to trauma from birth or early childhood that we don't even remember. And those first few years of development are very formative; our brains are already 80% of our adult size by the time we're three.

New research is even showing that sometimes our brains store traumatic memories that can only be accessed when the brain is in the same state as it was when the original trauma occurred. To explain how this works, there are two main neurotransmitters we have to discuss: gamma-aminobutyric acid, or GABA, and glutamate. GABA has many purposes, but its main purpose is to prevent overstimulation. Glutamate, on the other hand, is a neurotransmitter responsible for stimulation. GABA works by binding to a receptor, which prevents glutamate from increasing our stimulation. When our GABA levels are low, the high amount of glutamate in our system can result in us feeling overstimulated. People who experience post-traumatic stress disorder tend to have lower amounts of GABA in their brains than survivors of trauma who don't develop PTSD. Studies show that higher GABA levels may protect against the development of PTSD and help survivors recover from trauma even faster.

Okay, you might be thinking, "that's great, but what does it have to do with hidden traumatic memories?" Well, there are some GABA receptors that aren't focused on preventing overstimulation caused by glutamate. They're focused on changing our brain state—helping us regulate our mood, sleep, and attention. And according to a study out of Northwestern University, these extrasynaptic GABA receptors take information from a terrifying experience and store them as subconscious memories. In this study, mice were given a drug to stimulate their extrasynaptic GABA receptors, then were put in a box and given a mild electric shock. When these mice were put inside the same box the following day, they went about their business as usual and showed no recollection of the shock from the day before. But when these mice were given the drug again and then put back in the box, they froze, preparing themselves to be shocked again. This study shows that the mice could only access the memory of the shock when their brain was in the same state as when the shock originally occurred.

This state-dependent learning explains why we can't access some of our traumatic memories from our normal state of consciousness: They're only accessible when our brain is in the state it was when the trauma occurred. It also explains how environmental triggers that bring our brain back to the state it was in when the trauma occurred can result in us being flooded with fragmented memories of the pain we endured.

I remember going to work with the teachers of Marjory Stoneman Douglas one day a couple months after the shooting and having one of the teachers say, "Coming here today, I felt safe enough to wear flip-flops. It's the first time since the shooting. I was wearing sandals the day of the shooting and they were really hard to run in. It's been hard for me to put on anything but running shoes ever since." The reason I share this detail is that when we watch a traumatic event from the outside, we are often consumed by the big picture—the horror of what occurred. And yet, it is often the small details that affect trauma survivors the most. The smell, sounds, an image, a particular thought or fear in the moment. These are the imprints that can alter the way we think and act in the wake of a traumatic event. This is the way trauma can become insidious and can affect our entire lives.

We've also discussed that some of the effects of trauma, like flashbacks and hypervigilance, but there are many others as well. Trauma often disrupts our feelings of safety and trust. We can be left feeling as though the world is unsafe and no one can be trusted. We can feel unsafe in our environments and sometimes even within our own bodies. Safety and trust is such a large topic, we have a whole class on it later in this course, but the main takeaway about safety is this: When we feel safe, it is much easier to welcome and respond to what happens in our daily lives. When we don't feel safe, we can feel stuck in a constant state of looking for threats, making us unable to fully move through our trauma and heal.

Another common side effect of trauma is disassociation. When we disassociate, we feel like an outside observer of our body and our experience. We can be in disbelief and feel as though our experience is not real. We can literally feel detached, numb, or separate from our body. Our bodies hold physical and emotional memories, and trauma can make our body feel like an uncomfortable place to hang out due to that physical and emotional pain. Suppressing our thoughts and emotions, which can be done consciously or subconsciously, is another way we often try to detach from our experience. But suppression will only work for so long. Just as a balloon that's filled with too much air will pop, suppressed emotions are likely to get triggered and express themselves as anger, rage, or other reckless behavior. In order to heal traumatic memories, we need to allow our thoughts, emotions, and experiences to be expressed and acknowledged. That being said, we also don't want to feel overtaken by our experience. If suppression is one of the possible effects of trauma, fusion is another. In fusion, we fuse with our experience. We define ourselves by our trauma, or we feel like our lives and identities have been entirely overtaken by it. The trick is to find that sweet spot—to be curious about our thoughts and emotions without actually identifying with them.

Shame is another feeling that commonly comes after trauma, especially interpersonal trauma. According to renowned researcher Brené Brown, "Shame is the intensely painful feeling or experience of believing that we are flawed and therefore unworthy of love and belonging." Shame is the foundation of so many problems; addiction, violence, and codependency all have roots in shame. Shame is a vicious cycle; whenever we feel disconnected and isolated, we are likely to experience shame. And when we experience shame, we are likely to feel disconnected and isolated. Trauma can feel extremely isolating. When we experience trauma, it is common to interpret our internal distress as though something is wrong with us, but this is so far from the case. Distress is uncomfortable, but it is normal and even purposeful.

"Just get over it." "It's over now." "It wasn't that bad." "Be strong." All survivors of trauma are bound to have heard these words or similar ones at one point or another. Unfortunately, many people are uncomfortable with trauma and don't understand it, which is what results in statements like this. My hope is that if this class gets gets across only one thing, it's that our response to trauma is difficult, but it's normal. You're not weird, you're not crazy, you're not broken, you're having a natural response to a distressing event. When you aren't afraid of your response, it becomes easier to plan for how you will handle it if and when it comes up again. What will you do if something reminds you of your trauma? An important piece of this is to choose people who are willing to be there when you're reminded of your trauma. Find at least one person—a family member, friend, or professional—who won't tell you, "just get over it."

I know that the teachers I worked with who had a strong support system of people they trusted and whose lives were relatively stable before the shooting in general had an easier time moving forward than those with pronounced challenges and instability in their lives. The teachers who had pre-existing traumas they were dealing with had a much more difficult time, as new trauma often exacerbates pre-existing unhealed experiences. When we injure ourselves physically, we require a period of time to heal, and we often are left with a scar or a body part that's more vulnerable to pain. Do those sprained ankles ever really go away? And while this can be uncomfortable, we learn to adjust to our new normal. Emotional trauma works in the same way. Reminders of what happened might pop up now and again, but once you understand what's happening and learn how to manage it when your body responds, it becomes much easier to deal with.

Oftentimes survivors feel as though they have to choose between being vulnerable or being strong, but the truth is being vulnerable is being strong! Avoidance keeps us stuck. It holds us back. Being vulnerable opens you up to your whole experience. Acknowledging trauma can certainly be uncomfortable, but this, too, is normal. When you acknowledge the sensations, emotions, thoughts, and memories that are associated with your trauma, you're able to recognize them as little pieces of information that each have a message to share. You start to see that you are not your trauma—you just went through a traumatic experience. When you start to pay attention to how your experience has affected you, you're able to find the part of you that is unaffected, too—the part of you that is always healthy, whole, and complete—that is completely untouched by your traumatic experience.

In our next class, we're going to take everything from this class and put it into action. I'll be talking about post-traumatic growth, and we'll discuss not only how to move on from trauma, but how you can become stronger because of it.

Class 12

Discovering Post-Traumatic Growth

People do not become stronger, wiser, and more resilient in spite of their adversity. Rather, people become stronger because of adversity. This pattern was noticed by the researchers Richard Tedeschi and Lawrence Calhoun, who coined the term *post-traumatic growth* in 1995. The idea arose from their research on parents who were experiencing bereavement after the death of a child. While the parents suffered deeply after losing a child, they were also reporting many unexpected positive changes that occurred in their lives.

Trauma deepens one's ability to feel both pain and joy. Real compassion occurs when one feels the full spectrum of life so fully that one no longer suppresses pain. In many cases, the only choice after a trauma is to feel it. The result is that life opens up in new ways.

Five Areas for Growth

Over time studying a whole range of different traumas, Tedeschi and Calhoun noticed five important areas for growth that emerged in people who have experienced traumatic situations. These areas are:

1. Personal strength.
2. New possibilities.
3. Cultivation of meaningful relationships.
4. Spiritual change.
5. Appreciation for life.

This class will now take a look at each of these in turn.

Personal Strength

- Both individual and collective strength arise in unexpected ways after a trauma. The only way to really build strength is to be tested. When you want to build a muscle, you have to apply resistance. To build resilience, you need resistance as well.

- Psychologist Angela Lee Duckworth has done some fascinating research into this, showing that the most successful adolescents are not necessarily the smartest people or those with the most resources. Even when compared against many other success factors, including test scores and household income, the most successful young people are those who have the most grit, which Duckworth defines as the combination of passion and perseverance. In her best-selling book *Grit*, she encourages us step out of what is comfortable to discover what is possible through embracing adversity.

New Possibilities

- The second area for post-traumatic growth is the discovery of new possibilities. When you experience a trauma, it disrupts your worldview. You are forced to re-create your worldview and deepen your understanding of life.

- You try new things because the old ways don't work amidst your new reality. You become more creative as you try to process what has occurred. You try to reconcile your inner reality with your outside world, and a flood of new possibilities comes to the surface.

Cultivation of Meaningful Relationships

- The third area for growth after trauma is the cultivation of meaningful relationships. While some relationships may be challenged after a trauma, people will frequently bond more deeply with the people who shared the traumatic experience, or they will cultivate new relationships in the aftermath.

- Traumatic events tend to remind one of the importance of the people in his or her life. As a result, these events create opportunities for people to connect with others in new ways. People let themselves be helped, and they become more aware of the ways that they can help others.

Spiritual Change

- The fourth area for growth is spiritual change or existential exploration. Traumatic experiences can send you into a deeper exploration of your belief system. For some people, this can invite questions about if there is something transcendent that remains after the human form changes or is no longer.

- After experiencing a trauma, people often go through existential questioning about the nature of consciousness, whether they embrace a particular religion or not. The exploration often unlocks increased faith, meaning, purpose, and conviction. It can also help connect people with the part of them that is unchanging.

Appreciation for Life

- The fifth area of post-traumatic growth is appreciation for life. When people are reminded of the inevitability of their demise, they often appreciate their blessings even more.

- Traumatic events also make people want to get the most out of the time they have in life. For example, when someone close dies or you are reminded of your mortality in some way, you may find a new spark of life—that is, a new excitement for being present for the journey.

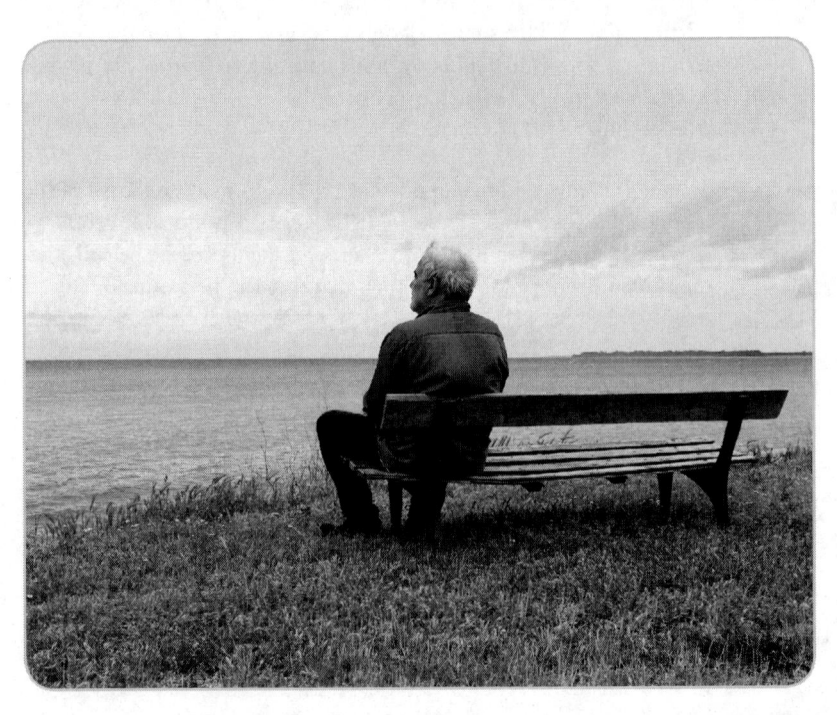

> **Victim, Survivor, and Changemaker**
>
> The five areas of post-traumatic growth form one window for observing the many positive things that can emerge from a trauma. This class now shifts to another way to look at post-traumatic growth—one that is more closely linked to the passage of time. This view looks at the three phases someone who undergoes trauma goes through: victim, survivor, and changemaker.

The Victim Phase

- When a person experiences a trauma, he or she can immediately start to feel under attack. Something happened that was out of the person's control. The body may start to feel like the scene of a crime, and it may feel like a person can no longer choose his or her path. This experience can leave the person feeling like a victim.

- Such an experience is entirely normal, and it can even be protective at times, but it can also be detrimental. It is important to feel what is present when you do find yourself in the role of the victim, but it is also important to not get stuck in that stage. You can't fully grow until you have the chance to move through the stage of being a victim.

- Signs that a person is in the victim phase include shame and blame creeping in with phrases like, "Why me?" or, "How could they have done this to me?" A person in the victim phase may feel powerless, under attack, and lacking control. The person may exhibit patterns of fear-based living, feeling afraid to confront things or engage in a fight.

- Taking on the role of a victim is an entirely normal response after a trauma. It can even feel good. There is some initial evidence that people actually get a temporary burst of positive endorphins from feeling like a victim. This is a dangerous moment of happiness that ultimately results in a letdown due to several key factors.

- Though receiving help from others can feel good, this can create a situation where codependency can easily develop. Additionally, the victim mentality can be a way to avoid personal responsibility and an excuse for not taking risks. It is possible to live an entire life as a victim by using the story as a reason why not to do something instead of using it as an opportunity for personal growth.

The Survivor Phase

- To move past the victim mentality, it is important to realize that one must give up the benefits of being a victim. Positive endorphin release can become a trap and a prison. At some point, to evolve, one has to shift from being a victim to being a survivor.

- The difference is that a survivor has choices, while a victim does not. Empowerment resides in having a choice. You may not be able to control your circumstances, but you can expand the sphere of what is actually possible to change. This can give us an intellectual framework that can carry us through to the other side.

- It may even be helpful to draw a picture of this out for yourself. Draw your current reality inside of an inner circle. For instance, your reality might be that you were recently diagnosed with diabetes. Then, outside the circle, write the possibilities that are immediately accessible to you to change your situation.

- This may simply be a change in mindset, or it may be an even bigger life shift, such as taking insulin, changing your diet, or visiting other doctors and specialists. Further possibilities could include joining a support group or awareness campaign, or writing articles about your experience. You can then keep expanding the possibility sphere out farther and farther to imagine what the ultimate possibilities are for you in this situation.

- A survivor also cultivates gratitude. Gratitude helps you see everything that is going right in your life instead of everything that is going wrong in it.

- You might even talk to your trauma and say, "You don't get the right to steal my future from me. I'm going to learn from this and move past it." From there, you can start finding solutions. Vulnerability still may be present, but this is when the notion that you are surviving and thriving begins to arise.

The Changemaker Phase

- Developing the notion of surviving and thriving is essential to reaching the third phase of post-traumatic growth: becoming a changemaker. A changemaker operates from an empowered view, realizing the changemaker has the capacity to create meaningful change—in both the changemaker's life and those of others.

- Moving from a victim mentality to a changemaker mentality may seem impossible or scary, and sometimes you will fail. However, you will never find your best if you don't try.

- Post-traumatic growth happens when you lean into your journey and discover how to live at the fullest potential of your true self. For some people, a trauma can transform from feeling like the worst thing to the best thing that ever happened to them because it started them on their way.

Suggested Reading

Falke and Goldberg, *Struggle Well*.

Hedrick, *Harriet Beecher Stowe*.

Rendon, *Upside*.

Tedeschi and Finch, *Posttraumatic Growth*.

Tedeschi and Moore, *The Posttraumatic Growth Workbook*.

Activities

- Which of the five areas for growth did you resonate most with? How so?

- Think of a difficult situation in your life. Draw your current reality inside of an inner circle. Then outside the circle, write the possibilities that are immediately accessible to you to change your situation.

- Watch the post-traumatic growth interview with Suzi Landolphi (Class 13).

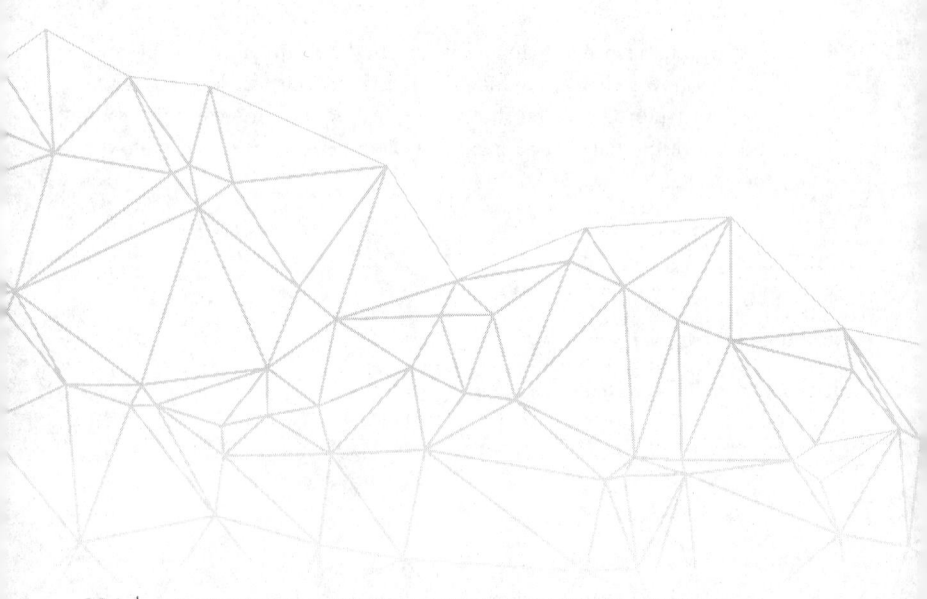

Class 12 Transcript

Discovering Post-Traumatic Growth

Harriet Beecher Stowe, you may remember, is the famous American abolitionist and author of *Uncle Tom's Cabin*, which many believe was a tipping point that brought the realities of slavery into the average American home in a way that made them realize it had to end. Legend has it that when Stowe visited the White House, Abraham Lincoln said to her, "So you're the little woman who wrote the book that started this great war." That is a serious impact for a piece of literature.

So let's step back and put these events into context. How does a woman in the mid-1800s write a book that helps change the course of history? Keep in mind, this is a time when most women had no formal education. Women would not get the right to vote for another 70 years. It was exceedingly rare for a woman to earn a living and almost unheard of for a woman to be a thought-leader. At the time, women rarely published articles or books in their own name. In fact, when Stowe began writing, she published articles under her brother and husband's names and used a pseudonym before finally stepping into her own unique voice and not only using her own name but also becoming an outspoken abolitionist.

So how did Harriet Beecher Stowe break through all of these societal confines to become someone who helped end the barbaric institution of slavery? Trauma. Trauma was what forced her to feel so fully that she had to do something about it. Stowe gave birth to seven children. She often wrote in letters and journals about how she loved her children deeply. She also wrote about the incredible toll it took on her body amidst the colossal responsibility of caring for so many children, often with very few resources or assistance. Amidst the challenge, a life-changing trauma occurred. Her beloved son Samuel Charles Stowe died.

She would often write about this as the biggest loss of her life and yet also one of the most important moments.

"Never give up," she wrote, "for that is just the place and time that the tide will turn." In the midst of this loss, she was living close to the Mason-Dixon line in Cincinnati, Ohio, which was a big stop on the underground railroad. She got to know many slaves and also let some stay in her home as they made their way to freedom. She often attributed her ability to feel deeply to the profound loss she endured. She said, "Any mind that is capable of a real sorrow is capable of good." She also said, "Having experienced losing someone so close to me, I can sympathize with all the poor, powerless slaves at the unjust auctions." It is clear in her writings that she realized that the plight of an educated white woman was not the same as the plight of the slaves. Yet she used the pain she experienced through losing her son to cultivate empathy for slaves. She saw it as a call to action.

Her pen became her voice and the way she carved a path to freedom for so many. In many ways, the realities of being a female writer forced her to be an even stronger writer. She knew her writing had to be exceptional, but it also had to be deeply heartfelt to accomplish her mission. She was capable of being both. *Uncle Tom's Cabin* became a masterpiece that served as a tipping point in a nation that was trying to reconcile its values against the institution of slavery. It helped people experience that slavery was everyone's problem, not just those directly involved in it. Stowe became a leader in the abolitionist movement, and along the way, she evolved profoundly as a person, growing wiser and deepening in her faith. For all of these reasons, she is a model of what has come to be known as post-traumatic growth.

While Stowe's life contains every aspect of post-traumatic growth, the term was not used during her time. Some doctors' notes during the Civil War show signs of soldiers exhibiting physiological responses to stress that they referred to as soldier's heart. During World War I and II, people began referring to the symptoms as shell shock. And of course, it's not just war veterans who experience trauma. It was only later when veterans' groups, feminist organizations, and Holocaust survivor groups began advocating for the cluster of symptoms we now refer to as post-traumatic stress disorder to have a diagnosis all its own.

Certainly, naming something is the first step to beginning to understand the full breadth of the experience. The problem with the term *disorder*, however, is that the symptoms that occur after we experience a traumatic event are actually the way our body is designed to handle stress. As we discussed in the class on trauma, the problem occurs when the body and mind cannot find their way out of the sympathetic nervous system response after the trauma is over. A lot of what this course is about is how to find our way through traumatic or stressful events without becoming "disordered" in our response, but instead stronger. That is the essence of resilience. In fact, because of the stigma implied by the word *disorder*, several years ago many people advocated for the dropping of the "D" and just calling it post-traumatic stress.

I know I felt that way when I was diagnosed with post-traumatic stress disorder. In the year 2000, I was in a near-death car accident in New York City that crushed my cab driver. I was trapped in the car with him for more than an hour. It took me years to recover physically from the accident in which I fractured my spine, sternum, and skull. It took much longer to recover mentally from the experience. The definition of *post-traumatic stress* read like a personal description of my mental state. Up to that point, I had, for the most part, a peaceful and happy life. I remember getting the post-traumatic stress disorder diagnosis and saying to the psychologist, "I don't have a disorder! I just went through something really difficult, and I need some help processing it and finding my way out again!" When I tell that story to trauma survivors, I always see people nod their heads in agreement. Why does something challenging happening to you have to result in a disorder? The answer is that it doesn't. As we often say in the realm of post-traumatic growth, it's not what's wrong. It's what happened. As humans, we often attempt to outthink the trauma. The mind wants to know why something happened, but really, we should be asking, "now what?" This empowers us to manage our response to the trauma rather than feeling like a victim of circumstance.

The reality is that we do not become stronger, wiser, and more resilient in spite of our adversity. We become stronger because of adversity. This pattern was noticed by Drs. Rich Tedeschi and Lawrence Calhoun, who coined the term *post-traumatic growth* in 1995. The idea arose from their research on parents who were experiencing bereavement after the death of a child. For most parents, the horrific thought of a child dying invokes more fear than even the thought of their own death. And yet, what the doctors noticed was that while of course parents suffered deeply after losing a child, they were also reporting many unexpected positive changes that occurred in their lives.

And why is that? Trauma deepens our ability to feel both pain and joy. Real compassion occurs when we feel the full spectrum of life so fully that we no longer suppress our pain. We have no choice in many cases after a trauma but to feel it. The result is that our life opens up in new ways. Over time studying a whole range of different traumas, Drs. Tedeschi and Calhoun noticed five important areas for growth that emerged in people who've experienced traumatic situations. These are personal strength, new possibilities, cultivation of meaningful relationships, spiritual change, and appreciation for life. Let's take a deeper look at each of these.

The first is personal strength. Drs. Tedeschi and Calhoun use the somewhat paradoxical phrase "more vulnerable yet stronger." We can see this happen on the news after nearly every major traumatic experience, whether terrorist attack, mass shooting, or natural disaster. The nature of the trauma brings forth the reality that we are, in fact, vulnerable in every moment. And the truth is that we always have been. Nothing has changed. We just experienced a glimpse into how vulnerable our lives actually are through the traumatic event. At the same time, though, we also witness how the traumatic experience brings people together. As author Brené Brown puts it, "In our culture, we associate vulnerability with emotions we want to avoid such as fear, shame, and uncertainty. Yet we too often lose sight of the fact that vulnerability is also the birthplace of … belonging … and love."

Both individual and collective strength arises in a whole myriad of unexpected ways after a trauma. The only way to really build strength is to be tested. When you want to build a muscle, you have to apply resistance. To build your personal strength—to build resilience—you need resistance as well. Psychologist Angela Lee Duckworth has done some really fascinating research into this, showing that the most successful adolescents are not necessarily the smartest people or those with the most resources. Even when compared against many other success factors including test scores and household income, the most successful young people are those who have the most grit, which Duckworth defines as the combination of passion and perseverance. In her best-selling book *Grit*, she encourages us to step out of what is comfortable to discover what is possible through embracing adversity.

The second area for post-traumatic growth is the discovery of new possibilities. When we experience a trauma, it disrupts our worldview and, in many ways, breaks apart our previous paradigm. We're forced to recreate our worldview and deepen our understanding of life. Our beliefs often get challenged and we see the way our core values rise to the surface to support us through the process. We try new things because the old ways don't work amidst our new reality. We get more creative as we try to process what has occurred. We try to reconcile our inner reality with our outside world and a whole flood of new possibilities comes to the surface. This is absolutely what happened with the teachers and students at Marjory Stoneman Douglas High School after the mass shooting in 2018. Suddenly they were planning marches, speaking on the news, singing at the Tony Awards, and creating art, music, and poetry out of their tragedy. While of course they suffered and are still suffering, they also have grown stronger and more self-confident, passionate, and inspired. They see the world in a bigger context, and by pursuing the new avenues that trauma has opened up, they are becoming an increasingly important part of that world.

The third area for growth after trauma is the cultivation of meaningful relationships. Oftentimes, in the wake of trauma, people report an increased sense of closeness with others. While some relationships may be challenged after a trauma, people will frequently bond more deeply with the people who shared the traumatic experience, or they will cultivate new relationships in the aftermath. Traumatic events tend to remind us of the importance of the people in our lives, and as a result, these events create opportunities for us to connect with them in ways we never did before. Not only do we let ourselves be helped, we may also become more aware of the ways that we can help others. Like Harriet Beecher Stowe, we may have a greater degree of compassion and empathy, which can connect us more fully with others. After experiencing the depths of pain ourselves, we become more sensitive to the pain of others and want to alleviate it if at all possible. We may also unite with others to create change in the aftermath of a traumatic event. And this process can open our hearts in new ways, unlocking the true power of community.

The fourth area for growth is spiritual change or existential exploration. Whatever our particular pathway to God or perhaps scientific understanding of consciousness may be, traumatic experiences can send us into a deeper exploration of our own belief system. It can change the way we perceive ourselves, often forcing us to look at our own existence in relation to something larger than the self. For some, this can invite questions about if there is something transcendent that remains after the human form changes or is no longer. One of the double amputees that I've worked with for many years, Hal, described this experience in a rather macabre but also very powerful way. Hal said:

> Who am I really? I lost one of my legs and part of [the] other leg in an IED blast, but did I go away? No, I'm still here. Then the docs had to start cutting my other leg down shorter because of the infection and it started going necrotic. Like I could see a part of my body dying before my very eyes. It's a weird thing to watch. But did I go away? No, I was still here. So that got me thinking. What if they cut off my arms? Nope, still here. What about an ear? Nope, [still here.] … Still here. Still the same.
>
> At some point in body-part elimination, my body would die. The point is that after losing limbs, I get that something in me is not these legs or arms or body. Something in me is so much more than this. Now, I'm not much for religion. But I know one thing. I am not just this body. This body is a temporary hangout for something larger than all of this. I don't even need a name for it because I can feel how real it is.

After experiencing a trauma, people often go through existential questioning about the nature of consciousness, whether they embrace a particular religion or not. The exploration often unlocks increased faith, meaning, purpose, and conviction. It can also help people connect with the part of them that is unchanging, just as my veteran friend Hal experienced.

There is nothing like being reminded of the vulnerability of life to help us remember how fortunate we are, which brings us to our fifth area of post-traumatic growth: appreciation for life. When we are reminded of the inevitability of our own demise, we often appreciate our blessings even more. We also want to make the most of the time we have in life. When someone close to us dies or we're reminded of our own mortality in some way, we find a new spark of life—a new excitement for really being present for the journey.

Last time I was home visiting my parents, my mother said to me, "I realized the other day that I probably have 25 more years to live if I'm lucky. I only see you four times a year. It struck me that I may only see you 100 more times. Please can we spend really meaningful time together during these trips and try to get together even more?" At first, I found her comment odd and was also shocked that my mother, who still seems very young and vital, was thinking in this way. I can't imagine thinking of life in these terms, like every time we go to visit thinking, "Well, mom, we only have 95 more trips left." But then I realized that in some way, she was right. I found myself putting my phone away while we were together and letting those work emails wait until after she went to sleep at night. I also found myself being more present with her in our discussions and wanting to plan fun outings that I knew we would enjoy together. Who knows how much time we have left together, and who knows how healthy we will be along the road. It felt important to make the most of what we had, which was the present moment.

I hope that learning about these five areas of post-traumatic growth will give you a window for observing the many positive things that can emerge from a trauma. But now let's shift to another way to look at post-traumatic growth—one that's more closely linked to the passage of time. Victim > Survivor > Changemaker is a way to describe the three phases a trauma survivor passes through in the post-traumatic growth process. Let's use the rest of this class to break down each of these phases.

When we experience a trauma, we can immediately start to feel under attack. Something happened to us that was out of our control. Suddenly our body may start to feel like the scene of a crime where we've lost our ability to choose the path in front of us. This experience can leave us feeling like a victim. In some situations, we may actually and actively be the victim of someone or something, as is experienced in the case of physical and mental abuse. In these cases where we are not able to make choices for ourselves, securing our safety becomes paramount. If you are actively the victim of physical or mental abuse, we have a whole list of references in the guidebook that can help you get the help you need to have choices once again. Please reach out.

Now, before we go more deeply into this topic, please keep in mind here that there is a spectrum of victimhood. Along this spectrum, there is a difference between being a child sex slave who's experiencing daily torture and perhaps someone who's the victim of a car accident that no one willfully or intentionally caused, similar to my situation. Clearly the role of the victim is quite different in both of these situations. Yet believe me, I was quite good at playing the role of the victim for many years after my car accident. Even now, nearly two decades later, I have to be watchful that the victim mentality doesn't creep in when I encounter something I can't do physically because of my injuries. The fascinating thing is that I've seen survivors of the child sex trade have less of a victim mentality than I once had because of my car accident. And let me tell you, it was a huge wake-up call. Seeing this reality is one of the things that helped me move past the victim phase.

In reality, we all play the role of the victim in one way or another. We have victim moments, most of us on a daily basis. We can feel like the victims of a political leader we don't like, victims in a traffic jam, victims of a long line at the grocery store, victims of someone's gossip, or perhaps victims of a difficult family member or coworker. This experience is entirely normal. It can even be protective at times, but it can also be detrimental. It is important to feel what is present when you do find yourself in the role of the victim, but it's also important to not get stuck in that stage. We can't fully grow until we have the chance to move through the stage of being a victim.

How can we identify when we're experiencing a victim mentality? The first sign is to notice that we don't feel like we have choices for one reason or another. We may feel denial or disbelief that something occurred. We may feel powerless, under attack, or that we don't have control of our lives. We may notice patterns of fear-based living where we're feeling afraid to confront things or engage in a fight. The phrase "why me" is another surefire way to identify the victim mentality. We also may start questioning our faith or feeling helpless, wounded, and broken—perhaps a feeling of hopelessness that we will never be able to get over what has happened. Oftentimes self-righteousness arises, a feeling that we are right and the other person is wrong. Shame and blame can also creep in: phrases like "It's my fault," or "How could they have done this to me?"

So why do we take on the role of the victim? Really, it's an entirely normal response after a trauma. It can even feel good. There is some initial evidence that people actually get a temporary burst of positive endorphins from feeling like a victim. This is a dangerous moment of happiness that ultimately results in a letdown due to several key factors. When people are concerned about us, they treat us with kindness and help out. And let's be honest, it feels great when people show up to help you out. We feel loved and cared for. And that said, there is usually an end to how long this lasts. It also creates a situation where codependency can easily develop. The victim mentality can also be a way to avoid personal responsibility. It's easier to make excuses or blame others for our actions when we're actively feeling like a victim. It can also be an excuse for not doing what we need to do in life and can prevent us from making decisions. Victimhood can also be an excuse for not taking risks. We do this at the cost of our own well-being. It is possible to live our whole lives as a victim by using our story as a reason why not to do something instead of using it as an opportunity for personal growth.

To move past the victim mentality, it is important to realize we must give up the benefits of being a victim. Positive endorphin release can become a trap and a prison. At some point if we want to evolve, we have to take a step and shift from being a victim to being a survivor. What is the difference? A survivor has choices. A victim does not. Empowerment resides in having a choice. We may not be able to control our circumstances, but what we can do is expand the sphere of what is actually possible to change. This can give us an intellectual framework that can carry us through to the other side.

It may even be helpful to draw a picture of this out for ourselves. Draw your current reality inside of an inner circle. For instance, your reality might be that you just got diagnosed with diabetes. Then outside the circle, write the possibilities that are immediately accessible to you to change your situation. This may simply be a change in mindset, or it may be an even bigger life shift. For instance, it might include taking insulin; changing your diet; exercising; losing weight; visiting other doctors, nutritionists with special expertise, or specialists who may have some special insights; joining a diabetic support group; participating in diabetes awareness campaigns; writing articles about your experience; changing your mindset around the disease; observing mental changes you can make to befriend your body; noticing the positive changes that have come out of the experience; helping someone else with diabetes who may be in a worse position than you; and even the experience to explore your faith in a deeper way.

You can then keep expanding the possibility sphere out farther and farther to imagine what the ultimate dream of possibilities are for you in this situation. When we do this, we take responsibility for our lives. We make a commitment to not let the things that have happened to us limit us. We open up the possibilities regarding what we can do about our reality. We open up to the belief that something needs to change; something is going to change, and we have to initiate it. When we do this, we step into our own power. We begin to get proactive with our challenges, and we open the door to find our peace in the midst of them.

A survivor also cultivates gratitude. Gratitude helps us see everything that is going right with our lives instead of everything that is going wrong in it. We can even talk to our trauma and say, "You don't get the right to steal my future from me. I'm going to learn from this and move past it." Then we start finding solutions. We learn from our strengths and weaknesses to find how we can thrive in life. There are ways to tell if we're doing this that can support us along the way.

Oftentimes when we're feeling like a victim, we can find ourselves never completing anything. While stepping into being a survivor, we sometimes have to work hard to complete what we start. If it feels difficult to tackle something large, we can start with something small but make sure we always finish. The ability to complete things relates to our sense of self-worth and confidence.

Vulnerability still may be present, but also the notion that I'm surviving and thriving begins to arise. Doing this is essential to reaching the third phase of post-traumatic growth: becoming a changemaker. A changemaker operates from an empowered view where we realize our capacity to create meaningful change in our own lives and in the lives of others. We see the value of our wisdom, the resources available to us, and we naturally begin to share them with others.

Suddenly, it's just not about us anymore. It's about being a part of something larger than ourselves and doing what we can to affect change. Over time, we learn to scale our impact and keep evolving our mission to dream bigger and bigger. Scarlett Lewis is a shining example of this. Her young son Lewis was killed in the Sandy Hook massacre, but before he died, he tried to save the lives of other children. She was so inspired by her son that she created the Jesse Lewis Choose Love Movement, which is a non-profit organization that's devoted to providing children with social and emotional learning—the type that the shooter, Adam Lanza, perhaps didn't have. Scarlett said:

> After Jesse's death, I knew that if Adam Lanza had been able to give and receive nurturing, healing and love, that the tragedy wouldn't have happened. [She went on to say,] I believe that the tragedy started with an angry thought in Adam Lanza's head. And an angry thought can be changed. So I asked everyone to start changing one angry thought into a loving thought every day. I said, "By doing that, you will positively impact yourself, those around you, and through the ripple effect, you will make a more peaceful and loving world."

Moving from a victim mentality to a changemaker mentality may seem impossible or scary, and honestly, sometimes you will fail. But you will never find your best if you don't try. Post-traumatic growth happens when we lean into our journey and discover how to live as the fullest potential of our true selves. Who knows—it may seem like a leap of faith now, but perhaps someday, this trauma that happened to you that seemed like the worst thing that ever occurred will transform into being the best thing that ever occurred because it cracked you open. It started you on your way.

Class 13

Suzi Landolphi on Post-Traumatic Growth

This class consists of an interview with Suzi Landolphi, a leader in the post-traumatic growth movement. For over 10 years, she has been providing horse-inspired growth and healing as well as other therapeutic activities for many different community, social service, and clinical organizations. She currently works at Boulder Crest Retreat in Bluemont, Virginia, as a PATHH Guide. PATHH— or Progressive and Alternative Training for Healing Heroes—is a quickly expanding

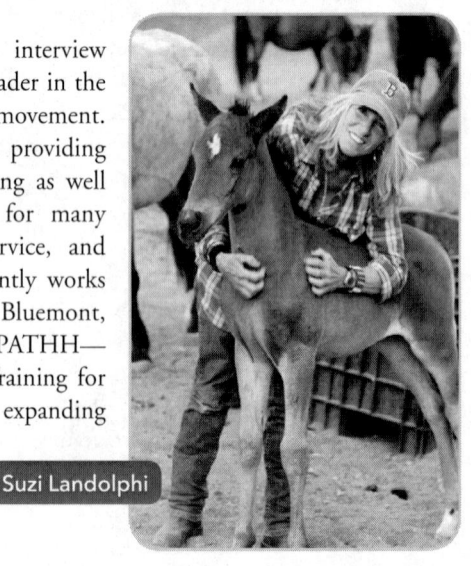

Suzi Landolphi

retreat program created by and for combat veterans that is based on 30 years of research on post-traumatic growth.

This guidebook chapter contains summarized information from Landolphi's interview. To see or hear the full interview, refer to the audio or video class. If you have obtained a transcript book, you can also read the full interview there.

The Idea of Post-Traumatic Growth

- According to Landolphi, the idea of post-traumatic growth has always been around. Ancient and indigenous peoples have always known about the idea that what doesn't kill you makes you stronger, and that you get gifts from trauma. The idea of the multigenerational transmission of trauma also points to the idea of multigenerational transmission of growth and gifts.

- While researchers Richard Tedeschi and Lawrence Calhoun were studying the idea of where wisdom comes from, they were asked to go to a support group for parents who had lost their child. They started to hear about how these parents had formed deeper relationships—that they created, for instance, a foundation to build baseball teams in inner cities because their son loved baseball. They had great personal strength, a great appreciation for life, and an understanding that life has a spiritual existence.

- Of course they would want to have their child back. However, their trauma actually brought them some great wisdom and growth.

Boulder Crest Retreat

- Boulder Crest Retreat was founded by US Navy veteran Ken Falke and his wife Julia. Their inspiration came while visiting wounded veterans who handled explosive ordnance disposal. Eventually, the couple formed Boulder Crest Retreat to help such veterans.

- Landolphi soon began working with the retreat. She and the Falkes found that the veterans who suffered the most from post-traumatic stress disorder also had the worst childhoods.

- For example, a person could have a horrific childhood, grow up, use the gifts of trauma to become a great soldier, suffer a wound in the line of duty, and then return home to the site of their original trauma. Their home may be a place a trauma occurred that the veteran never disclosed.

- At Boulder Crest, emotional regulation is a large focus. Specific techniques used include archery and transcendental meditation.

- Another important idea is that you can only control your own life; however, when other people see you change, they may change as well. If you appreciate life more and appreciate new possibilities, there is a high likelihood you will develop a deeper or better connection with the people around you.

- Those people who cannot change have the right not to do so. However, you also have a right to not be close to them and set boundaries.

Creating New Possibilities

- Landolphi points to a person's principles as a great tool for creating new possibilities for oneself. Keep in mind that principles are very different from your personality. In essence, principles are true guidelines that you will not cross. Moreover, you will not cross them

> **Forgiving Your Imperfections**
>
> An additional idea espoused by Landolphi is to accept imperfections. An attachment to perfection will lead to suffering. If you make a mistake, accept it and move on. You can always go back and apologize. This plays into the definition of *success* at Boulder Crest Retreat, which is "to be better than I was yesterday."

because you believe in them. They honor yourself and everything you care about.

- Try coming up with three to five principles that you will use every time you make a decision. For instance, if you are faced with a choice where one option goes against your principles, then making your decision should become easier. Examples of principles include integrity, kindness, and honesty.

Suggested Reading

Falke and Goldberg, *Struggle Well*.

Hedrick, *Harriet Beecher Stowe*.

Rendon, *Upside*.

Tedeschi and Finch, *Posttraumatic Growth*.

Tedeschi and Moore, *The Posttraumatic Growth Workbook*.

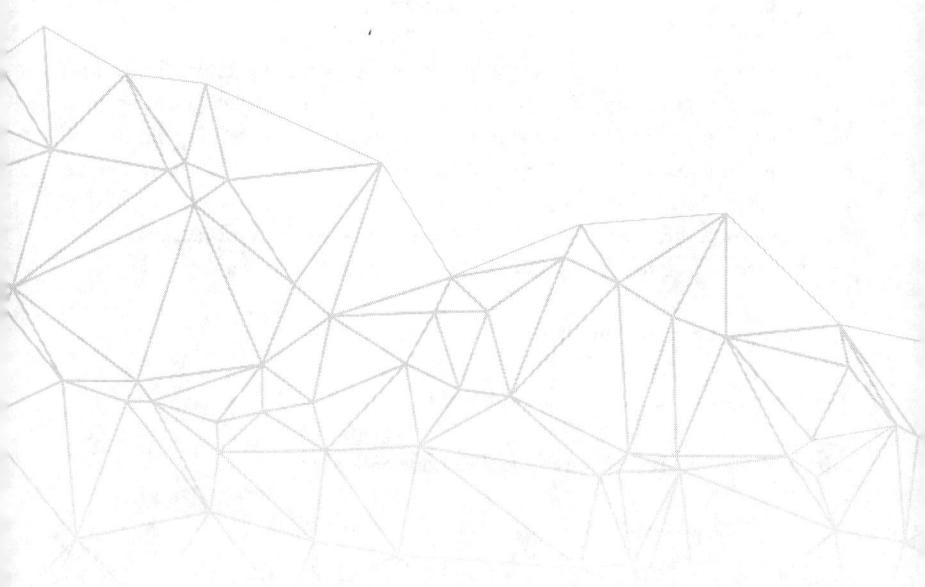

Class 13 Transcript

Suzi Landolphi on Post-Traumatic Growth

Molly Birkholm: Hello and welcome. I'm joined today by Suzi Landolphi, who is a true leader in the post-traumatic growth movement. Thank you so much for joining us today Suzi.

Suzi Landolphi: I love being here with you.

Molly: Suzi, just to let you know a little bit about Suzi, she currently works at Boulder Crest Retreat in Bluemont, Virginia as a PATHH guide. She has a long history of doing all sorts of other things. PATHH, just to give a little bit of background is Progressive and Alternative Training for Healing Heroes. It's a quickly expanding retreat program created by and for combat veterans and it's based on 30 years of research on post-traumatic growth.

So, before coming to Boulder Crest Suzi cofounded the Big Heart Ranch and Farm where rescued animals and humans support each other's healing. Suzi began her own healing journey many years ago learning to gentle wild horses. She's now a member of the board of directors of Lifesavers Wild Horse Rescue and facilitates Wild Horse Warrior Journey retreats for veterans. On top of that Suzi has hosted her own TV and radio talk shows. She's published two books and has been a frequent guest on *The Oprah Winfrey Show*. Thank you so much!

Suzi: I'm tired just hearing that.

Molly: Oh, my gosh! What a life you've had.

Suzi: I should not be here anymore. I've done enough.

Molly: No! We need you! You're not allowed to leave.

Suzi: That's the nice thing about, hopefully, what happens is you do and then you teach, then you share and you hopefully you become a wise elder. We need them. That's important.

Molly: Well, you have one of the youngest spirits I know. But I also consider you a wise elder.

Suzi: Thank you.

Molly: She counsels me all the time, too, so…

Suzi: Doesn't need much.

Molly: I need plenty, I assure you!

Suzi: (Inaudible) Once in awhile.

Molly: Oh, we just had a whole class on post-traumatic growth so I feel like this interview is the perfect thing to follow so people can really hear and interact with how this plays out in the real world, because it is something that happens in the real world. So, if you could just start out a little bit and tell us more about the post-traumatic growth movements.

Suzi: So, it actually started, it's always been around. Let's just put it that way. We just don't know about things until we put a name on them and then we kind of put it in in some kind of clinical terms. Then all of a sudden it seems to be more real or more valuable. But, you know, ancient peoples, indigenous peoples, have always known about post-traumatic growth. You know, that idea that doesn't…what doesn't kill you makes you stronger. And that you get gifts from trauma and that if you believe in historical trauma, which we all do, if you believe in multigenerational transmission of trauma, then you have to believe in multigenerational transmission of growth and gifts. It just makes sense.

So, Richard Tedeschi and Lawrence Calhoun 30 years ago or more were studying this idea of where does wisdom come from? And they were asked to go to a support group for parents who had lost their child. And they sat there, as every good psychologist should, and keep their mouth shut while they're in a support group. And they started to hear some things they couldn't believe. They started to hear about how these parents had formed deeper relationships; that they built, say, a foundation to build baseball teams in inner cities because their son loved baseball. They had great personal strength, a great appreciation for life and an understanding that life has a spiritual existence.

Now do they really, and would they really want, to have their child back? Of course, but the fact is they couldn't deny that this trauma, this horrible thing that has happened, actually brought them some great wisdom and growth.

That's really where it came from.

And just to add to that, when they did start to talk about post-traumatic growth, or give it a name if you will, they went back and looked in history to see what they could find, if anybody had written, and of course, all kinds of people had written about this idea of strength. All religions have it. The idea that people who went through the Holocaust, Victor Frankl's *Man's Search for Meaning*.

An amazing book that changed my life when I was in my teens, *Lessons from the Hanoi Hilton*, which are the POWs of the Vietnam era. And we've been blessed at Boulder Crest to meet several of them and they also came back with post-traumatic growth. Although I'll tell you the psychologist told the families that don't expect them to be able to be the same man that came, that went, that's coming back. They probably will be institutionalized, that they will not be able to function because of the trauma they've gone through. Everybody expected all of them to come back 100% with PTSD. And 4% came back with PTSD.

Molly: Incredible.

Suzi: And those 4% were in the POW camp the shortest amount of time.

Molly: Unbelievable.

Suzi: It's unbelievable, isn't it? And they came back. We have senators and businessmen and all kinds of wonderful careers that these men have carved out for themselves based on post-traumatic growth.

Molly: What do you think made them so strong after that experience?

Suzi: Well, it's funny. We can only interview them. They've been interviewed every year since they've come back. And so, we just had them at Boulder Crest Retreat and we talked to Charlie Plumb and Gerald Coffee and Everett Alvarez, and he was the very first POW. And we asked him about that, and certainly other people have to, and what they actually said was it was their connection, the connection to one another that they were absolutely committed to:

It was called return home with the honor.

Now most of them during their torture told anything that they knew, and they felt terrible. They felt like they had totally let down everybody, including themselves, the country and their other men. And when they all shared that they had all done that, then Stockdale their leader said, "So, did I. And that doesn't matter. What matters is that we return home with honor. That we support one another now, and forever and that we go." So, that purpose, that passion for something greater than yourself, so you can either sit around beating yourself up or you can decide to do something that's better for some somebody else and something else.

So, connection by far was the first thing that they were going to hold each other up. They were going to help one another.

Molly: And that vulnerability, that disclosure peace, feels so important to be able to bear those dark parts of yourself.

Suzi: I think that's true for all of us. And post-traumatic growth tells you that. It says that if you continually educate yourself about what happened to you, not what's wrong with you, but what happened to you. And understand more about any kind of healing opportunity when you emotionally regulate, when on a daily basis, you take some deep breaths. You decide that you're going to respond versus react. So, emotional regulation, which you do all the time.

Yoga, Irest, any of those opportunities to take our central nervous system and calm it down and our emotions.

Disclosure is the third part. The third thing that we can do on a regular basis if you disclose everyday a little bit about what happened to you that day in order to be able to get up the next day and do better than what you did yesterday, that's part of facilitating post-traumatic growth. And you know that after that you get to create a new story. So, I get to create a new story every day, every minute of every day. I can choose to do something different and do it in a way that creates the life I deserve.

And the last is what you're doing right now, which is you're sharing with other people. That you're an expert guide. That you make sure that people get to know the wisdom that you have experienced from any trauma that you have experienced and come out on the other side.

Molly: Thank you. Now, Suzi and I have worked together at Boulder Crest Retreat Center. This is such a special place. Could you please share with everyone more about Boulder Crest Retreat, both how it was started? What happens there, the whole experience of being a part of Boulder Crest?

Suzi: So, Ken Falke, Ken and Julia Falke. He is a 22 years Navy EOD, retired. He was going to Georgetown to get a master's in public policy. He kept hearing about the men and women in the EOD community, stepping on IEDs, getting hurt. He was going to Walter Reed everyday after school and it was just horrible what was happening. And he realized that the families didn't have enough resources to actually go to DC and spend months there with their loved one. So, as only Julia and Ken will do, is they invited them back to their home, their estate called Boulder Crest Estate, and they would stay in their house or in their two little cabins on the property.

And Julia and a bunch of women friends were sitting around having a glass of wine. And they wrote on a napkin, "You know we could build some cabins down there so the families could come and stay." And they donated 37 acres and the first million dollars and built what they thought was going to be two cabins until Ken kept realizing that this high suicide rate and this PTSD rate was just epidemic proportions. So, he and Julia decided to actually form a retreat.

Once they did that it was very clear to Ken that what we were doing wasn't working. Meanwhile, on the other coast, I'm doing these retreats with veterans at the same time realizing that the clinical work that we were asked to do doesn't always work in the way that we want it to. So, we were experimenting with what else we could do. And even though we didn't know about post-traumatic growth at that time, which is bizarre that as a therapist you don't get taught about that, you don't, that's not part of your education. We called it strength based and solution focus. That we're not going to go back in just, you know, go back over the problem all the time or keep exposing you to the problem. What we're going to do is keep looking for your strength and your solutions.

The thing that happened was when we went out to Boulder Crest and I was there the first day it opened and we talked to Ken. He was wide open to the idea that just maybe, just maybe, it wasn't all the trauma on the battlefield that was causing this. By his own experience on the battlefield, that wasn't the worst thing that's ever happened to him. It was bad. Horrible things happen. You have to do some horrible things. You also have a tremendous purpose. Now we're going back to the POWs. You have tremendous purpose you have a brotherhood and a sisterhood and you are doing some amazing things that most of the population could not do, would not do.

So, we decided take a look at what else happened. We looked through the rucksack of life and what we discovered was that the men and women that suffered the most, combat veterans from PTSD, also had the worst childhoods.

Molly: Mmm.

Suzi: So, now we've got a whole new way of looking at it. What makes it so special at Boulder Crest is that we look at everything that happened. There's nothing wrong with you. It's what happened if you had a horrific childhood.

And a lot of trauma, you probably had all those symptoms of PTSD as a child. You leave your home at 17. You go into the military and those gifts or those results of trauma at home actually make you a great soldier. Right?

So, then now they use them. They become a great soldier. They get hurt and they get sent back home to, I say, well I've coined "the scene of the crime," a crime that they've never disclosed and that's what you just brought up, this idea of disclosure. So, Boulder Crest we emotionally regulate. We have TM. We do all kinds of things that…

Molly: TM meaning Transcendental Meditation.

Suzi: Transcendental Meditation. We do archery. We do a lot of these emotional regulation practices and we educate them about what happened and then how to make those choices in order to create that life and definitely take their strengths. I mean you can only imagine what combat veterans and first responders have for training and strength. They just forgot. They forgot.

Molly: In the whole notion of post-traumatic growth there's this profound welcoming of our humanity. You know, the humanness of what we all share. There's such a freedom in not having to be perfect, of being able to say, "I'm not perfect" and that feels like such a liberation to know that we can find our peace and our freedom, not in spite of what happened to us, but actually because of it.

Suzi: That's true. You know, I think people that have gone through horrific trauma, we talked about the Holocaust and POWs and indigenous people already know this; that that idea of perfection was actually, they laughed. You know, I hung out with a lot of my Native American friends. And I was welcomed into a culture to teach me more about what's truly important, like what's important now.

And I was with a bunch of Navajo wonderful women who were weaving. And I watched them, literally watched them, teach younger women how to weave. And it was perfect. I mean they could make rugs that were absolutely perfect and they chose not to. They taught these young women how to make a mistake, to choose a mistake and to put it into each rug that they make. And the young girls were kind of horrified at the beginning, in fact, why would I do that? Because we don't want you to ever think you have to be perfect. Life is not perfect. Nothing's going to be perfect. So, why are you striving for something that doesn't have to be? It's only going to cause you suffering.

You may think the Buddhists say that very well. You know when you are, have attachment to perfection you're going to suffer a lot. So, I revel in my imperfections. In fact, I have a whole bunch of family and friends that constantly remind me about how imperfect I am.

Molly: What a gift!

Suzi: What a gift! The horses will let you know! You know, if you're looking for it, then people will feel safe enough to tell you. And then if you can have a bit of a lightness about you, about yourself, if you can say, oh yeah, these wrinkles I got these by living. Oh, my hair is kind of messy. I mean if we could do that and be okay with that and then you could say, "And yeah, I made a mistake today. Got grumpy at someone. I said something I shouldn't have." You know you always have the opportunity, it sounds bizarre, but can always go back and apologize. I mean you literally could do that.

Molly: Yeah, what a revolutionary concept.

Suzi: What an idea! "I'm sorry, I messed up." And then not beat yourself up about it because then that makes it about you again. And we have a definition of success at Boulder Crest and its…the definition actually is, "To be better today than I was yesterday."

Molly: Mmm.

Suzi: I mean, just that. Just a little bit better today than I was yesterday. So, I won't see anything there about perfection or accomplishment or anything like that. And to me resilient means that I don't have to go way down or way up.

Now things are going to happen without any of your input at all. My grandson contracted leukemia twice. We battled it for eight years. We didn't do anything to make that happen. Life happens. You know it's interesting, though Molly. Because my daughter and I have been doing these practices and understanding that there's going to be some gifts with this horrible thing that's happening, we have so many moments of post-traumatic growth. We did use our resilience, and then we went beyond.

Molly: Wow.

Suzi: And he's my grandson is amazing. I mean he's just… has so many gifts and he has some definitely some effects from it. There's no question about it. But you can not negate the gifts that he has and the growth that he has. And that's when I say gifts, I mean growth.

Molly: So, when you go through an experience like that, and thank you so much for sharing, you know just, this ability to be able to be present in your own trauma and stress in the midst of being someone who heals others and sometimes we feel like, "Oh, I can only go and do that thing that I really want to do when my life is perfect." But as you just illustrated, that day probably will never come.

Suzi: I haven't seen it yet. My clock's ticking. I don't know how much longer I'm going to be here.

Molly: We've got you for a while. But yeah, I mean, just to be able to say, yeah I'm going to get up and go. My life's not perfect. I'm not perfect.

Suzi: That's right. No.

Molly: I'm going to get up and make a difference.

Suzi: And I'm not going to be a victim and I'm not going I'm not going to stay in victimhood. Sometimes things people do things to me that I didn't ask for, that I didn't bring on. That's just because I live in a herd. So, that's going to happen. I'm not going to stay in victimhood. That's what I choose not to do.

Molly: So, when we go, start going about our own healing journey and post-traumatic growth journey, a lot of times we start working on ourselves, but we still live in a home with other people who might not be doing that at all, or have families we don't necessarily live with, or friends or colleagues and we're still bouncing off them and interacting with them. So, how does that play out?

Suzi: You know one of the things we say at Boulder Crest, we talk about that. We say, you know your family didn't come here, although we do family retreats, which is quite amazing. And the kids always get all of this quicker than the adults. We say when you change, when you change, when you make it about you first, keep the focus on yourself, there is a high likelihood that others around you will not only notice that change, but actually participate in their own change. If you try to change them, I can guarantee you that's probably going to go bad. It's a battle. It's probably not going… I know I've seen me do it.

So, the idea is that it always starts with us. I have no control over anybody else. Only me. And what I do know though is if I work those emotional regulation practices, if I appreciate life more, if I believe in new possibilities, all those things that post-traumatic growth tells me can happen when I do these practices, there's a high likelihood that I will have a deeper connection or a better connection with those people. And those people that cannot change, they have a right not to change and I have a right not to be that close to them. I just do. I have to set those boundaries.

Molly: Could you speak more about boundaries and the process of remaining resilient or becoming resilient?

Suzi: You know I find it interesting that emotional boundaries are so hard to construct and practice, yet, boy do you know where your yard ends and someone else begins. We actually have fights over that, right? You know where your car ends and someone else's car doesn't. Because when I open the car door and bang your car I have not honored the boundary. And I think that what happens is again our fear and sadness are wanting to be so connected to other people, our need to be connected and wanting to be loved, we absolutely have these porous boundaries that cause so much myth and misconception around relationships.

And I thought, I was thinking about this the other day, actually. You know I worked with a bunch of people this is very intense work. It's joyous works sometimes and difficult work. And the staff and I were joking the other day, we're all talking about the fact that we say something and we still misconstrue it. It's like well, you know, someone said to me the other day, "Suzi, please stop." And I was like, "Oh, that's a boundary. Funny I didn't notice that." You know, because I was so thought I was like, Oh no, they need and I want to… ah that's that old thing I have to watch out for. That's that thing that I have to manage, where I am not in charge of what somebody else likes, dislikes, does, wants to do. It's not my right. Not my need to tell them what it is or to continue to even offer it on them, unasked for advice is criticism.

So, those boundaries are important. And if we believe in them in other places, I can't go into your checking account, although I might like to because I don't what you… I might want to do that. I can't! Right? Therefore, I can't just tell you what to do, when to do it and how to do it. I can't cross over those boundaries. They're important. They keep us safe. They actually keep us more connected. Boundaries actually help with connection.

Molly: This is essential.

Suzi: Listen to, absolutely.

Molly: Could you speak about codependence?

Suzi: So, let me tell you a funny story. So, Melody Beattie who wrote the bible on codependents called *Codependent No More*. She was living near where we lived and she has a daughter and I have a daughter and as life would have it they hung out. That was so hard because, of course, they would, you know, talk and go, oh my mother is so codependent she wrote the book. And then at first my daughter would say, yeah, my mother's like, if you look up codependents, her pictures in the dictionary. It's a hard one you know, it's because, I think it's because of how we are raised. I mean it just truly is. I think our whole culture now is very codependent.

Again, indigenous peoples knew about interdependence. There's no such thing as independence. I didn't make my boots. I didn't make this. I didn't do any of this on my own. So, I'm truly not independent on any level. And, that.

opposite of that would be codependent, where I need you to do and make me feel everything: my value, my love, I mean, everything about and that I'm going to react to everything that you do as if I have to do something about it.

That's codependence it's at its worst.

And interdependent means that I would love it if you and I got along really well and you respected me and you cared for me and I'm going to do a lot to try to make that happen. Except I'm not going to give up my own self-worth for that. I can't. And if someone asks me to then they don't really care about me. So, codependence is this inability to be able to hold your own self-value in that if someone is mad at me I absolutely believe that somehow I've lost all my value, when that's just not true. They are mad at me and maybe it has something to do with that happened to them a long time ago and I'm just bringing it up again by accident even.

So, I think we have to be real careful. We are interdependent, which I love. So, when you came to Boulder Crest you helped us. I can help you and back and that is that wonderful thing that says I honor you. I honor that we lived in this culture together, this world together, that you are my friend. And at the same time I honor that you, Molly, you get to make your own decisions. You get to live your life, you get to create it the way you want and that's not a reflection on me.

Molly: So, Suzi as we start to wrap this amazing time up together, I want to ask you a question. And that is, how do we go about creating new possibilities for ourselves to create a future that we really want? And how can we be sure that we stick to this no matter what happens to us in the process?

Suzi: Wow, that's a great question. I would have to say, first and foremost, our principles. If you base your life on principles and not your personality that will help and your personality, I know lots of people believe, oh, I'm an introvert and this, no, we're everything. Everybody's everything.

Principles are very different than your personality. What they are, they are true guidelines that you will not cross. You will not cross because you believe in them and they hold a sacred value. And they are absolutely those things that honors, not only yourself, but everything you hold near and dear. And they actually honor life itself.

So, if you come up with some principles, three to five principles, that you're going to use every time you make a decision, that will help you because I don't know about you, but for me, because of how I was trained, sometimes my thoughts are not true. And they're not helpful and sometimes my feelings are not facts and they're not helpful.

So, if I make every decision on how I feel and what I think, I'm going to make some very poor decisions. If I bring in some principles and I say, well, that feeling and that thought, but it doesn't match my principles. What I want to do about that goes against everything I believe in, in terms of my principles: like integrity, kindness, honesty, whatever they are; I get to take a deep breath and go, I'm going to have to say it, I'm going to have to do this. Even though I'm afraid, even though I might lose something, even though I might even make someone upset, I have got to make those decisions based on my principles first.

Molly: Mmm. Thank you so much, Suzi. I truly appreciate our time together.

Suzi: I can't thank you enough for inviting me. I learn a lot every time I'm with you. We have these deep conversations. It's important because we inspire one another to do our best, to be a little bit better today than we were yesterday.

Molly: We do. We all need each other.

Suzi: We do.

Molly: And we have fun together, too!

Suzi: We do this alone, that's true.

Molly: Now what you won't see as we'll have a dance party afterwards.

Suzi: Yes!

Molly: Thank you all so much. Hope you enjoyed it as much as I did.

Class 14

Cultivating Community and Connection

It is normal to feel lonely once in a while, but feelings of persistent loneliness are unfortunately increasing in society. The antidote to loneliness is genuine connection with others. This class looks at several methods to help you build those connections.

Fostering Connection

- Humans are wired for connection. Research on babies shows that they need touch for cognitive development. Even more, all humans have mirror neurons that mimic the emotions and behavior

> There is a difference between being lonely and being alone. A person living alone might not feel lonely because of the quality of their friendships, whereas a person surrounded by people all day could still feel lonely because those relationships lack connection.

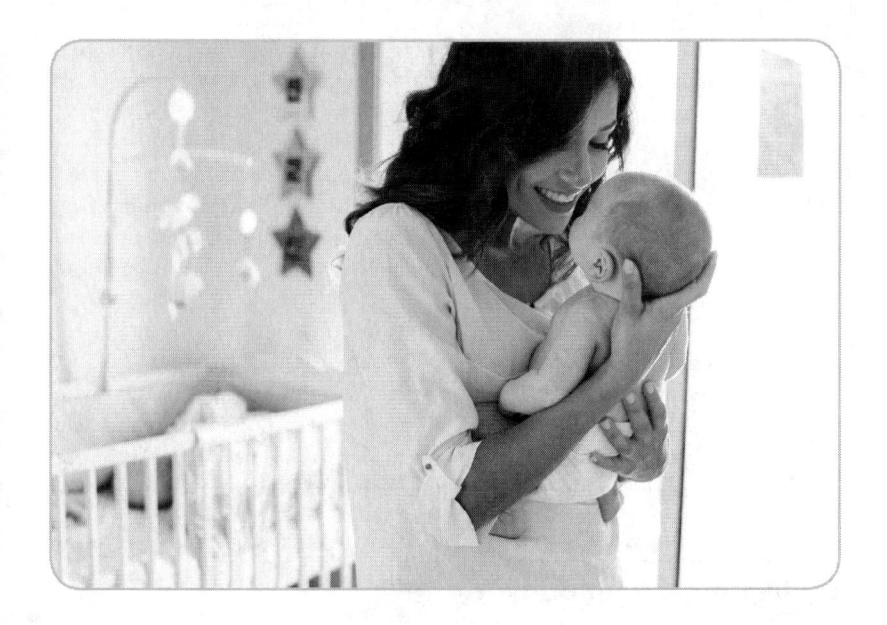

of people they interact with. People learn how to be human from other humans. That's why friendships and other relationships are central to your ability to thrive and be resilient.

- Connections start with trust. Trust happens when you feel that a person genuinely cares about your well-being. When people feel mutual concern for each other's well-being, that creates true friendship.

- This doesn't mean that you have to be a social butterfly. Having four to five very close friends is more effective than having lots of casual friends. The most important factors in a friendship include trust, dependability, and genuine enjoyment in your friend's company.

- Ultimately, much of one's ability to connect comes down to belief systems and attitude. If a person judges or rejects those who are supposedly different, those people will shut down, and the rejector will ultimately feel more separate and isolated. If one wants to truly rid society of loneliness, one has to open up to genuinely connecting with others. The more compassionate a person is of others, the easier it is to connect.

- It is also possible—and sometimes even easier—to form meaningful connections with animals, especially mammals. Horses and dogs are commonly used in trauma treatment to help clients develop a sense of connection and safety. Service animals, support animals, and pets can also be dependable friends.

- Community group practices like group chanting, breathing, singing, and dancing are also extremely effective at fostering connection with others, in part due to their ability to regulate bodily states and help process experiences. These practices are less common in the West, but they are seen quite prominently in other traditions and cultures.

Cultivating Community

- To cultivate your sense of community, you can start by nourishing the important relationships you already have. For example, you might reconnect with an old friend and devote the time and space to really listening to what they have to say. If you're looking to expand your community, see if you can create opportunities to spend time with people who share a mutual interest, such as joining an exercise group, volunteering on a political campaign, going to dog parks, starting a book club, and so on.

- Remember that what you put into your relationships and community is what you'll get out of it. Many people complain they don't have community, but at the same time, they haven't done much to create or nourish their community. It's also important to pay attention to what you choose to do with your community. For instance, does getting together always mean drinking together, or can you connect over other interests?

Co-Meditation

- Co-meditation is a powerful and practical tool that you can use to strengthen your relationship and connection with others. It is a great way to practice deep listening and being truly present with the people in your life.

- Co-meditation is a partner practice that is easy to do and takes a surprisingly short amount of time to bring you fully into the present moment. Once you've found someone to try this with, decide who is going to start as the giver of undivided attention and who will be the receiver of undivided attention.

- You'll switch halfway through, so each person will have the opportunity to practice both supporting someone and being supported. The only real instruction is this: Sit across from each other and see what happens.

- You can sit there until each person's turn reaches its natural end, or you may want to set a timer, perhaps between 15 and 30 minutes per person, so that you are not distracted by trying to keep track of time during the meditation. Some people prefer to go back and forth multiple times at shorter intervals, like two or five minutes, rather than each person taking a prolonged turn. Choose whatever feels right for you.

- Once you are sitting across from each other, let the receiver of undivided attention lead the way. He or she might want to sit there in silence, with eyes open or closed. Alternatively, this could be used as an opportunity for the recipient to take a look at and share what is going on in their inner world.

- If the recipient would like to spend their time diving into self-inquiry, the person giving attention can start by asking the recipient to let attention wander throughout their body to see if there are any feelings, emotions, or beliefs that are calling their attention. Allow your partner to verbally and nonverbally explore what comes to the surface.

- Throughout the experience, the person giving attention can ask the recipient the following three questions: What do you notice? Where in your body do you feel this? Can you say anything else about that? These questions can be asked as many times as necessary until the person receiving attention feels as though they've processed whatever has come up.

- The listener can also take notes on what the person sharing has to say. These notes can be a powerful tool for self-reflection after the meditation is over. At the end, ask the recipient if there are any takeaways. Also ask if there is anything he or she needs to feel complete in that moment.

Giving Back

- Another way to benefit from connection is to give back to your community. A study on 750 former prisoners of war found incredible resilience among these veterans. Once they were released from imprisonment, they avoided developing depression and PTSD, two diagnoses that are very common among veterans. Results from the study showed that altruism was one of the most important characteristics that set them apart and resulted in their impressive resilience.

- Giving back through money and time obviously benefits the recipients of help, but numerous studies also show significant benefits for the giver. Additionally, according to neuroscientist Richard Davidson, the brain has four circuits that impact one's sense of well-being: one for maintaining positive states, one for bouncing back from negative states, one for attention focusing, and one entirely devoted to generosity.

- Studies have shown that as a person spends more money on others, the spender experiences more happiness. Functional MRI scans show that giving money to charity activates brain regions associated with pleasure and reward, like the ventral striatum.

- The research isn't limited to the effects of giving money. Research also shows that volunteering one's time results in improved happiness as well. Some research even suggests that volunteering reduces the likelihood of developing depression, improves physical health and reduces cognitive decline as a person ages, and lowers the likelihood of early mortality.

- People can be both intrinsically and extrinsically motivated. Extrinsic motivation involves something from the outside influencing one's behavior, such as working to earn money, attending a lecture to get free food, or studying to avoid failing a test. Intrinsic motivation comes from within—that is, doing something because it is personally rewarding.

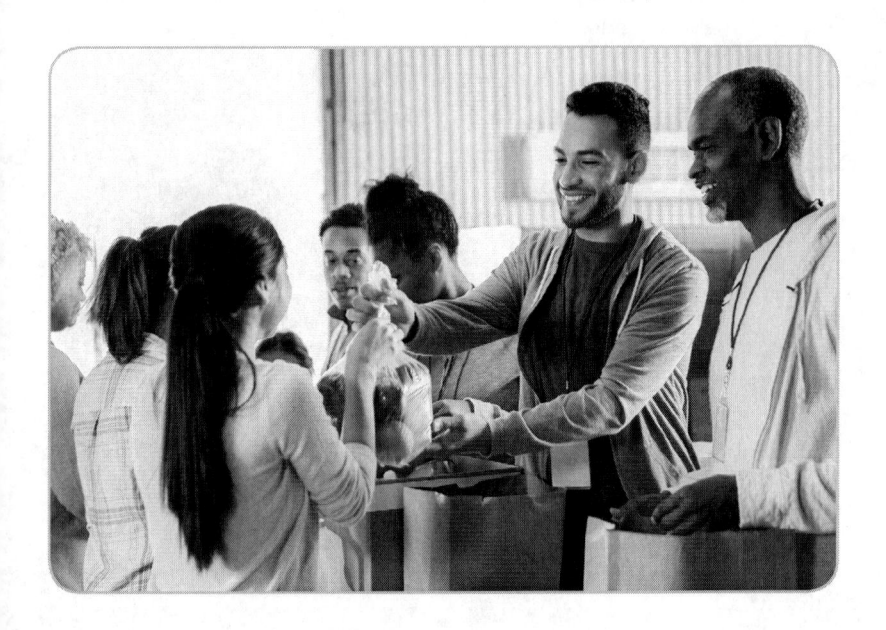

- Intrinsic motivation leads to higher life satisfaction. Studies show that volunteers typically choose to give back due to intrinsic motivation as opposed to extrinsic. People who value their intrinsic life goals derive more benefit and satisfaction from volunteering than people who are more focused on their extrinsic goals, like social standing and career status.

Suggested Reading

Beattie, *Codependent No More*.

Kristof, *Half the Sky*.

Activities

- Focus this week on establishing community or deepening your connection within your current community.
- If you have a willing partner, try a co-meditation.
- Give back to someone, a group of people, or an organization in a way you've never done before.

Class 14 Transcript

Cultivating Community and Connection

Welcome! So far in this course, we've spent a lot of time exploring the personal and lifestyle choices that can help us cultivate resilience. But we need to remember that relationships matter too. In fact, some of the biggest factors that determine our resilience include our connections with other people in our lives. Having dependable relationships; a strong, stable community; and ample opportunities to give back can transform the way we navigate both the good and the challenging moments of our lives. There's even strong evidence that links personal longevity to social bonds. The global life expectancy averages 71.4 years, but in the world's five Blue Zones, the life expectancy is much higher. *Blue Zones*, a term first coined by Dan Buettner in 2005, are regions spread across the world, but they share characteristics that are thought to explain why these populations have a much higher life expectancy. Let's look at three of these zones to see what they have in common.

People from Okinawa, Japan attribute their longevity not only to having a close family and a community but also to having strong bonding within that community. Small, tightly bonded social circles called *moai* allow for everyone to have strong social support while lowering mental stressors and encouraging healthy behaviors. As a result, Okinawans have the longest-living women in the world, with many living to be over 100. Another Blue Zone is Sardinia, Italy, which has the highest concentration of male centenarians in the world. One of the main contributing factors is closeness with family. Men with daughters tend to live even longer than average within Sardinia due to the care they tend to receive from their daughters as they age. Finally, there's Loma Linda, California, the only Blue Zone in the United States. Loma Linda has a large Seventh-day Adventist population, and members of this group attribute their longevity in part to having a strong, shared set of values that emphasize community. They also maintain a Sabbath, or a day of rest, during which many people spend time bonding with each other.

More evidence along these lines can be found in Harvard University's Study of Adult Development. For more than 80 years, this study has followed the lives of 268 former Harvard students, a group that included John F. Kennedy at one time. You can imagine how much data researchers can collect across eight decades! So what did they find? Close relationships and community are what keep people the happiest and healthiest throughout their lives. The study's former director, George Vaillant, once summarized the research this way: "The seventy-five years and twenty million dollars expended on the [Study of Adult Development] points ... to a straightforward five-word conclusion: 'Happiness is love. Full stop.'"

Much of the modern world has been plagued by a terrible disease called loneliness, which is unfortunately on the rise. It's common to feel lonely in a new city or workplace, in the absence of a close confidant, or even when you feel different than those around you. It's normal to feel lonely once in a while, but feelings of persistent loneliness are unfortunately increasing in society today. Sociologist Lynn Smith-Lovin found that one in 10 people reported having 0 close friendships. Another study at Brigham Young University looked at the close link between loneliness and mortality. Researchers found that feeling lonely increased a person's risk of dying early by 26%. It turns out being lonely is even worse for the body than air pollution and obesity.

What is the antidote to loneliness? Not superficial conversation, not likes on social media, but genuine connection with others. When we're around other people we trust and feel comfortable with, we experience a sense of safety and security. I've seen this extensively with members of the military and veteran communities. Military teams get so close they often feel safer in a war zone amongst their peers whom they trust implicitly than they do when they return home to a suburban neighborhood, where they're statistically much safer but lack the strength of their community.

It's important to remember that there is a difference between being lonely and being alone. A person living alone might not feel lonely due to the quality of their friendships, whereas a person surrounded by people all day could still feel lonely because those relationships lack connection. Loneliness comes from feeling isolated and alienated. People who are lonely often lack social support, which is one of the most important safety networks any human can have. Social support can look different for each person, but what's important is that it makes you feel connected, meaning you feel truly heard and seen by others.

Humans are literally wired for connection. Research on babies shows that they need touch for cognitive development. Even more, all humans have mirror neurons that mimic the emotions and behavior we see in people we're interacting with. The truth is, we learn how to be human from other humans. That's why our friendships and other relationships are central to our ability to thrive as humans and to be resilient. One study even found that in our later years, having a strong friend group better predicted a person's well-being than having a strong family did. So how do we connect in a world that can sometimes seem so disconnected? It starts with trust. It is no question that trust is a complicated topic, and we'll dive deep into it during our class on safety, but in the most simple terms, trust happens when you feel that a person genuinely cares about your well-being. And when people feel mutual concern for each other's well-being, that creates true friendship.

This doesn't mean that you have to be a social butterfly. Having four to five close friends is more effective than having lots of casual friends. The most important factors in a friendship include trust, dependability, and genuine enjoyment in your friend's company. Think about the people you consider to be your friends and pay attention to any similarities you share with them. You might have similar lifestyles, interests, character traits, values, or some other connection that encourages feelings of trust and serves as the foundation of your friendship. Now think about the people you don't consider to be your friends. Do you notice differences in their lifestyles, values, or some other factor that causes you to view these people as different?

When we consider people to be different than us, we tend to see them as a threat. Brain research even suggests that our ability to be empathetic with someone doesn't turn on if we view that person as being an outsider or not part of our group. Think about that for a second. Think about the implications of this in terms of gender, politics, race, and religion. Psychiatrist Bessel van der Kolk goes further to explain the implications of this in-group bias in his book *The Body Keeps the Score*, saying, "Isolating oneself into a narrowly defined … group promotes a view of others as irrelevant at best and dangerous at worst, which eventually only leads to further alienation."

Ultimately, much of our ability to connect comes down to our belief systems and attitude. If we judge or reject those who are different, those people will shut down, and we find ourselves ultimately feeling more separate and isolated. If we truly want to rid our society of loneliness, we have to open ourselves up to genuinely connecting with others. The more compassionate we are of others, the easier it is to connect, and the happier and the more resilient we are. We also don't have to wait for others to take this first leap. By greeting people with kindness and genuine concern for their well-being, we build our own compassion muscles. Plus, people met with kindness tend to feel safe opening up in time, too. This is a phenomenon that Archbishop Desmond Tutu captures perfectly in *The Book of Joy*, a beautiful book that shares wisdom from both Tutu and the Dalai Lama. Tutu puts it this way: "We are wired to be caring for the other and generous to one another. We shrivel when we are not able to interact … We depend on the other in order for us to be fully who we are." This speaks to the heart of community and connection.

It is also possible, and sometimes even easier, to form meaningful connections with animals, especially mammals. Horses and dogs are commonly used in trauma treatment to help clients develop a sense of connection and safety. Service animals, support animals, and pets can also be dependable friends. Community group practices like group chanting, breathing, singing, and dancing are also extremely effective at fostering connection with others, in part due to their ability to regulate our bodily states and process experiences. These practices are less common in the West, but they're seen quite prominently in other traditions and cultures.

So let's talk about community and the power it has in cultivating genuine connection with others. There's a concept that comes out of southern Africa called *ubuntu* that beautifully describes the idea of community. *Ubuntu* means, "A person is a person through other persons." In other words, we were designed to have community and to be a part of that community. It is interesting to look at how people relate in the world around us. Most people today live increasingly isolated lives. Research suggests that people living in rural areas tend to have a stronger sense of community than those of us living in urban or suburban areas, and that families in these rural areas often feel more able to ask for help and more supported once they do. It's amazing that a person living in New York City could live surrounded by people, passing through crowded subways, and yet never feel connected to anyone, whereas an African tribe could literally have their lives depend upon each other while living nomadic lives in the middle of the Sahara Desert. Most people live somewhere in between.

So what can you do to cultivate your own sense of community? You can start by nourishing the important relationships you do have. Reconnect with an old friend and devote the time and space to really listen to what they have to say. If you're looking to expand your community, see if you can create opportunities to spend time with people who share a mutual interest, such as joining an exercise group, volunteering on a political campaign, going to dog parks, starting a book club, and so on. Shared interests are an easy way to find genuine connection with people. Remember that what you put into your relationships and community is what you'll get out of it. Many people complain they don't have community, but at the same time, they haven't done much to create or nourish their community. It's also important to pay attention to what you choose to do with your community. Does getting together always mean drinking together, or can you connect over other interests? It is said that we become the five people we spend the most time with, so it helps to be mindful of what it is that you and your community spend your time doing.

Studies on disaster response from across the globe have found that nothing protects against the stress and trauma that comes with disaster more than the support of others. And sometimes it seems to take a huge disaster for people to come together and support one another. Who here has ever rushed to make a donation to a group of people in crisis after a disaster—to a group of people we don't know, and who are often of a different race, religion, and on the other side of the world? I know that I have, and I'm sure that many of you have too. When this happens, we are relating to people on a human level, with no focus at all on differences. One human community.

Of course, we've all had feelings that run against community too. Feelings that break the bonds between ourselves and others. So what can we do if we find ourselves struggling with feelings of envy, judgment, or anger towards others? The Dalai Lama and Desmond Tutu suggest three things. First, we can make it a point to express gratitude, reminding ourselves that we're blessed to have what we do have. Second, we can employ the strategy of reframing, or asking yourself, "Why do I feel like I need this extra thing in the first place?" And third, we can challenge ourselves to broaden our perspective. Every situation is co-created; seeing how we have contributed to the situations that make us mad can often reduce those feelings of anger, as can recognizing the other person as just another human with their own pain, problems, and fear. Everyone struggles, and in a way, we're all united by this.

Remember, the purpose of community is not defined by sheer numbers, it is defined by the quality of connection. There is a powerful and practical tool that we can use to strengthen our relationship and connection with others called dyadic meditation, or co-meditation. Co-meditation is a great way to practice deep listening and being truly present with the people in our lives. So much of our time interacting with others is superficial or sometimes even self-focused. How often during conversations do you find yourself not really listening or not being listened to? How often do you find yourself focusing on what you're going to say next rather than on what the other person is saying? Being fully present, meaning we're not ruminating on the past or worrying about the future, is a key to genuine connection. Even the science supports the healing powers of being fully present. In 1994, Stephen Porges developed the polyvagal theory, which highlights the importance of social relationships in our ability to heal from trauma. The theory explains the connection between our experiences with others and our visceral reaction to those experiences. Experiences with others can include things like eye contact, voice modulation, and touch. According to the polyvagal theory, focused attunement with someone, like we create through co-meditation, can help us calm our body, emotions, and mind.

Co-meditation is a partner practice that is easy to do and takes a surprisingly short amount of time to bring you fully into the present moment. Once you've found someone to try this with, decide who's going to start as the giver of the undivided attention, and who will be the receiver of undivided attention. You'll switch halfway through so each person will have the opportunity to practice both supporting someone and being supported. Now here's the only real instruction: Sit across from each other, and see what happens! You can sit there until each person's turn reaches its natural end, or you may want to set a timer, perhaps 15 and 30 minutes per person, so that you're not getting distracted by trying to keep track of time during the meditation. Some people prefer to go back and forth multiple times at shorter intervals, similar to what we did in another class in terms of using a two- or five-minute timeframe, rather than each person taking a prolonged turn. Choose whatever feels right for you.

Once you are sitting across from each other, let the receiver of undivided attention lead the way. He or she might want to sit there in silence with eyes opened or closed, or it could be used as an opportunity for the recipient to take a look at and share what is going on in their inner world. If the recipient would like to spend their time diving into self-inquiry, the person giving attention can start by asking the recipient to let attention wander throughout their body to see if there are any feelings, emotions, or beliefs that are calling their attention. Allow your partner to verbally and nonverbally explore what comes to the surface. Throughout the experience, the person giving attention can ask the recipient the following three questions: What do you notice? Where in your body do you feel this? And can you say anything else about that? These questions can be asked as many times as necessary until the person receiving attention feels as though they've processed whatever has come up. The listener can also take notes on what the person sharing has to say. These notes can be a powerful tool for self-reflection after the meditation is over. At the end, ask the recipient if there are any takeaways, or if there is anything he or she needs to feel complete in that moment.

We benefit not only from having community but from giving back to our communities as well. A study on 750 former prisoners of war found incredible resilience among these veterans. Once they were released from imprisonment, they avoided developing depression and PTSD—two diagnoses that are very common among veterans. Results from the study on this remarkable group of humans showed that one of the most important characteristics that set them apart and resulted in their impressive resilience was altruism. Giving back through money and time obviously benefits the recipients of help, but numerous studies like the one I just mentioned also show significant benefits for the giver. According to Aristotle, each of us in life strives to achieve eudaimonia, which can be translated as a state of happiness or flourishing. Not all of us follow the right path to attain this desirable state, however. In fact, according to Aristotle, eudaimonia is only truly achieved when we actively fulfill our moral duties. Just ask anyone who devotes their life to giving back to others, and you'll likely find that many of them would agree with Aristotle.

According to neuroscientist Richard Davidson, the brain has four circuits that impact our sense of well-being: one for maintaining positive states, one for bouncing back from negative states, one for attention focusing, and one entirely devoted to generosity. Studies have shown that as we spend more money on others, we experience more happiness. This has been found to be the case both cross-sectionally and over the course of our lifetimes. Functional MRI scans show that giving money to charity activates brain regions associated with pleasure and reward, like the ventral striatum. In a 2007 study at the University of Oregon, participants were given $100 and were told they could keep it, give it to a food bank, or divide the sum of money in any way between the food bank and themselves. So what do you think the study found about those who donated the entire sum to the food bank? You guessed it: They had activation in their ventral striatum. In another study on prosocial behavior and happiness, it was found that, not surprisingly, prosocial spending increased feelings of happiness, whereas personal spending had no correlation to happiness, even when controlling for income. The research isn't only limited to the effects of giving money, either. Research also shows that volunteering our time results in improved happiness as well. Some research even suggests that volunteering reduces our likelihood of developing depression, improves our physical health as we age, reduces our cognitive decline as we age, and lowers our likelihood of early mortality.

People can be both intrinsically and extrinsically motivated. Extrinsic motivation involves something from the outside influencing our behavior—working to earn money, attending a lecture to get free food, or studying to avoid failing a test. Intrinsic motivation comes from within. It's doing something because it is personally rewarding. Guess which type of motivation leads to higher life satisfaction. That's right: intrinsic. And studies show that volunteers typically choose to give back due to intrinsic motivation, as opposed to extrinsic. We've all probably at some point or another experienced the warm glow that comes from helping a good cause or another person or even an animal. Watching others' welfare improve as a result of our efforts is inherently motivating. But watch what happens to that warm glow the moment that the purpose of giving back shifts to an extrinsic motivation, like building your network or gaining social approval. It might disappear, feel more like an ego boost, or evolve into other emotions. Research shows that people who value their intrinsic life goals derive more benefit and satisfaction from volunteering than people who are more focused on their extrinsic goals, like social standing or career status.

Now I want to shine a limelight on two friends of mine who've dedicated themselves to giving back and highlight how this has impacted their own resilience. Nikki McKean is a photographer, restaurant owner, and iRest Yoga Nidra teacher. She's also a wife and a mother of two young girls. Nikki is also living through her second cancer diagnosis and round of radiation treatment in two years. Talk about resilience. Nikki thanks cancer for helping her build a new community and giving her family even more quality time together, but she didn't stop there. In the two-week period between her diagnosis and the beginning of her second radiation treatment, Nikki created her Let's Radiate project, which is a card set that provides both daily inspiration and activities that connect you with yourself and others in your community. Prior to creating her project, Nikki said this: "Unimaginably beautiful things are happening every day, even in the chaos—the question is, what am I doing to contribute to that? How do I get through this and help teach others it's possible to heal through light and love in dark days?" It's an absolute inspiration to see how Nikki has come alive through an experience that may have otherwise left her feeling sick or broken. Instead, her experiences made her even stronger and more resilient. Nikki's experience is a beautiful example for us all to explore what happens when we welcome our experiences and use them to create genuine connection with others. If you're inspired and want to learn more about Nikki and the Let's Radiate project, you can visit www.feelthat.ca. The proceeds of the card deck are being donated to charity.

Another friend of mine who has devoted her life to giving back is Stacey Antine. Stacey is a registered dietician who epitomizes giving back. First, Stacey founded HealthBarn USA in 2005 as a way to combat obesity, heart disease, and diabetes in children. HealthBarn USA gives children the chance to grow their own food, learn how to cook, and understand the effect their food has on their bodies. Stacey has made her life's work giving back to society by normalizing healthy eating in children. She didn't stop at HealthBarn; she also founded Healing Meals, which is a nutritious food-gifting program. Through Healing Meals, nutritious food is provided at no cost to children receiving cancer treatment and seniors in need. Chefs, students, and other community members donate their time to create and prepare the food.

Stacey often shares how she used to walk past homeless people every day and drive past senior living facilities where the residents were malnourished and a children's hospital where children were trying to heal on over-processed hospital food. Meanwhile, she was eating a super healthy and organic diet. One day, she had the revelation that she could not feel fully nourished if the people who lived around her were going hungry. The realization propelled her into creating Healing Meals and provided the inspiration that got her community involved with the project. Stacey's work embodies the art of giving back and really the importance and benefit of community as a whole. Food is a powerful tool for creating connection—everyone eats! And the more we're connected, the happier and more resilient we are.

The Dalai Lama sums up the power of community, and I'm going to end today with some of his inspirational words:

If I relate to others from the perspective of myself as someone different—a Buddhist, a Tibetan, and so on—I will then create walls to keep me apart from others. And if I relate to others, thinking that I am the Dalai Lama, I will create the basis for my own separation and loneliness. After all, there is only one Dalai Lama in the entire world. In contrast, if I see myself primarily in terms of myself as a fellow human, I will then have seven billion people who I can feel deep connection with. And this is wonderful, isn't it? What do you need to fear or worry about when you have seven billion other people who are with you?

Thank you.

Class 15

Finding Safety

Safety is central to your ability to be resilient. Feeling unsafe keeps the brain in survival mode, but feeling safe promotes feelings of security, equanimity, and calm. This class explores the very fundamental need of safety. It starts by looking at childhood to see how a person's earliest experiences influence how safe the person feels in this world. Then, the class provides some internal and external strategies for promoting feelings of safety. The class ends by exploring the connection between safety and trust.

Attachment Theory

- A person's sense of safety and trust depends largely on circumstances and life experiences, especially those from the formative years of development. Attachment theory, developed by John Bowlby and Mary Ainsworth, delves into the importance of a person's earliest relationships.

- According to attachment theory, everyone has an attachment style, which describes how a person relates to others, especially how one responds when feeling hurt or threatened. This attachment style goes all the way back to experiences in childhood.

- Children form an attachment to adults out of a need for safety and protection. The way in which that need is met or not met affects people throughout their lives. A person's attachment style depends on the quality of the relationship the person had with his or her primary caregivers as a child. It can also be affected by trauma and other significant interpersonal events.

- Broadly speaking, attachment styles fall into two categories: secure and insecure. A secure attachment style occurs when parents are aware of their child's needs and consistently attend to these needs. In a secure attachment, a child seeks out his or her caregiver during times of distress, and the caregiver lovingly responds to the child's needs.

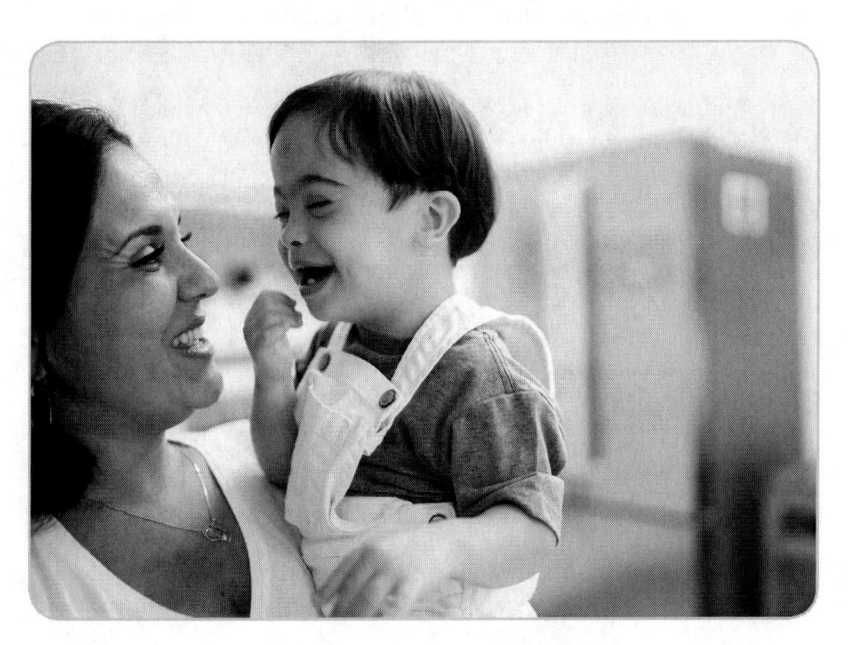

- Secure children generally feel safe and have trust in themselves and in the world. As a result, they begin to form attitudes and habits that can support resilience in later life. Secure children develop the ability to cope with stress, relate with others in a healthy way, and have a solid sense of self.

- An insecure attachment style occurs when caregivers are not physically or emotionally responsive to their child's needs. There are three main types of insecure attachment. One is characterized by ambivalent feelings toward caregivers. The second is characterized by dismissive feelings toward caregivers.

- The third is disorganized attachment, which is when parents essentially pass their own trauma to their children through fear tactics, causing children to feel afraid of the same person they seek safety from. Insecure attachment can cause children to have difficulty regulating their emotions, to see the world as being unsafe, to lack trust in people, to have low self-worth, and to believe that people—including themselves—aren't capable of meeting their needs.

- As you reflect on your own childhood experiences, you may find that they line up with an insecure attachment style. Luckily, change is possible. Positive relationships with other figures like mentors, friends, family members, and therapists can help change insecure attachment into more secure attachment. You can also learn important techniques to feel safe inside of yourself and to cultivate a sense of healthy, safe attachment with others.

Creating an Inner Resource

- Creating an inner resource is one technique for making an internal sense of well-being. Your inner resource is a haven of inner peace, safety, stillness, and serenity.

- Everyone has their own unique inner resource: It is already hardwired into your central nervous system, waiting to be called so that it can offer you feelings of ease and serenity. Your inner resource helps you combat negative experiences by allowing you to remember the unchanging wholeness and security that exists inside of you, no matter what is going on in your outside world.

- To find your inner resource, think back to a real or imaginary place or situation that evokes a feeling of well-being. It could be a home, a room, a place in nature, the night sky, or anything else that gives you feelings of ease and security. It might include loved ones, pets, a spiritual figure you connect with, or objects, such as a favorite stuffed animal. Some people prefer an imaginary inner resource, such as floating on a cloud.

- You can use the imagery and sensorial experiences to evoke an internal sense of well-being. As you continue to cultivate this internal sense of safety and well-being, you may not need the imagery any longer and can simply just drop back into an internal feeling of safety and security.

- You can return to your inner resource at any time, day or night. When you bring to mind your inner resource frequently—during both hard and good times—you'll be reminded that it is always there to support you.

The Spiral Technique

- Some types of mental health treatment use concepts similar to an inner resource, such as the safe place used in EMDR therapy. EMDR, or eye movement desensitization and reprocessing, is a form of psychotherapy that helps the body heal from unprocessed trauma. Another technique used in EMDR is the spiral technique, which is a way you can work with uncomfortable emotions.

- For this technique, start by bringing to mind an image that represents the uncomfortable emotion for you. As you do this, notice where in your body you have feelings of discomfort. Then take that feeling and pretend it is a spiral of energy, spinning in one direction or another. Is the spiral spinning clockwise or counter-clockwise? Depending on what you answer, gently try to change the direction that the energy is spinning in your body.

- While all techniques work better for some people than they do for others, those who find this technique successful will say that the uncomfortable emotions start to disappear when they make their spiral start to spin in the opposite direction. Similar to the inner resource, this tool can be used to bring you back to feelings of safety and calm.

Protective Factors

- Every person has risk factors and protective factors that affect their ability to bounce back from adversity. Naturally, risk factors are correlated with negative outcomes, and protective factors are correlated with more positive outcomes. Some examples of risk factors are child abuse and neglect, poverty, neighborhood violence, parents who use substances or who have mental health issues, and limited economic opportunities.

- Conversely, you can increase the number of protective factors in your life to increase your sense of safety. Think about what gives you a sense of protection and safety, and consider how you can build up these factors. It can be helpful to make a list and then create a timeline for when and how you are going to increase these protective factors in your life.

Prevention Strategies

- Another way to promote safety is through the use of prevention strategies. Prevention strategies involve setting yourself up for success. It can be easy to think of prevention strategies that help with physical safety—regular car maintenance, using seat belts, and so on—but prevention strategies can be used to support your sense of emotional and interpersonal safety, too.

- Using your inner resource is an example of an emotional prevention strategy. When you use your inner resource after noticing the first signs of a trigger, you are preventing a larger emotional reaction by calming yourself and focusing on your inner resource.

- Boundary setting is another prevention strategy. If you struggle with asserting or sticking up for yourself, it can be helpful to enter situations with a plan for how you will respond if someone tries to cross your boundary. In order to do this, you'll have to establish what your boundary is ahead of time, too.

- One method is to establish a plan to make sure you're not left alone with someone who scares you. Another tactic is to think ahead of time about what you'll say and do if someone treats you disrespectfully.

Safety and Trust

- Trust is the foundation of your ability to feel safe. When you feel safe, you feel protected from harm, meaning you trust the people and things that are there to protect you.

- Understanding how you trust—in other words, understanding what it is that causes you to give trust and to whom—is key to promoting personal safety and resilience. When you are aware of your own trust patterns, it becomes easier to capitalize on what works and change what is holding you back, allowing you to navigate relationships and evaluate your feelings of safety with more ease.

- To understand your own trust patterns, think of a person that you trust or don't trust. Ask yourself questions to dig into why it is that you do or don't trust them. Examples of such questions include:

    1. Do you trust their dependability?

    2. Do you trust their physical, emotional, and intellectual capability?

3. Is their behavior consistent?

4. Do they have and live by a moral code, even when times get hard?

5. Do they have genuine care for your well-being, or does their interaction with you seem to be self-serving or transactional in nature?

6. Do they try to understand you, or do they judge you and impose their own beliefs on you?

- Run through this list of questions a few times, each time with a different person in mind. See if you can notice patterns for when you do or don't tend to trust someone in the various circumstances of your life. Think about the role that these patterns play in your life, especially in terms of your own personal resilience.

Trusting Yourself

- Trusting yourself is an important part of your ability to be resilient. You might feel entirely safe and secure one moment, only to be hit by a natural or personal disaster that eradicates those feelings of safety. The only thing you truly have full control over is yourself, which makes trusting in yourself paramount.

- The best way to do this is to practice having consistent feelings of safety and trust in yourself and in your purpose. It can be helpful to evaluate how much you trust yourself, which can also give you clues as to how trustworthy you appear to others, too.

- To conduct that self-evaluation, here are a few questions that may be helpful:

    1. Am I dependable?

    2. Do I have and live by a moral code, even when times get hard?

3. Do I understand myself, or do I judge myself and hide who I really am?

4. Do I genuinely care about my well-being?

5. Do I trust in my ability to keep working toward my higher goal and purpose?

- If your answer to any of these questions is no, try not to worry. You may have just unearthed something that will ultimately help you boost your sense of trust in yourself and your resilience.

- If you feel comfortable doing so, do some self-investigation into what lies beneath your lack of self-trust, looking for where it comes from, what contributes to it, and what you can do to develop self-trust. Support is paramount to safety, so if the thought of this self-investigation is overwhelming, think about reaching out to a mental health professional who can help support you through the process.

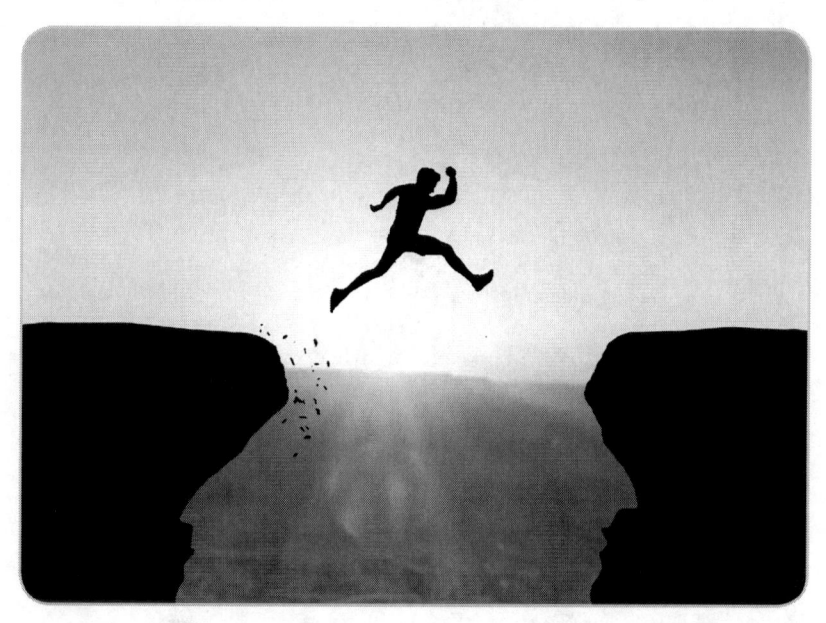

- Another way of measuring how much you trust yourself is to keep a record of the lies you tell. Lies distance a person from living a complete, peaceful, authentic life. People typically lie when and where they feel the most vulnerable. You can learn a lot about yourself by becoming conscious of the times you lie.

- To do this, use a small journal or your phone, and start to write down every time that you lie. Look through your list and ask yourself why you told each lie. See the places where you're going away from the truth. See what patterns emerge. This activity acts as a mirror that reflects the places where you're suffering in life. The ultimate goal is to make the person in the mirror look the same as the person you see inside.

- Feeling safe with yourself creates a healthy place for you to reside. It also creates the opportunity for others to feel safer with you. When you're able to be authentic—speaking your truth rather than living behind a façade—you liberate others to be authentic with you, too.

Suggested Reading

Miller, *The iRest Program for Healing PTSD*.

Activities

- Establish an inner resource.

- Answer the following:

    » What type of attachment style do you think you have? How does this manifest throughout your life?

    » What are your protective factors?

    » What does trust mean to you?

- Think or write down the name(s) of at least one person you can count on for support. If you are unable to do this, consider establishing a relationship with a professional for support.

- Complete Practice Class 7 (Class 23), titled "Finding Safety with Yoga Nidra."

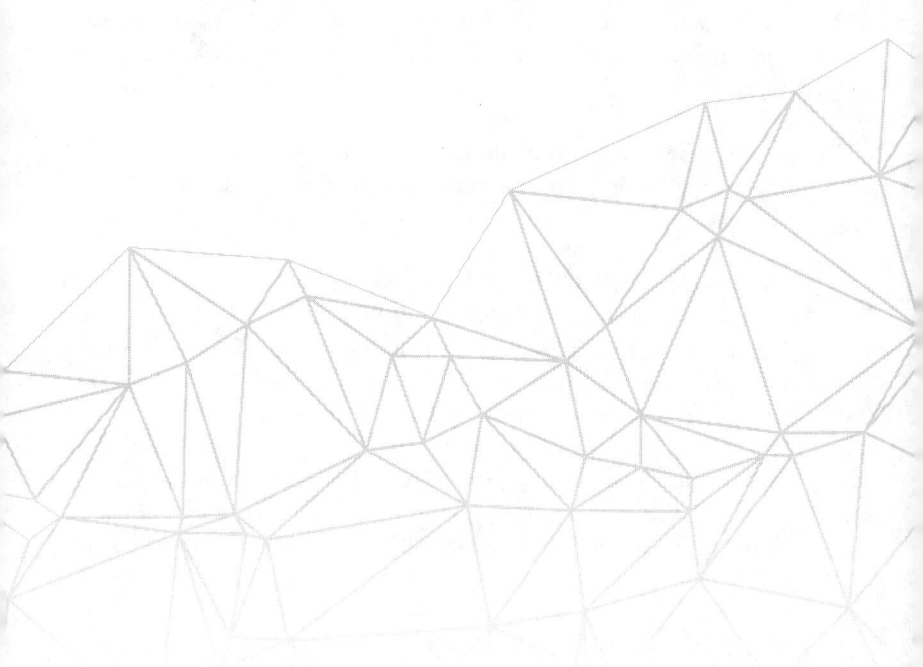

Class 15 Transcript

Finding Safety

One of my favorite jobs is when I go to do resilience training for the Special Operations troops in the US Military. While I go to teach them about how yoga, breathing, Yoga Nidra, and meditation can make them more resilient, I always learn so much from them about what makes them hold up under some of the most stressful conditions anyone could ever face. Everything they do revolves around safety in one form or another, from endless rounds of physical and mental training to the careful creation of a close-knit community. You will rarely find people more deeply connected than a team that has gone to war together. Why? Because their safety—their lives—depend upon each other. They do one of the most dangerous jobs on this earth, and if they're going to survive and accomplish their missions, they have to maximize their safety.

I asked a Marine who has been deployed a double-digit number of times to share with me his insights into the role safety plays in resilience. It's interesting because his answer reflects many of the points we're going to talk about today:

> Bet you didn't think you'd hear a Marine say this, but safety starts in here [he says, pointing to his heart]. You've got to feel safe inside. You've got to know why you're doing something. You've got to really believe in it and you've got to really believe in the people you're doing it with; otherwise you will not feel safe. Safety is something you carry around inside. It's an inside job.
>
> Safety is also about knowing how to chill and process. After an op, you've got to have a way to deal with what's going on between your ears. It can't just be drinking your old friend Jack from the bottle or something like that. That's where

meditation and Yoga Nidra kick in. Getting out for a hike can help. Talking to [someone]. It's better to deal with it. Otherwise it builds. Then you break.

Over the years, I've seen that man grow more and more resilient, wise, and thoughtful the more missions he does. He has one of the least safe jobs on the planet, but he continues to rise. It's not that he doesn't have challenges as a result of his wartime experiences because he readily admits that he does. The difference is that he knows how to deal with it. He is living proof that resilience is possible and that safety is a huge part of it.

So how does this apply to our lives? His response reveals several aspects we will discuss both in this class and throughout the course. Safety is central to our ability to be resilient. When we feel unsafe, our brains are stuck in survival mode, or the sympathetic nervous system response, and we have very little access to our higher cognitive functioning. Feeling stuck in this survival mode prevents us from being able to move forward. When we feel safe, by contrast, we experience a sense of security, equanimity, and calm. We can respond rather than react to what life throws our way. Instead of focusing on what could go wrong, we focus on what could go right, opening us up to options that make it possible for us to work towards and reach our goals.

The importance of safety is demonstrated in many psychological theories, such as in Maslow's hierarchy of needs, where safety is considered to be one of the most fundamental needs we have as humans. In today's class, we're going to thoroughly explore this very fundamental need. We'll start by going all the way back to childhood to see how our earliest experiences influence how safe we feel in this world. Then we're going to look at some internal and external strategies for promoting feelings of safety. We will end this class by exploring the connection between safety and trust and analyzing what it actually means when we say we trust someone.

Feeling safe means we feel protected from danger or harm physically, emotionally, and mentally. And feeling protected from danger or harm requires having trust in the people and systems in our lives. Our sense of safety and trust depends largely on our circumstances and life experiences, especially those from our formative years of development. In fact, there is a whole theory on the importance of our earliest relationships and the impact that these relationships have on us for the rest of our lives. This theory is called attachment theory, which was developed by John Bowlby and Mary Ainsworth from the mid- to late 1900s.

According to attachment theory, everyone has an attachment style, which describes how we tend to relate to one another, specifically how we respond when we feel hurt or threatened. And this attachment style goes all the way back to our experiences in childhood. Children form an attachment to adults out of a need for safety and protection. The way in which that need is met or not affects us throughout our lives. Our attachment style depends on the quality of the relationship we had with our primary caregivers as children. It can also be affected by our traumas and other significant interpersonal events we experience in our lives. Our earliest interactions with our parents and caregivers set the groundwork for our belief system, which includes our thoughts, emotions, and expectations about ourselves and the world around us. Our attachment style is deeply embedded in that belief system.

Receiving love from our caregivers is how we learn to see our own value and how to give love to others. People who learned early to attach with others have an easier time connecting with people in all sorts of contexts. Of course, it is also possible to form healthy attachments even if we did not grow up in the most ideally loving household, but it's important to acknowledge when and how it didn't occur. There are lots of reasons why caregivers might be unable to bond with their children. Perhaps it's due to their past relationships with their own caregivers, or maybe they've experienced trauma in their lives. Unfortunately, the lack of consistent, quality connection between parents and children can have long-term repercussions. Often those children will grow into adults who feel not wanted, not worthy of love, untrusting of the world, and as though something is wrong with them.

Broadly speaking, attachment styles fall into two categories: secure and insecure. A secure attachment style occurs when parents are aware of their child's needs and consistently attend to these needs. In a secure attachment, a child seeks out his or her caregiver during times of distress, and the caregiver lovingly responds to the child's needs. Secure children generally feel safe and have trust in themselves and in the world. As a result, they begin to form attitudes and habits that can support resilience in later life. Secure children develop the ability to cope with stress, relate with others in a healthy way, and have a solid sense of self.

An insecure attachment style occurs when caregivers are not physically or emotionally responsive to their child's needs. There are three main types of insecure attachment. One is characterized by ambivalent feelings towards caregivers. One is characterized by dismissive feelings towards caregivers and disorganized attachment, which is when parents essentially pass their own trauma to their children through fear tactics, causing children to feel afraid of the same person they seek safety from. Insecure attachment can cause children to have difficulty regulating their emotions, to see the world as being unsafe, to lack trust in people, and to have a low sense of self-worth, as well as to believe that people, including themselves, aren't capable of meeting their needs.

Now as you reflect on your own childhood experiences, you may find that they line up with an insecure attachment style. Does that mean you're stuck? Not at all. Because luckily, change is possible! Positive relationships with other figures like mentors, friends, family members, and therapists can help change insecure attachment into more secure attachment. We can also learn important techniques to feel safe inside ourselves and to cultivate a sense of healthy safe attachment with others. We can't control our upbringing, but as adults, we can control what we choose to do with the life we've been given. So let's discuss some ways we can improve the feeling of safety in our lives and in turn improve our resilience.

We're going to start with one of my personal favorite techniques for creating an internal sense of well-being, and that's creating an inner resource. We will use this tool again when we do our Yoga Nidra practice and in some of the other practice sessions. Your inner resource is a haven of inner peace, safety, stillness, and serenity. Everyone has their own unique inner resource. It is already hardwired into your central nervous system, waiting to be called so that it can offer you feelings of ease and serenity. Your inner resource helps you combat negative experiences by allowing you to remember the unchanging wholeness and security that exists inside of you no matter what is going on in your outside world. While most of us are not living in immediate danger, we all have fears that can cause strong, uncomfortable, or sometimes even scary reactions in our body and mind. Everyone has their own triggers or perceptions that cause us to feel strong fear, sadness, or anger. When we become triggered, or we are about to become triggered, we can use our inner resource to bring us back to feelings of well-being. Your inner resource is a tool to help you regain control during challenges and recover more quickly once they've passed.

To find your inner resource, think back to a real or an imaginary place or situation that evokes a feeling of well-being. It could be a home, a room, a place in nature, the night sky, or anything else that gives you feelings of ease and security. It might include loved ones, pets, a spiritual figure you can connect with, or objects such as a favorite stuffed animal, a cherished item, or a picture. Some people prefer an imaginary inner resource, such as floating on a cloud. You can use the imagery and sensorial experiences to evoke an internal sense of well-being. As you continue to cultivate this internal sense of safety and well-being, you may not need the imagery any longer and can simply just drop back into an internal feeling of safety and security no matter what is happening around you. Personally, my inner resource is the feeling I have when I meditate. It feels like peace without an opposite, and nothing can feel more safe and secure to me than this.

You can return to your inner resource at any time, day or night. When you bring to mind your inner resource frequently—not only during hard times, but during good times, too—you'll be reminded that it is always there to support you. Over time, you won't have to call for it, and it will just naturally appear. It will do so on its own, providing an internal feeling of safety and security. It will hopefully start to arise naturally the moment you start to sense stress or tension so that you're held through your experience. Sometimes we say, "at first you remember your inner resource, and then your inner resource remembers you."

Some types of mental health treatment use concepts similar to an inner resource, such as the safe place used in EMDR therapy. EMDR, or eye movement desensitization and reprocessing, is a form of psychotherapy that helps the body heal from unprocessed trauma. And as we've learned, trauma and a perceived loss of safety go hand in hand. Another technique used in EMDR is called the spiral technique, which is another way we can work with uncomfortable emotions. For this technique, start by bringing to mind an image that represents the uncomfortable emotion for you. As you do this, notice where in your body you have feelings of discomfort. Then take that feeling and pretend it's a spiral of energy, spinning in one direction or another. Is the spiral spinning clockwise or counter-clockwise? Depending upon what you answer, gently try to change the direction of that energy and experience how it's spinning in your body. While all techniques work better for some people than they do for others, those who find this technique successful will say that uncomfortable emotions start to disappear when they make the spiral start to spin in the opposite direction. Similar to the inner resource, this tool can be used to bring you back to feelings of safety and calm.

Every person has risk factors and protective factors that affect their ability to bounce back from adversity. Naturally, risk factors are correlated with negative outcomes, and protective factors are correlated with more positive outcomes. Some examples of risk factors are child abuse and neglect, poverty, neighborhood violence, parents who use substances or who have mental health issues, and limited economic opportunities. The Adverse Childhood Experiences, or ACE, Study is a monumental research study conducted in the 1990s by the CDC and Kaiser Permanente. The ACE Study measured the effects of risk factors in childhood on over 17,000 study participants and found that for each adverse experience a child has, the child's risk of negative health and well-being outcomes increases. Not only that, but for each adverse experience the child has, the negative outcomes become increasingly more intense.

Risk factors imply a lack of safety in a person's life. Fortunately, the negative effects of risk factors can be mitigated by protective factors, which help to improve a person's sense of safety more quickly after enduring the trauma or stress caused by the risk factors. Some examples of protective factors are access to health care; stable housing; community support, such as social services or religious institutions; and stable, caring relationships with parents or other adults, such as teachers, even if that means having just one person in your life you can trust and count on. Knowing this, we can increase the number of protective factors we have in our life to increase our sense of safety. Think about what gives you a sense of protection and safety and consider how you can turn up the volume on these factors to help you feel more stable and secure in the areas of life where you feel the most fearful or tense. It can be helpful to make a list and then create a timeline for when and how you're going to increase these protective factors in your life.

Another way to promote safety is through the use of prevention strategies. Prevention strategies involve setting yourself up for success. It means preparing yourself ahead of time so that you can either prevent problems or be equipped to handle problems when they do arise. Did you ever ignore your mom's suggestion to bring a coat or an umbrella, only to find yourself shivering or soaked later in the day? It can be easy to think of prevention strategies that help with our physical safety—regular car maintenance, using seat belts, and so on—but prevention strategies can be used to support our sense of safety and emotional and interpersonal safety too. In fact, using your inner resource is an example of an emotional prevention strategy. When you use your inner resource after noticing the first sign of a trigger, you're preventing a larger emotional reaction by calming yourself and focusing on your inner resource, keeping you and potentially others safe.

Boundary-setting is another incredibly useful prevention strategy. When we struggle with asserting or sticking up for ourselves, it can be helpful to enter situations with a plan for how we will respond if someone tries to cross our boundary, and obviously in order to do this, you'll have to establish what your boundary is ahead of time too. This could be establishing a plan to make sure you're not left alone with someone who scares you or thinking ahead of time about what you'll say and do if someone treats you disrespectfully. It might be to walk away from the situation, to ignore an antagonizing comment rather than falling into a heated argument, or letting someone know you'll talk to them once they're able to talk to you with respect.

It is important to keep in mind that our sense of safety is relative. It is impossible to eliminate all risk. As mentioned in previous classes, ultimately, all we can really control is how we react to what happens that is out of our control. The goal of safety is not to eliminate all risk but to keep risk low and have as much control over it as possible. There is also a difference between feeling uncomfortable and feeling unsafe. When we feel unsafe, we feel like we're at risk of real harm. This often puts us in a fight-or-flight mode, which activates the older, more primitive parts of our brain, as opposed to our prefrontal cortex. When we don't feel safe, it's hard for us to focus on anything aside from what is causing us to feel unsafe, which makes learning near impossible. On the other hand, feeling uncomfortable occurs when we venture outside of our bubble but don't feel like we are at risk of real harm. Unlike feeling unsafe, feeling uncomfortable is oftentimes where we learn best. Even though it feels just that—uncomfortable—being outside of our comfort zone exposes us to new experiences and ideas that help us learn, grow, and improve our performance and creativity.

As I mentioned earlier, trust is the foundation of our ability to feel safe. When we feel safe, we feel protected from harm, meaning we trust the people and things that are there to protect us. We are constantly giving our trust to people and things, oftentimes without the conscious awareness that we're doing so. We trust that the chair we sit on won't collapse. We trust that the restaurant server we hand our credit card to won't keep our credit card information. We trust that our employer will pay us for the work we've done. When we don't trust someone or something, it is often the result of an experience in which we gave our trust and then were harmed anyway—something that happens to everyone over the course of a lifetime. Ultimately, we should trust people who deserve our trust and people who have earned it.

There are many components to trust. We confide in people when we trust they won't share what we've told them. We trust that our partner and friends understand our wants and needs. We trust that those closest to us will tell us the truth. On the whole, trusting someone means we believe they will act in our best interest and won't take advantage of us. But our interests change depending upon the circumstance or situation; the way we trust our husband or wife is most likely going to be different than the way we trust our dentist. Just as there are many different ways to define what it means for something to be in our best interest, there are many different ways we can decide who we trust.

Researchers and professionals have developed multiple ways to define the different ways we can trust someone. One study divides trust into three different categories: economy-based trust, information-based trust, and identification-based trust. Economy-based trust is trust that is connected to some sort of economic benefit and oftentimes exists out of fear of loss or punishment when that trust is violated. Economy-based trust largely determines our trust in systems and businesses. Information-based trust is trust based on the information we have about another person and their behavior. Are they predictable? Are they dependable? Do they live with integrity? Our answers to these questions often point to how well we trust someone. Identification-based trust is based on emotional bonds. We feel identification-based trust when someone genuinely cares for us and understands our needs.

Trust is not simple. It is dynamic, and our ability to trust changes throughout our friendships, relationships, and lives. How we trust or don't trust people is heavily affected by our life experiences, and we weigh different types of trust differently in different situations. We feel safe when the type of trust we value the most is met in any given situation. For example, you might not trust that a family member is always honest with you, but you know that when push comes to shove, you can depend on them if you need help, and that causes you to feel safe with them. Or on the other hand, you might trust a doctor's integrity but question their capability, which might cause you to feel unsafe in their care.

When our trust has been violated, it is natural for us to become skeptical. Our brains are programmed to detect danger and to use our experiences to help us evaluate what is dangerous and what's not, which helps us to ensure our survival. Sometimes, though, this mechanism can cause problems, such as when we become hyper-focused on looking for reasons why we can't trust someone. This can result in difficulties connecting with others, a tendency to push people away, and other interpersonal problems. As we discussed in the self-care class, everyone lies in some form or another. So does that mean that no one can be trusted? Of course not! Oftentimes the intent behind someone's behavior is more telling than the actual behavior itself. The truth is, we could not survive as a species without at least some reliance on each other, and reliance requires some form of trust.

Understanding how you trust, or in other words, understanding what it is that causes you to give trust and to whom, is key to promoting personal safety and resilience. When you are aware of your own trust patterns, it becomes easier to capitalize on what works and change what is holding you back, allowing you to navigate relationships and evaluate your feelings of safety with more ease. To understand your own trust patterns, think of a person you trust or don't trust, and ask yourself questions to dig into why it is that you do or don't trust them. Do you trust their dependability? Do you trust their physical, emotional, and intellectual capacity? Is their behavior consistent? Do they have and live by a moral code even when times get hard? Do they have genuine care for your well-being, or does their interaction with you seem to be self-serving or transactional in nature? Do they try to understand you, or do they judge you and impose their own beliefs on you? Run through this list of questions a few times, each time with a different person in mind. See if you can notice patterns for when you do or don't tend to trust someone in the various circumstances of your life. And think about the role that these patterns play in your life, especially in terms of your own personal resilience.

Our ability to trust others is one component of determining how safe we feel, but the ability to trust ourselves is just as important, if not more important, in determining our feelings of safety and our ability to be resilient. Change is constant. People disappoint us. We could feel entirely safe and secure one moment, only to be hit by a natural or personal disaster that eradicates those feelings of safety. As we've talked about multiple times, the only thing we truly have control over is ourselves, which makes having trust in ourselves paramount. To be resilient is to endure change, including changes in our perception of safety in our outside world. The best way to do this is to practice having consistent feelings of safety and trust in yourself and in your purpose. If we are able to maintain an internal sense of safety and trust in ourselves knowing we can always count on ourselves during hard times, this can act as a buffer when we encounter setbacks. Oftentimes, evaluating how well we trust ourselves gives us clues as to how trustworthy we appear to others too.

To conduct that self-evaluation, here are a few questions that may be helpful: Am I dependable? Do I have and live by a moral code, even when times get hard? Do I understand myself, or do I judge myself and hide who I really am? Do I genuinely care about my well-being? And perhaps most importantly in terms of resilience, do I trust in my ability to persist? Do I trust that no matter what, I can and will keep working towards my highest goals and purpose? If your answer to any of these questions is "no," first of all, try not to worry, because you may have just unearthed something that will ultimately help you boost your sense of trust in yourself and your resilience. If you feel comfortable doing so, do some self-investigation into what lies beneath your lack of self-trust. Where does it come from? What contributes to it? And what can you do to develop self-trust? As we've discussed, support is paramount to safety, so if the thought of this self-investigation is overwhelming, think about reaching out to a mental health professional who can support you through the process.

Feeling safe with yourself not only creates a healthy place for you to reside, it also creates the opportunity for others to feel safer with you. When you're able to be authentic, speaking your truth rather than living behind a façade, you liberate others to be authentic with you too. Honesty and vulnerability can be hard, but they're brave, and they open doors for you to live as your most authentic self. And when you're living authentically, you're living your truth. And when you're living your truth, you can trust that you're doing what is right for you. And when you trust that you're doing what is right for you, you're well prepared to manage and recover from life's challenges, even the biggest challenges you may never expect.

Thank you.

Class 16

Opening to Joy and Gratitude

Everyone wants to feel happy, but people often spend more time chasing it outside of themselves than they do cultivating and nourishing an internal experience of joy, peace, and happiness. True, authentic joy arises from a deep connection with who you truly are and how that truth expresses itself in the world. Moreover, joy is an essential part of resilience, so this class looks at ways you can open yourself up to experiencing joy.

Desmond Tutu on Joy

On the subject of joy, South African cleric and activist Desmond Tutu has this to say: "Joy is much bigger than happiness. While happiness is often seen as being dependent on external circumstances, joy is not. ... [As] we discover more joy, we can face suffering in a way that ennobles rather than embitters. We have hardship without becoming hard. We have heartbreak without being broken."

Perspective

- To find joy, perspective is essential. Typically, if a person has a narrow or small view on life, the person will descend into judgments, anger, and fear. A broader view helps one realize that while problems may be present, they are not the only things that are present.

- Part of broadening your perspective includes taking responsibility for your joy and peace, rather than depending upon it to come from outside of yourself. A willingness to participate in life is a form of taking responsibility for your experience. The power is in your hands to choose how you meet this life.

- Blaming other people or circumstances for one's misfortune is a sure sign that a person's perspective has grown too narrow. When blaming starts, people automatically put themselves in the role of the victim, and then everything brings them down because they feel like life is happening "to" them. It is a sign that they are trying to source joy outside of themselves.

- Sometimes the world may leave you feeling powerless and like life is shooting arrows at you. In some sense, you may externally be powerless, but you can affect your internal experience. When those arrows start to fly, you can shift your perspective from what is coming at you to an internal space of wholeness and then focus on what you are putting into the world. When you do this, you take your power back.

Experiencing Challenges

- Please keep in mind that experiencing authentic joy does not mean you override the challenges you are feeling. Experiencing joy doesn't mean forcing yourself into a false sense of optimism or positivity. Rather, you are setting yourself free to experience everything that is present. When resistance drops, joy arises.

- There is a huge sense of freedom and relief found in not trying to keep all of the difficult emotions and memories buried somewhere deep inside. When you feel connected to life and safe in yourself, it allows you to feel emotions like anger and fear without getting hijacked by them, because that deeper sense of well-being is also present. This is where the resilience resides.

Mindfulness and Joy

- This kind of connection can be cultivated through mindfulness practices, which recognize that authentic gratitude and joy contains all emotions, even sadness and anger. Authentic gratitude and joy honors and holds a person's full experience.

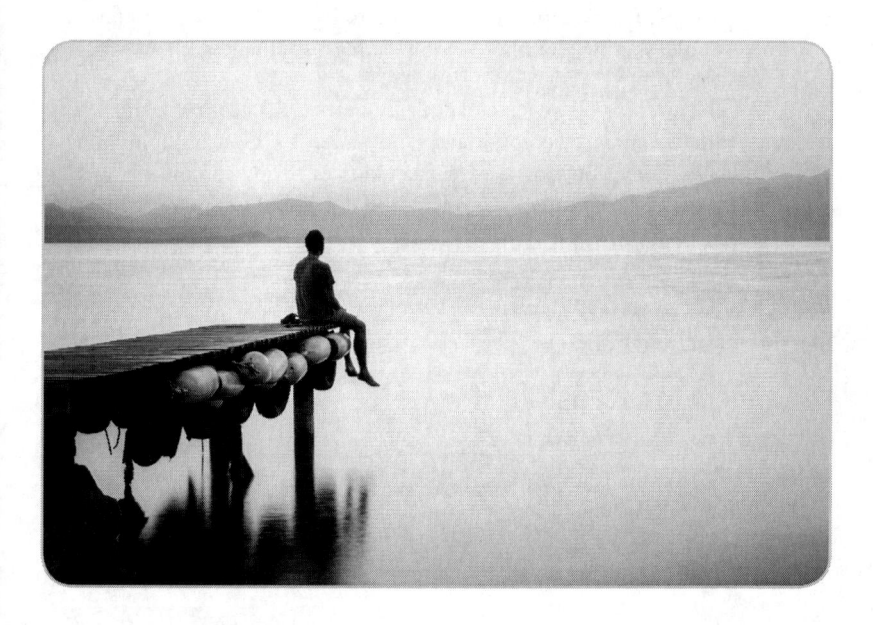

- When you think your life is only going to be happy, peaceful, or prosperous, you put yourself in a trap and place conditions on your well-being. Keep in mind that every moment brings the possibility of experiencing joy. Gratitude and welcoming open the door to this possibility.

- When people are caught in a storm of emotions, they often try to pull something closer or push something else away. This pulling and pushing actually takes people farther and farther away from the happiness that they seek. The reason for this is that true, lasting joy is not dependent upon anything outside of yourself. True joy is an internal experience.

- When there is a willingness to meet life and all of your emotions, there is joy in the midst of it. Cultivating traits like forgiveness, compassion, and generosity supports your ability to experience this unchanging, internal joy.

- Internal joy can arise through having deeper connection and gratitude, but you can also use external joy to help evoke a sense of internal joy. External joy is the type of joy that is evoked from things outside of yourself. For example, it is delightful to be together with your favorite people, sharing a meal or accomplishing a goal together.

- The problem with external joy is that if that source of joy goes away, the joy starts to go away, too. Even so, by using mindfulness techniques, you can use external sources of joy to connect with a deeper sense of internal joy. For a brief mindfulness practice, refer to the audio or video class.

Suggested Reading

Dalai Lama and Tutu, *The Book of Joy*.

Gilbert, *Stumbling on Happiness*.

Williams, *The Nature Fix: Why Nature Makes Us Happier*.

Activities

- Practice feeling gratitude simply for being alive. See what happens to feelings of joy.

- Set yourself free to experience everything that is present in your body and mind in this moment.

- Try to unlock joy through practicing forgiveness, compassion, or generosity. You might try writing a letter of forgiveness, practicing a loving-kindness meditation, or helping out a family member, friend, or stranger.

- Practice the guided meditation at the end of this class as much as you'd like.

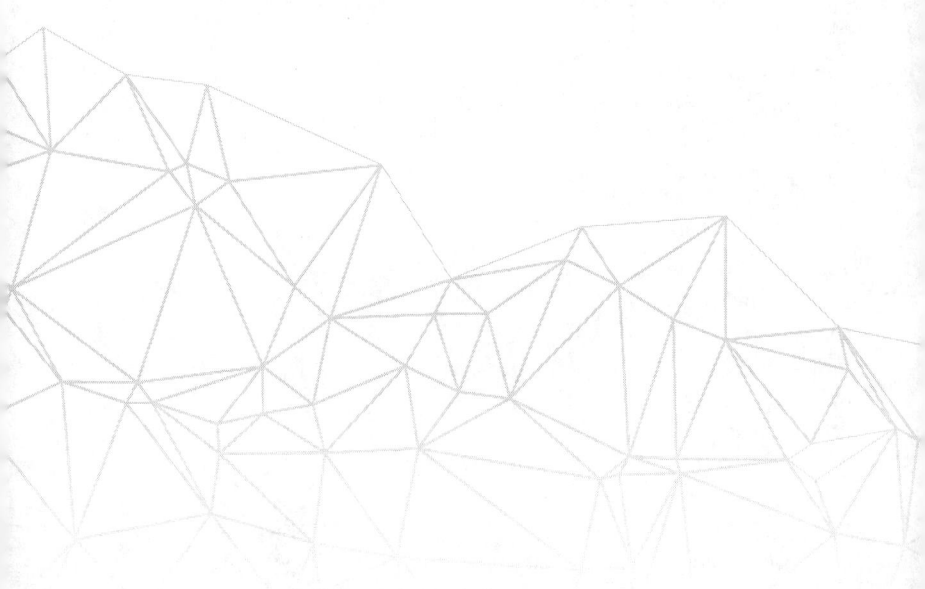

Class 16 Transcript

Opening to Joy and Gratitude

This may sound like a crazy thing to do, but I would like to start this class on joy and gratitude with a poem on sadness that I wrote during a very challenging moment of my life. Please trust me for a moment because by the end, I hope you will see why it relates to the true way that joy and gratitude arise to bring resilience to our lives.

You arrive like an unwelcome visitor.
Sometimes by storm, other times
by slow-building clouds
that finally
must
rain.

You pour down anger,
fear, grief, and frustration.
Intrusive.
Disrupting.
Leveling.

You have a cruel way of
showing me what I love
and value
most of all
by taking it away.
Or threatening to.

And that makes me want to hate you.
It makes me want to send you away
as
fast
as
possible.

That's the storyline we learn from birth:
"Don't cry, baby."
Then as we age, the grown-up version of this arises:
"Here is a tissue,"
or a hug,
or a drug,
or whatever you need to stop making you and everyone around you feel
so
damn
uncomfortable.

Numb it.
Hide it.
Make it go away fast,
because if you sit there being
so vulnerably sad,
you might make me feel the sadness
that I've worked
so desperately
to bury,
deep inside.

It is true, sadness.
You are the storm no one wants,
yet we all need.
Because when we numb you, sadness,
we also numb joy,
and love,

and connection,
and everything we want most in life.

Try as we might to avoid you,
we
do
also need you.

There is no poem without you.
No love song.
No epic story to be told.
No hero awakening.

You give life meaning.
Depth.
Purpose.

And if I really listen to you
with my whole heart,
I find,
in all your darkness
and haze,
the lessons I have to learn,
and the wisdom I can only learn by feeling
you.

So here I am,
standing in the rain.

All are welcome to join me.
You, survivors of trauma and tragedy.
You, with the broken heart.
You, who isn't even sure why you're hurting.
You are welcome here,

either by choice,
or in the moment when life doesn't give you a choice.

I stand with you because I've lived through this storm before and I know,
deep in my cells,
just as you do, that
it is only because of darkness that we know what light is.
It is only through this
wild
shattering
storm
that we find the part of ourselves untouched by any of it.

It is not in spite of you, sadness, that I know what joy is.
It is because of you.

Even in the moment
when the depths of sadness feel unbearable,
if I really listen,
if I really feel,
joy is here too.
Real joy.
Joy that doesn't need a reason.
Joy that arises as an expression of the peace
that exists,
at the center of my being,
untouched by
anything
that has ever happened in this life,
or anything that ever will.

It is you, sadness, that brings me into the power of this present moment.
So fully connected to this precious human life,
real and vulnerable,
full of love and pain.

Understanding what authentic humanity
really
is.

And that,
that makes me move a little.
That makes me put down the umbrella.
That makes me start to look up
from the ground
to see,
feel,
smell,
hear, and
taste
how beautiful the rain actually is
as it pours down on me.

You, sadness.
You make me feel alive.
Cold, yes.
And wet.
And afraid.
But here.

So fully here.

In this profound
welcoming
of what really is,
I find my freedom.

So really, sadness is the gatekeeper to uncaused joy. Living in a world free from personal struggles or global adversity is not where we will find our joy. We will not learn to be resilient by insulating ourselves or hiding out far from any challenges or ugliness we find in the world. I get this goes against everything that marketing campaigns tell us about thinking our way to a happier life or buying something that will instantly alleviate our pain. How is it possible to be authentically joyful in a world that is constantly challenging us and pushing us to our limits? Is it possible? I certainly hope so! And I sincerely believe it is possible. Every one of us innately wants to be joyful and happy. If you ask just about anyone what they want out of life, that almost always makes the list. Yet according to the 2017 Harris Poll Survey of American Happiness, just 33% of Americans say they're happy. That's right, only a third. Clearly there is something missing.

We all want to feel happy, but then we typically spend more time chasing it outside of ourselves than we do cultivating and nourishing an internal experience of joy, peace, and happiness. We discover authentic joy when we welcome life fully, especially all the parts of ourselves that were previously kept buried deep inside: our trauma, our shame, our hurt, our feelings of inadequacy. We find authentic joy through deep connection with ourselves, people, and the world around us. Joy arises when we connect completely with the places that previously felt cut off or disconnected. There is joy to be discovered around you everywhere, right now in this moment. It's floating around us constantly. The potential for joy is present in every interaction, every step, every bite, every moment of life. Not just in the quote-unquote happy moments of life but in the challenging moments too. True authentic joy arises from deep connection with who we truly are and how that truth expresses itself in the world.

Why is this important for resilience? Because joy is an essential part of resilience. You can even think of it as "Vitamin J keeping the doctor away." When we feel joyful, our whole perspective changes. Think about how much smaller all of your problems feel when you're really in a joyful state of mind. To get a better handle on this, let's listen to what Desmond Tutu says about the difference between joy and happiness. Tutu is a sincerely joyful person, which is even more astonishing given the life of tremendous hardship he's lived through, surviving assassination attempts and leading the anti-apartheid movement in South Africa while Nelson Mandela was in prison. He says:

Joy is much bigger than happiness. While happiness is often seen as being dependent on external circumstances, joy is not. Discovering more joy does not save us from the inevitability of hardship and heartbreak. In fact, we may cry more easily, but we will laugh more easily, too. Perhaps we are just more alive. Yet as we discover more joy, we can face suffering in a way that ennobles rather than embitters. We have hardship without becoming hard. We have heartbreak without being broken.

So if joy does not come from outside of ourselves, where does it come from? We first have to look at our perspective. Typically when we keep a narrow or small view on life, we descend into judgments, anger, and fear. Oftentimes if we just look up and then broaden our view, we find a whole world around us where our problems may be present, but they are not the only things that are present.

Through my work as cofounder of Warriors at Ease, I've spent a lot of time at Walter Reed National Military Medical Center. For those of you who don't know, Walter Reed is one of the primary hospitals where service members are brought after injury for rehabilitation. During my last visit, I was noticing how inside of each room we went into in the trauma unit, there was a different story. The service member's perspective on their experience had such a direct effect on their state of being. In one room, there was a man who was blinded by an explosion and severely depressed. Physically, aside from the blindness, he was relatively fine. Mentally, he was in a deep hole. He had little interest in learning anything that might help improve his mindset.

In the next room was a big burly guy with a bald head and a long brown beard, as well as a 1,000-watt smile. He shared openly that his legs, penis, and testicles had been blown off in an IED explosion. Despite losing half of his body and after more than 50 surgeries, he pronounced to us, "My main job around here is to go up and down the halls and cheer everyone up because basically I'm worse off physically than most of them. I tell them, 'I'm okay because of what's in here," he said, pointing to his chest, "not what's down there," he said, pointing to the place where his lower half of his body used to be.

In the next room, we found a handsome, young helicopter pilot with his beautiful, young fiancée curled up next to him on the bed and bridal magazines spread everywhere. The room was thick with young love. "He got shot in the butt through the floor of the helicopter!" the young woman proclaimed with a laugh. And then she said, "At least now he's out of combat, and now we can plan our wedding." He smiled and they snuggled in next to each other.

You can see here three different people whose experiences were entirely different based upon their perspectives. We will all suffer in life in our own ways. The choice is how we will respond to it. If you go down your street or apartment building, you will find much the same experience. The lens through which we view our lives plays a huge role in determining our potential for experiencing true joy.

Part of broadening our perspective includes taking responsibility for our own joy and our peace rather than depending upon it to come from outside of ourselves. Our willingness to participate in life is a form of taking responsibility for our own experience. The power is in our own hands to choose how we meet this life. Blaming other people or circumstances for our misfortune is a sure sign that our perspective has grown too narrow. When blaming starts, we automatically put ourselves in the role of the victim, and then everything brings us down because we feel like life is happening to us. It's a sign that we are trying to source our joy outside of ourselves. Sometimes the world may leave us feeling powerless and like life is shooting arrows at us. In some sense, we may externally be powerless, but we can affect our internal experience. When those arrows start to fly, we can shift our perspective from what is coming at us to an internal space of wholeness, and then focus on what we're putting into the world. Immediately when we do this, we take our power back.

We are in charge of our own hearts and minds. As Gandhi so famously said, "Be the change you wish to see in the world." We have the choice each moment to shift the way we see and participate in the world. I learned this lesson most strongly from the survivors of human trafficking I've worked with over the years. In case you don't know, there are over 40 million people living in modern-day slavery in the world. That's more than at the time we consider abolition in the mid-1800s. Millions of these modern-day slaves were sold as young children into the sex trade. They survived the unimaginable, sometimes for many years. I work together with some of the survivors in safe houses where they stay during their transition from their former lives into their future selves. We use the same practices I'm sharing with you with them as well.

One woman in the safe house shared, "I survived by knowing that they could hurt my body, but they couldn't break my spirit. I'm stubborn as hell. That's how I survived. And I'm glad I did because a lot of the girls wanted to die. I never did. Now I have a second chance at life." Working with these inspirational women and men has taught me countless lessons, including the relativity of the problems I personally face as a human being, and also that our perspective in life has a huge part to play in our resilience. When we meet adversity and say, "I'm not going to be the victim," a whole new world of possibilities opens up. Joy naturally starts to arise. We do not need to be a victim of circumstance. We can be proactive in cultivating joy by shifting our internal perspective, broadening our horizon, and seeing what is right about our lives, the lessons that are there in the challenges, and the joy that is present in every moment when we experience deep connection.

Your willingness to show up as authentic and at the same time joyful and grateful is a gift you offer to the world. When you really own your own experience and are not a victim of circumstance, you take back your own joy and in the process, shine that light out for other people as well. Your own life can become an inspiration for others to discover hope and possibility. Please keep in mind that experiencing authentic joy does not mean we override the challenges we're feeling. We aren't forcing ourselves into a false sense of optimism or positivity. Rather, we are setting ourselves free to experience everything that is present. When resistance drops, joy arises.

There is a huge sense of freedom and relief found in not trying to keep all of the difficult emotions and memories buried somewhere deep inside of ourselves. When we feel connected to life and safe in ourselves, it strengthens us in a way that allows us to feel emotions like anger and fear without getting hijacked by them because that deeper sense of well-being is also present. This is where the resilience resides. And as strange as it may sound, the more fully we connect with these emotions—all of our emotions—the more we will feel connected to ourselves and the world around us. The kind of connection I'm talking about can be cultivated through mindfulness practices like Yoga Nidra, which recognizes that authentic gratitude and joy contains all of our emotions, even sadness and anger. Authentic gratitude and joy honors and holds our full experience.

Have you ever noticed when you really sit with a challenging emotion, like sadness or anger, and perhaps have a good cry or primal scream, that the emotions may hurt, but there is often also a subtle or obvious sense of joy present because you are feeling so fully? Have you ever laughed in the middle of your tears? I have! Quite honestly, it happened last week! How is that possible if joy is not also present amidst the other emotions? When we think our life is only going to be happy, peaceful, or prosperous, we put ourselves in a trap and place conditions on our well-being. This moment—every moment—has the possibility of experiencing joy. Gratitude and welcoming opens the door to this possibility.

When you look at the sky, some days it's crystal clear. Other days, it storms like crazy with lightning and thunder. You don't see the sky refusing clouds or looking for shelter from the storm. The sky is not limited by the storm or the sun or the clouds, just as your joy does not have to be limited by the circumstances of your life. We are the sky. Our true nature is peaceful and joyful. We can look for the places where we still have resistance, or clouds, to discover what is keeping us from peace and joy—the parts of ourselves that need to be felt, seen, and heard. We can watch as we feel the rain and snow, and then we can watch as it passes and the sun comes out again. Often after the storm passes, we appreciate the sun even more.

When we are caught in a storm of emotions, we are either trying to pull something towards us or push something else away. This pulling and pushing is actually taking us farther and farther away from the happiness that we seek. The reason for this is that true, lasting joy is not dependent upon anything outside of ourselves. True joy is an internal experience. When there is a willingness to meet life and all of our emotions, there is joy in the midst of it. Cultivating traits like forgiveness, compassion, and generosity supports our ability to experience this unchanging, internal joy. Suffering comes from resistance. It comes from wanting life to be different than what it is. It comes from our attachment to a desired outcome. When we take responsibility for our joy and our peace, we suddenly experience a sense of proactivity in how we engage with emotions. And then that starts to reveal that there is a sense of well-being and peace present. Then you feel more empowered to open up to your own authentic voice because you are being held by this deeper experience of peace.

We've been talking a lot about how internal joy can arise through having deeper connection with gratitude, but we can also use external joy to help evoke a sense of internal joy—a direct experience of well-being. That joy doesn't need a reason or a destination. As we said before, authentic internal joy arises as a result of feeling close to who we truly are. External joy is the type of joy that's evoked from things outside of ourselves. It is, of course, a delightful thing to celebrate all the amazing aspects of life: being together with your favorite people, eating your favorite food, watching a gorgeous sunset, sunrise, or accomplishing a goal. The problem with external joy is if that source of joy goes away, the joy starts to go away too. It may linger for a little bit of time, but then it starts to dissipate.

Even so, by using mindfulness techniques, we can use external sources of joy to connect with a deeper sense of internal joy. To see how this works, let's do a brief practice together now. Psychologist Paul Ekman has identified several states of being that are associated with joy. We're going to use these states, or emotions, in a guided meditation practice. As I'm describing them, watch if a memory, thought, or image comes to mind. If an opposite emotion arises, you are entirely welcome to feel whatever is present. The more fully you connect with the experience, the more potential the practice has. Approach it with openness and curiosity.

Feel free to close your eyes and take a moment to feel your present experience. How does your body feel? Observe your breath. Notice as you're breathing: are there any feelings, emotions, or thoughts that are present? Welcome yourself just as you are.

First, bring to mind a feeling of amusement. Amusement includes something entertaining that gives you anything from a chuckle to a deep belly laugh. You can think about something that you really had a good laugh about. Think about how that feels in your body when you just can't stop laughing. What feeling is present in your body when you absolutely cannot stop laughing? Experience this. Sense and explore the feeling of amusement.

Now notice a feeling of relief. Relief follows another emotion, such as fear, anxiety, and even pleasure. It's an experience of noticing joy again after a challenging emotion has passed. It may help to think of a time when you were really worried about something, like a test result or a work project, and then it passed. Notice what your body feels like as that tension just drains away and a sense of calm arises once more.

Observe now a feeling of contentment, a calmer kind of satisfaction where it feels like everything is just as it should be. What does it feel like when you don't want to change anything? Sense and explore a feeling of contentment, noticing what your body feels like as it rests in the fullness and stillness of the present moment.

Now observe if a feeling of pleasure is present. Pleasure is based on joy derived from the five senses. Think of a time when you felt pleasure. Notice what is present as you feel this experience. Observe what physical sensations are here now.

Next, bring to mind a feeling of wonder. Wonder occurs in the midst of something astonishing and admirable. What brings you to a state of awe or an experience that you have to recalibrate your understanding of the world to assimilate it? This could be perhaps a place you've experienced in nature, an experience of an infinite starry sky in the desert, or watching someone win a gold medal they've worked their whole entire lives for. Once you evoke this feeling of astonishment, notice what this feels like in your body. What arises?

Now evoke a feeling of excitement, which is a response to a novelty or challenge. Perhaps its experiencing something you always wanted to experience or doing something new for the first time. This may evolve into a feeling of rejoicing or celebrating happiness. What brings you a feeling of life and vitality, the thrill of excitement, and perhaps the celebration it evokes? What does this feel like in your body?

Now experience the feeling of elevation that arises as you witness an act of kindness, compassion, or generosity. What do you feel when you experience the open heart of yourself or another through an obvious or subtle act of kindness? Notice what experience this evokes in the body. Feel this for a few moments.

Now observe a feeling of gratitude. It may help to remember a time when you felt a true sense of appreciation for being the beneficiary of something helpful, or gratitude can arise for just being fully open to this present moment. Notice what happens in the body as you open up to all of the blessings in life, both the obvious things that make you thankful and even the challenges that are here teaching you valuable lessons. Sense and explore the feeling of gratitude, a profound welcoming and reception of life just as it is.

Now observe any feelings of ecstasy, the bliss of an experience that transports us outside of ourselves, where you lose the confines of your physical body and feel an innate sense of connection with everyone and everything your consciousness encounters. Maybe this arises naturally, and if not, imagine what it feels like to experience your entire perception of reality become a celebration. Like there is nothing keeping you from experiencing the bliss of your true nature. Everything your consciousness touches feels like it touches back in the warm embrace of true connection. Feel how separation dissolves in this embrace. Stay with this for a moment, and notice what this feels like in your body. Is there separation between you and the world around you? Or can you actually feel out into the space around you, exploring how the only limits are those we impose with our minds. Stay with this.

Watch as this may start to settle into a deeper experience of stillness. As you feel this interconnectedness. Feel how this deep connection reveals radiance, a serene joy that arises from experiencing our inherent well-being and benevolence. Our interconnection with all of life itself. Feel a part of the whole and a part of the stillness. Watch how from the stillness, an experience may arise. Welcome this. Feel it fully. Then watch as it drops back into the place from which it came:

your true nature. Healthy, whole, and complete just as you are. Stay with this experience, resting in your true nature. When you come back to life, notice if joy comes back with you. Make an intention to nourish this joy with every thought, word, and deed.

Thank you.

Class 17

Practice 1: Building Resilience

This practice class is focused on building resilience through yoga, and this guidebook chapter provides background information on the practice as well as images of the poses. Refer to the video class for additional guidance on the class's poses, including chair variations.

If you are using a chair, make sure it is a steady one. Do not use a chair that could move around or slip on the floor. Some people like putting their chair on a yoga mat or a non-slip surface.

Keep in mind that yoga is a nurturing practice. It should make your body feel good. If something doesn't feel right for you, don't do it, or find an adaptation that does feel good to you. If you have any doubts about if your body is capable of doing the activities in this class, please consult your doctor first.

Breathing

- Throughout the practice, you'll be using a technique called *ujjayi* breathing, which is an inhalation and exhalation through the nose. This is designed to warm the breath, which helps the body warm up as well.

Pose Information: Sun Salutations

- This class's first pose involves sun salutations. You can think of sun salutations as yoga warm-up exercises. Sun salutations have historic roots back in the Himalayas, where people would go on pilgrimage to a sacred temple or site. They would take 10 steps and then bow down, performing an act of prostration or gratitude to give thanks for all the blessings in their life. They would also give thanks for the sun, the ultimate source of life, which is why the practice is called sun salutations, or *Surya Namaskar* in Sanskrit.

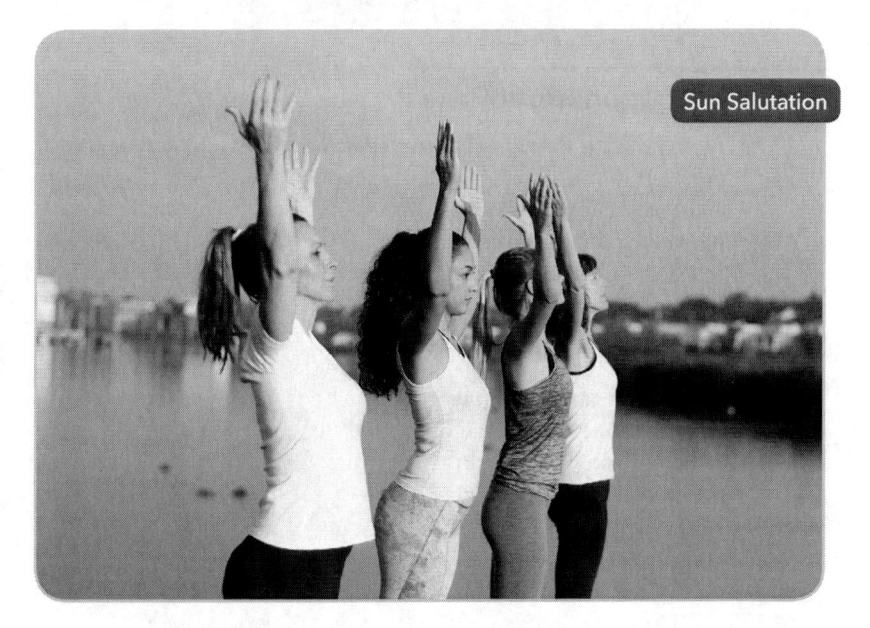

Sun Salutation

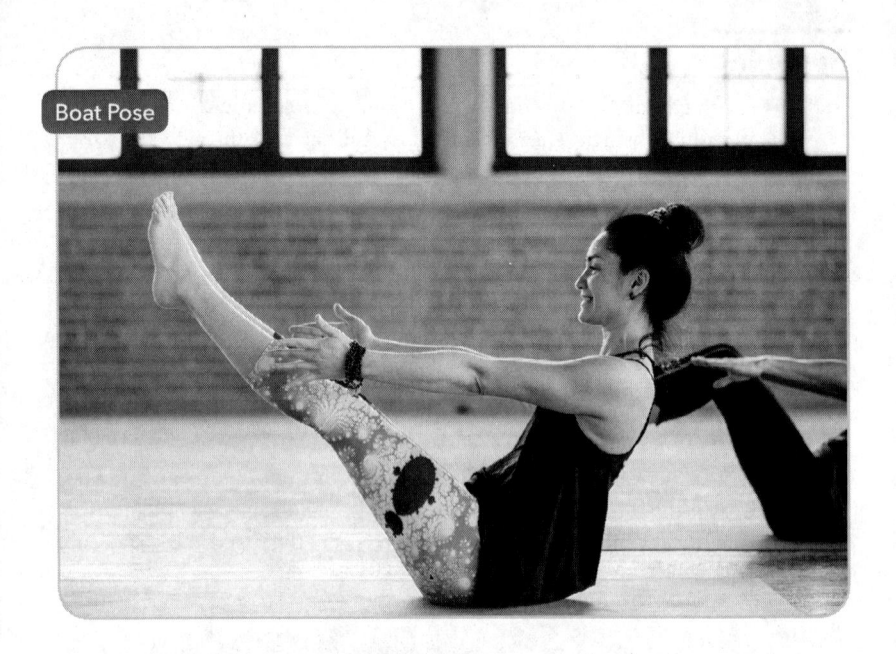

Pose Information: Boat Pose

- After working through sun salutations, the class turns to the boat pose. For the boat pose, if you're in the chair, you can lift your legs up and then bend your knees so that your knees are coming in toward your body. You can either hold behind your thighs and lift up, or you can start to straighten the legs. You should be using your abdominal strength here.

- If you're on the ground, there are two variations. You can bring your knees up, bent, and bring your arms out alongside the calves. If you need to, you can hold on behind the legs. For a more advanced variation, you can extend the legs out and extend the arms, keeping the spine straight. This pose builds core strength. It is also a nice balance pose.

Pose Information: Child's Pose

- From the boat pose, you will lower and rotate yourself around into the child's pose. If you're sitting in a chair, you can relax the head down for a moment, with the hands in a comfortable neutral position. If you're on the ground, you can either have your knees together or separate. You can have your arms straight out, or you can relax them back by your feet. Do what feels best to you.

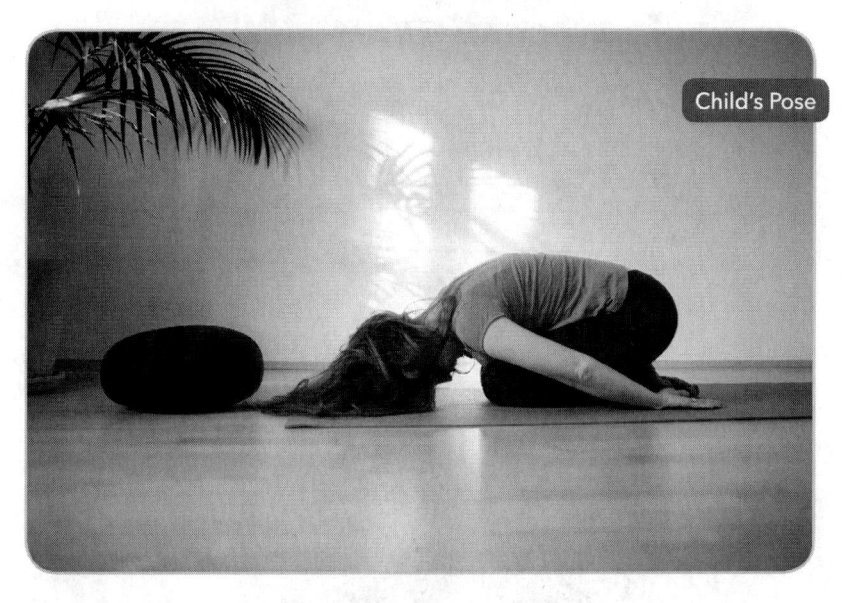

Child's Pose

Pose Information: Dolphin Pose

- Next up is the dolphin pose. For the dolphin pose, if you're in a chair, put your hands on the arms of the chair. Try to keep the elbows in as you lift your body up and then place it back down again. You can do this several times, but take a break at any point you need to. If you'd like to increase the challenge, you can hold yourself up in the position.

- For the floor version, position your elbows under the shoulders, and then interlace your hands in front of you. This may be as much as you want to do, and that's fine. This pose is a way to build strength in the upper body and abdomen.

- If you would like to go farther, you can bring the chin down, and then lift the back up before coming back down. Exhale on the downward movement and inhale on the upward movement. Try not to drop the hips when you come down, instead keeping the back straight.

- If this is too hard, you can also bring your knees down onto the mat, and then do the same position, swimming like a dolphin dives: down and up. You can do about 10 repetitions of this pose in whatever style you'd like. When you're finished, come back into the child's pose.

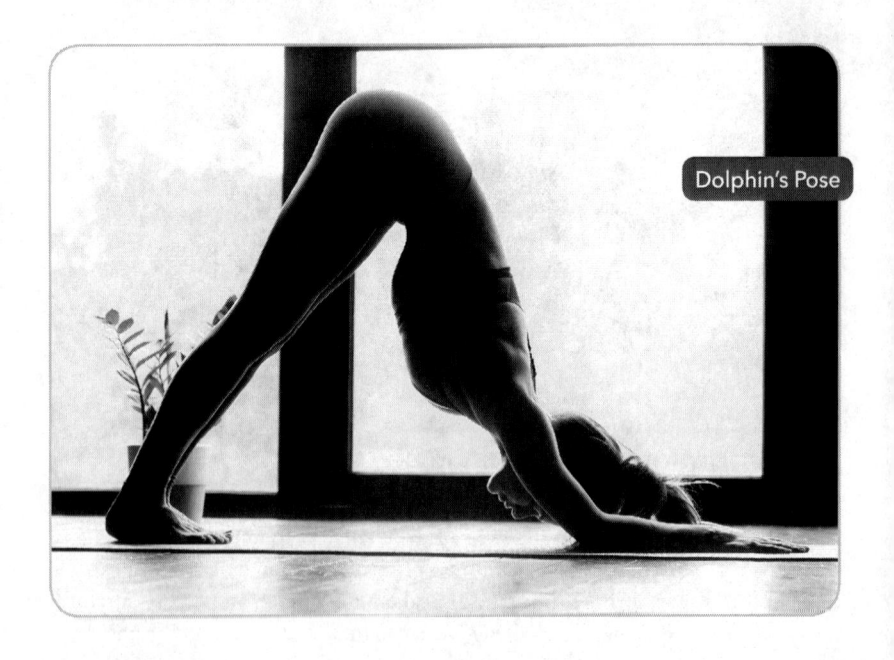

Dolphin's Pose

Pose Information: Tree Pose

- After returning to child's pose, the practice shifts into standing poses, starting with the tree pose. If you don't have a chair and you would like extra support, you can always use a wall.

- For the tree pose, find a position where your left foot can root down. Put the heel down and then slowly spread out the toes. Next, bend into the knee. You should feel like you have roots extending down from your foot into the earth. Keep in mind that balance is in large part a function of your gaze. When you're doing the tree pose, make sure your eyes are fixed on a stationary point on the floor.

- After rooting down through the left foot, a couple of variations are available. You can tuck the right foot gently up into the inside of your left leg, or you can draw it up a little farther onto your calf.

- Never put the foot right on the knee. This could damage the knee. However, you can bring the foot up into the inside of the thigh, or you can bring the foot all the way up into a half lotus pose if you are confident that you can hold the pose in that position.

- Bring the hands up into a prayer position if you're standing. If you're using a chair, you can you leave your hand on the chair. If standing, you can lift the arms up, though this is optional.

- If your hands are out, slowly bring them back into the prayer position. Next, release the hands and release the leg down. Wiggle your arms and legs, shaking out the body.

- Next, bring the right foot forward. Spread out the toes, and then root the foot down. You should feel the thigh muscles start to engage. Bend into the right knee, and then slowly find your position with the left foot, sliding it up any amount onto the right leg. Again, hold onto a wall or a chair if that's helpful for you.

Tree Pose

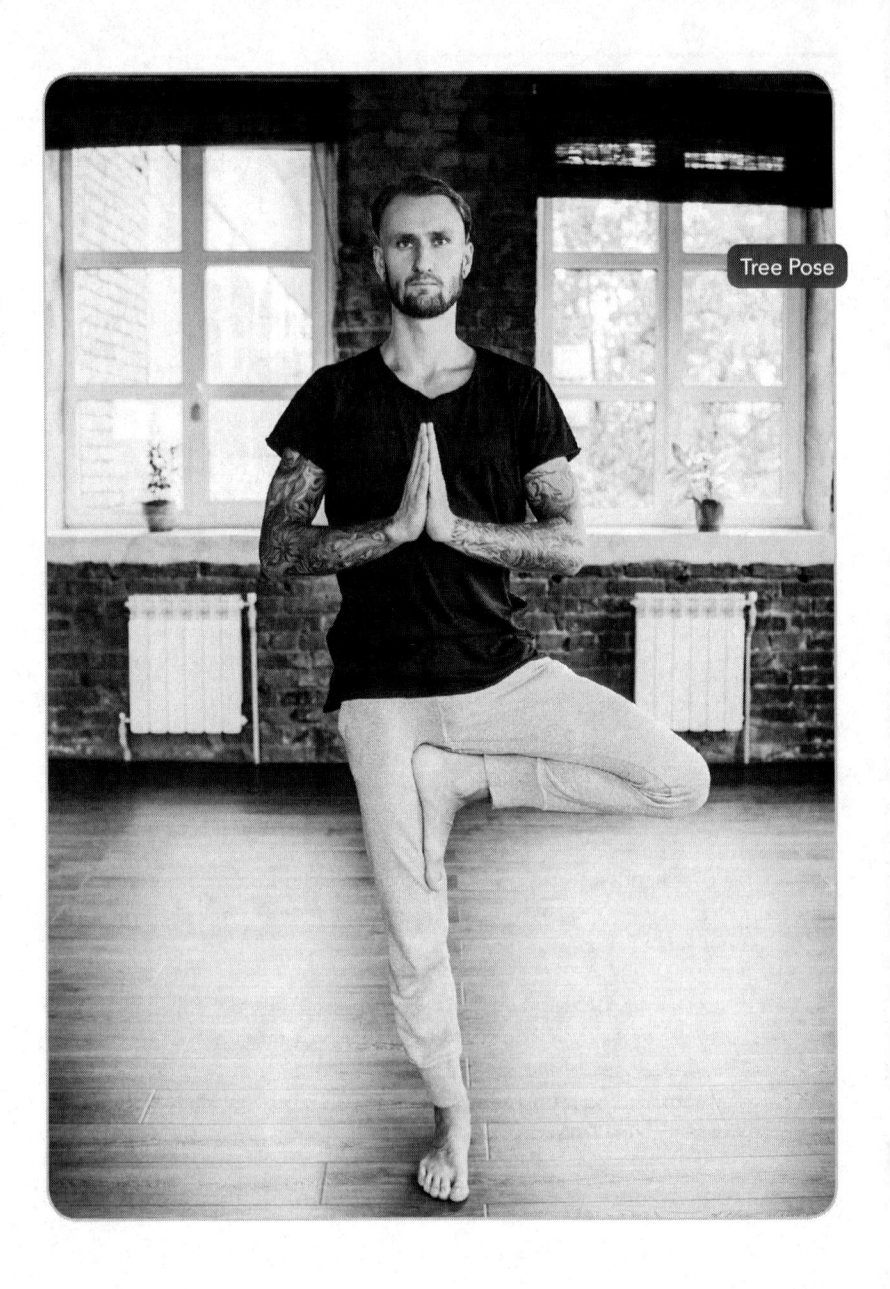

- If you'd like, you can elevate your arms up. Breathe and keep rooting down through the foot as the head lifts up toward the sky. Slowly, on a deep inhalation, draw the hands into your heart. Release the arms and relax, and then shake everything out again.

Pose Information: Triangle Pose

- Next up is the triangle pose. You can put your right hand on a chair for support, or place it on your thigh. Separate your legs. For this pose, you will want the foot that is facing out to be pointed directly out. The foot on the backside should be pointed slightly in.

- If your hand is on your thigh, slide your hand down the leg, and then bring the right arm out in front of you and swing it up over your ear. Try to make your body flat. If it's not, you can also take the back foot out a little bit more. Once you practice, you'll find the right distance for you.

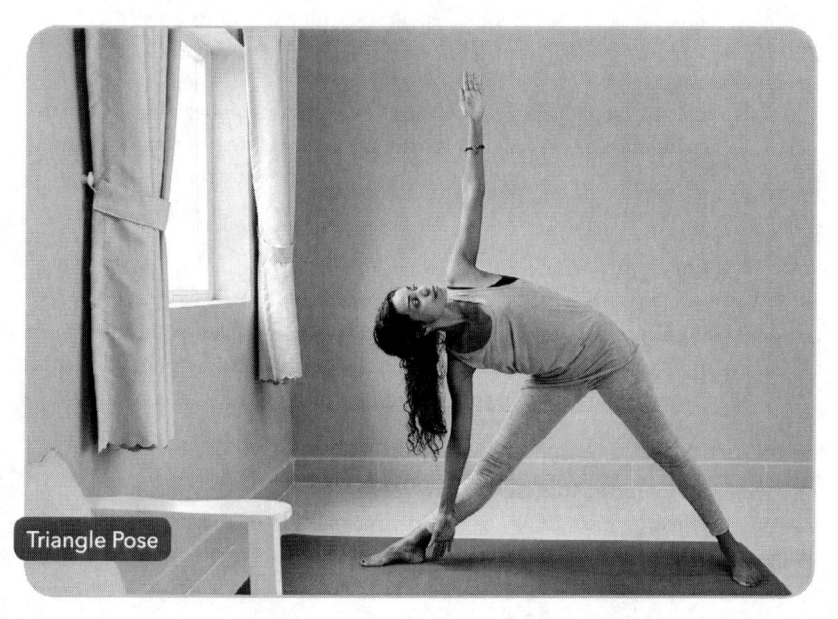

Triangle Pose

- The other option is to swing the arm up and around, and then tuck your chin into your chest, pressing into the feet for strength and lifting the body up. After that, switch sides. If you're using the chair, turn your body so that the left foot is facing forward and the left hand is on the chair.

- If you're on the ground, turn the left toes out and the right toes in. Bring the left hand onto the thigh or chair, and then bring your right arm up and slide yourself over. If desired, you can swing the right hand up and over the ear. Breathe deeply.

Pose Information: Warrior Pose

- Next, slowly come up and prepare for the warrior pose. Separate your feet a bit wider than they were during the triangle pose. As you come down, bend into your right knee, then look down. You want your knee to be over your ankle. Once you're in position, tuck your tailbone under and then inhale, extending your arms out. Place your gaze over your right middle finger.

- You should feel like you're sitting your hips down as the head lifts up. If you're using a chair, your arm can be extended out, and the eyes should be focused outward. If you need to come out of the pose at any point, do so.

- When you're ready, slowly come up and step your left foot forward. Bring your right leg back. Once again, make sure your feet are wide, and bend into your front left knee. Look down and make sure your knee is right over the ankle. The right toes should be pointed in at a 45-degree angle. Tuck your tailbone under.

- Extend your arms out, and gaze over the left middle finger. Keep dropping the hips down and elevating the crown of the head. Next, step your foot up to the top of your mat; if you're using the chair or have otherwise modified the move, you can sit down once more.

- If you are not using a chair, the next phase involves coming down onto the ground. Lift your arms up parallel with the ground. Start to sit down, and then slowly use your hands to lower yourself down. This will lead to a reclined spinal twist if you're on the ground.

- If you're in a chair, start by bringing your left hand onto your right knee. Then, you can place the right hand wherever it feels good to you. It can go on the arm of the chair or behind your back to perform a final twist.

- If you're on the ground, lift up your right foot and place it just above the left knee. Place your left hand on the right knee and pull it gently over to the side. The right arm extends out. Gaze toward your right arm. Start breathing up and down the spinal column. Feeling with each breath that you're soothing your nervous system, releasing any tension in the spine.

- Next, if you're in the chair, bring your right hand on your left knee, bring your right hand onto your left knee and twist your body to

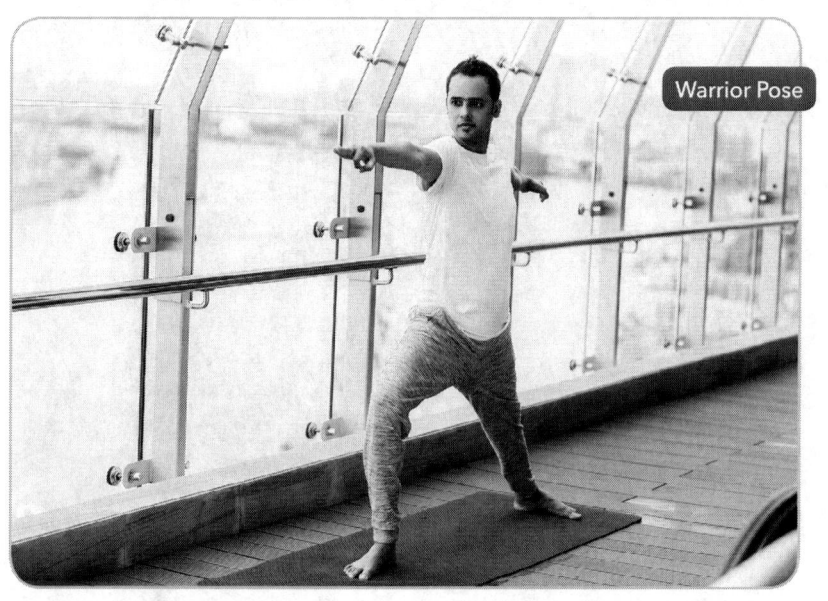

Warrior Pose

the left side. If you're working from the ground, bring the foot just above the right knee, moving the left knee over to the right. The left arm extends, and your gaze will go over to the left. Once again, take long, deep breathes up and down the spine, feeling as if each breath is nourishing your spinal column.

- Come back to center and extend the leg out. If you're lying on the ground or working from the chair, you can give your body a hug. Give yourself credit for nourishing your body and mind.

Pose Information: *Shavasana*

- This class's final relaxation pose is called *shavasana*. If you're in a chair, feel free to scoot toward the back of the chair and make any adjustments you need to be comfortable. If you're on the ground, bring your feet about mat-distance apart and let the toes fall out to the

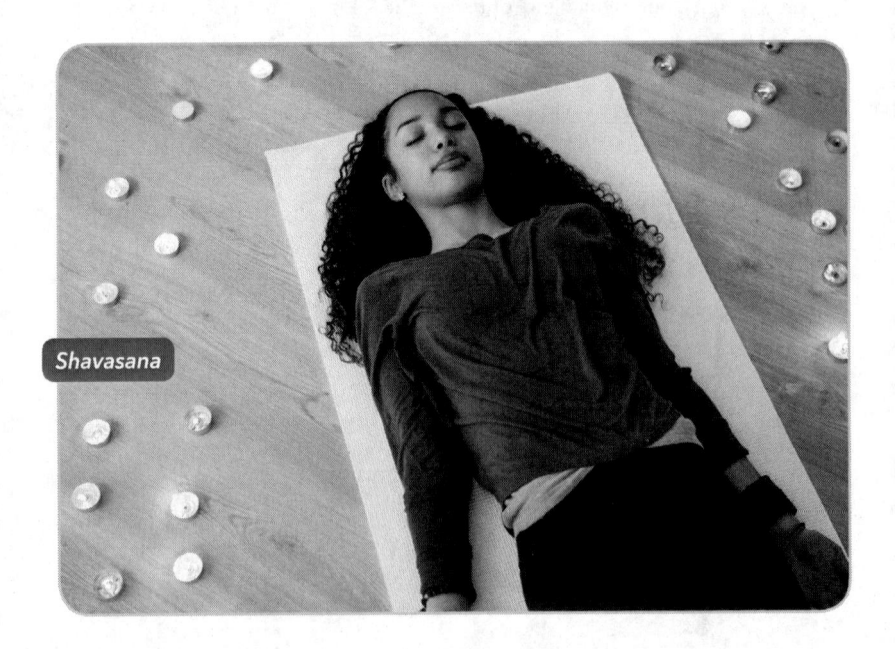

Shavasana

side. Roll the shoulder blades back and down together. Let the palms face up in an open, receptive position.

- If there's any tension in the neck, you can turn your head to the right and the left a couple of times. When you've released the neck tension, tuck your chin into your chest to elongate the backside of the neck, and then let your neck find a neutral position. Feel the whole plane of contact between the body and the surface beneath you.

- Observe the experience of your physical body, noticing all the physical sensations that are present. Then, if you'd like, take a few long, deep breaths to release any lingering tension that may be present in your body. Observe the state of your mind, welcoming any feelings or emotions and beliefs.

- Fill your heart so that it feels soft, open, alive, strong, and peaceful at the same time. You're welcome to stay here as long as you would like, resting in the stillness. When you're done, take a break of 5 to 10 minutes before returning to your day.

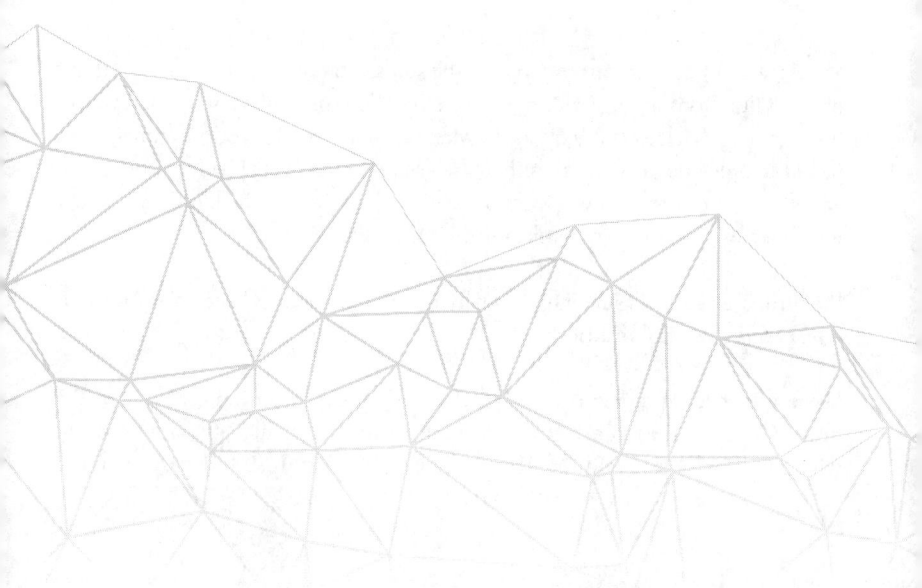

Class 17 Transcript

Practice 1: Building Resilience

Hello and welcome to the building resilience practice class. I'm joined today by two friends, Emma, who is going to be demonstrating the four versions of the poses. And Randy, who will be demonstrating the chair variations of the poses.

Please keep in mind that yoga is a nurturing practice. It should make your body feel good. So, if something doesn't feel right for you, please don't do it, or find an adaptation that does feel good to you. Also, if you have any doubts about if your body is capable of doing the practice as we do, please consult your doctor first.

All right, so are you ready to dive in to our building resilience practice? Here we go.

So, we're going to start out today with the sun salutation practice. You can think of sun salutations as yoga warm-up exercises. The sun salutations actually have historic roots back in the Himalayas where people would go on pilgrimage to a sacred temple or site. They would take 10 steps and then they would bow down and an act of prostration or gratitude to give thanks for all the blessings in their life. They would also give thanks for the sun,

the ultimate source of life, which is why the practice is called sun salutations, or *Surya Namaskar* in Sanskrit.

We're going to start out with our hands in a prayer position in front of the heart. Close the eyes and just take a moment to give thanks, giving thanks for whatever is present in your life that feels like a blessing. Thanks for this day and life, the people who make our lives possible. And even giving thanks for the challenges that are here teaching us valuable lessons.

As we move through the sun salutations, also give thanks to your body. All the good work it does keeping you healthy and alive.

Throughout the practice we're going to be doing a breath called *ujjayi* breathing, which is an inhalation and exhalation through the nose. This is designed to warm the breath which helps the body warm up as well. Hands in prayer position, take a deep inhale and exhale. Inhale, extend your arms above your head, separate your hands. If you're standing, press your hips forward. If you have a healthy neck, you can relax your neck back a little. If not, keep your chin gently tucked.

Now, extend the arms out and down as you bring your hands down towards the ground, feeling that nice flow of blood to the brain, helping concentration and memory. On an inhalation bring your right leg back if you're working on the floor, and if you're in the chair lift your right leg up, and you can hold on behind the thigh or just let your muscles keep the leg up.

Now on a breath retention bring the left leg back to meet the right. If you're in the chair you can continue to hold the leg. Coming into a plank position, feeling the strength of the hands on the floor, pressing back through the heels. The head is in alignment with the spinal column. On an exhale, drop the knees down onto the mat, leave your butt up in the air. Keep the elbows pinned into the rib cage as you bring your shoulders down, and your chin down onto the mat like an inchworm.

If you're in the chair roll the shoulders down, look towards your belly button. And now, slide the chest forward and up through the hands, roll the shoulders back and look up.

On an exhalation curl your toes under if you're on the floor and slide back into the inverted V or downward facing dog, as you may know it. If you're in the chair you can lift your legs up and reach down for your toes. If that's too much for you, you can just reach the arms out. While you're here take a few deep breaths and you can alternate the heels a little bit. If you have lower back issues it may feel better for your back to keep your feet together. If it feels better, you can keep the feet apart. Everyone needs to find what's best for their body.

Now, on an inhale, bring the right leg forward; if you're in the chair bring the legs down. And lift the right leg up once again, and then bring the left leg forward to meet the right. The head comes down towards the knees and you lift the tailbone up, even a fraction of an inch. If you're in the chair bring the leg down. And then everyone together we'll inhale lift their arms up, gently arched back once more, softening the heart. Exhale, drawing the hands in prayer back to the heart and then down by her side. Exhale completely, inhale and exhale the hands into a prayer position in front of your heart.

Inhale, extend the arms up, separate the hands and gently arch back. Exhale, extend the arms out and down, coming down. Bringing your fingertips in line with your toe tips, if possible. And if you don't make it all the way to the floor you can leave your hands on your shins. This time inhale and bring your left leg back. Drop the knee down, look up, if you're in the chair lift the left leg up.

Retain your breath as you come back into the plank position. Bringing the leg down and then on an exhalation, knees, chest and chin come down in the chair. Roll your shoulders down, look down at your belly button. Inhale. Roll those shoulders back. Look up. Exhale, curl the toes under, press back into inverted V or extend the legs out and reach down towards your legs.

Inhale, bring your left leg up between your hands, drop the right knee down, look up. If you're in the chair lift your left leg up. Exhale, bring the other leg forward, head comes down towards the knees, lift the tailbone up. Inhale, extend the arms out and up; if you're in the chair bring the leg down. Lift up, gently arch back. Exhale, drawing the hands into the heart and then relaxing them at your side.

We'll move through this a couple more times. If at any point it's too much for you, you can just stand in a neutral position or come to a seated position.

Inhale. Exhale, hands into prayer position in front of the heart. Inhale, extend the arms up, separate the hands, gently arch back. Exhale, extend out and down. Bring your fingertips in line with your toes. Inhale, bring the right leg back, drop the knee down, look up or lift your right leg.

Retain your breath as the left leg comes back to meet the right. Feeling the strength in the plank position, on an exhalation drop your knees and chest and chin down, or roll your shoulders down towards your knees. Inhale, slide the head forward, gently roll the shoulders back and up. Exhale, press back into an inverted V or reach for your feet.

Take a deep breath here and a long stretch. Now, inhale, bring the right leg forward up between your hands. Left knee down. Look up. Retain the breath, bring the left leg up to meet the right. Lift your tailbone up. And then inhale, extending the arms out and up. Lift the arms up, gently arch back. Exhale, drawing the hands into prayer in front of the heart. And then relaxing them at your side. Inhale. Exhale. Hands in prayer position.

Inhale. Lift the arms up, press the hips forward, gently arch back. Exhale, extend the arms out and down, coming down. Inhale, bring the left leg back this time, drop the knee down. Look up, retain the breath. Bring the right leg back to meet the left, feeling your plank position here. Strengthen from the body. And then on an exhale, drop the knees down, leave your butt up in the air, bring your chest and shin down between your hands, keeping your elbows pinned into the ribs, roll the head down if you're in the chair and then inhale, slide the chest forward and up, open up through the chest. Tuck your toes under and press back into the inverted V.

Take a deep breath here. Now on an inhale bring the left leg forward, drop the right knee down. Look up. Exhale, bring the other leg forward. Head comes down to the knees. Inhale, extend the arms out and up, lift up, gently arch back. Exhale, bring your arms by your side.

And now, separate the feet, hip distance apart if you're standing; if you're in the chair, you can bring them just a little wider. Then a choice here. If you're standing you can start to swing the arms side to side, releasing any tension in the spinal column. Finding a nice rhythm for the body. And if you don't have low-blood pressure you can start hinging at the hips and coming down. If you're in that chair you can swing gently side-to-side.

Feeling the spine loosening up, letting go of any tension. Slowly coming back up to a standing position. And now if you're standing, lift your arms up, parallel with the ground. Start sitting the hips down while keeping the spine long. It's okay if you can't make it all the way, and then bring your hands down. Perfect. And come on down.

Now the next thing we're going to do is called the boat pose. So, for the boat pose, if you're in the chair you can lift your legs up and then bend your knees, so your knees are coming in towards your body. And then you can hold either behind your thighs and lift-up. Or you can start to straighten the legs. So, a little more than you were doing on our downward dog adaptation. So, you should be using your abdominal strength here.

If you're on the ground, there's two variations. You can bring your knees up, bent, and bring your arms out alongside the calves. If you need to you can hold on behind the legs, or if you want a more advanced variation, you can extend the legs out and extend the arms, keeping the spine nice and straight. Can see this really builds that core strength. Also, a nice balance pose. Take one more deep breath here.

And then slowly come down and rotate yourself around coming into the child's pose. If you're sitting in a chair you can just relax the head down for a moment with the hands in a comfortable neutral position. For the child's pose, you can either have your knees together or separate. You can have your arms straight out or you can relax them back by your feet. Again, everybody is different, so do what feels best to you.

For the dolphin pose, if you're in the chair, we're going to put our hands on the arms of the chair. If you are using a chair, make sure you have a nice steady chair. You don't want to use a chair that could move around or slip on the floor. So sometimes people even like putting their chair on a yoga mat or on a no-slip surface.

So, Randy here is going to demonstrate. You're going to try to keep the elbows in as you lift your body up and you mount from the chair and then place it back down again. You can do this several times and at any point when you're ready to take a break, you can take a break. If you'd like to increase the challenge you can hold yourself up in that position.

And now, Emma is going to demonstrate the dolphin pose on the floor by first taking the elbows right under the shoulders, measuring the distance by holding on to the outside of the elbows, then interlacing hands in front of you.

This may be as much as you want to do and that's fine. It's a great way to build strength from the upper body and abdomen. If not you can exhale, bring the chin down and then lift the back up, the butt up and keep exhaling down, inhaling up. Exhaling down, inhaling up. Try not to drop the hips when you come down, but to keep the back really straight.

Of course, that makes it harder. If for whatever reason this is too hard for you, you can also bring your knees down onto the mat and then do the same position, swimming like a dolphin dives, down and up. We're doing what Randy is doing here, lifting himself up and down. You can do about 10 repetitions of this pose in whatever style you'd like. When you're finished come back into the child's pose.

So, it's a great pose that you can do for a really efficient exercise. So, if you have a day where you don't have enough time to exercise, the dolphin is a pose where you can really work the backside of your arms. You can work your upper back, your lower back, your abdomen. It's a really integrated pose that you get a lot of benefit from.

Once you're done come into the child's pose. If you're sitting in the chair you can gently tuck the head and relax for a moment. Take a deep breath here. Feeling the comfort of the practice, how deeply it nourishes your body.

Now, to prepare for this standing poses Randy is going to stand up and move his chair around a little here. If you don't have a chair and you like a little extra support with your balance poses you can always use a wall. And again, whatever you use make sure it's very stable on the floor so it doesn't slide out away from you.

The first pose we're going to do here is the tree pose, which is a balance pose. You'll notice in yoga that we work three main areas: strength, flexibility, and balance. So, in any practice you'll find a combination of those. For the tree pose you're going to want to find a position where your left foot can really root down. So, put the heel down and then slowly spread out the toes, placing the pinky toe and then all the way across down onto the ground. And then bend into the knee and really feel like you have roots extending down from your foot into the earth. So, you really grounding down here feeling solid, like the earth is holding you in this pose.

Now, balance is in large part a function of our gaze or our vision. So, when you're doing the tree pose make sure your eyes are fixed on a stationary point on the floor. For instance, you could pick a little knot on the wooden floor or a place on the carpet if that's where you're working. Keep your eyes locked there. You'll see it can really help you stay balanced. Same applies in life. So again, route down through that left foot. There's a couple of variations here. You can tuck the foot, just gently up into the inside of your leg, or you can draw it up a little farther on to your calf.

Never put the foot right on the knee because it could damage the knee, but you can also bring the foot up into the inside of the thigh or you can bring the foot all the way up into a half lotus pose if your really confident that you can hold the pose in that position. If you have on slippery pants like mine or you might be hard to keep the foot there.

But, you'll bring the hands up into a prayer position if you're standing, or if you're using the chair or you can you leave your hand on the chair. And it's interesting to play with this here. If you feel really confident in your balance you may want to start talking, because you can see that can agitate balance or you can see what happens if you close your eyes. If you'd like and you're standing you can open up the limbs of your tree and lift their arms up.

If you fall, it doesn't matter. Balance is a practice of finding how we're always moving, always seeking balance and each moment. It's only through cultivating balance that we're able to maintain it for longer and longer periods of time. Life is just like that.

Slowly if your hands are out, bring them back into prayer, draw them into your heart. Release the hands, release the leg down. Now wiggle out the arms and legs a little bit, shake out the body. You'll remember for one of our lectures that shaking out the body is a great way to relieve stress and tension. So, kind of do a little wiggle worm dance.

All right, so now that we're all wiggled out, we're going to bring the right foot forward. We're going to put the pinky down and then spread out the toes, then send down those roots into the earth, really ground the foot down. That helps so much and you'll notice how naturally the calf just starts to wrap right around the bone. All of a sudden the kneecap starts to lift up. You can feel the hamstrings and all of your thigh muscles start to engage.

Bend into the right knee and then slowly find your position with the left leg, sliding it up any amount onto the leg. Again, holding onto a wall or a chair if that's helpful for you. Coming into your pose. If you'd like you can elevate your arms up. Have fun with it, challenge yourself. Breath, keep rooting down through the foot as the head lifts up towards the sky. And slowly, on a deep inhalation, draw the hands into your heart. Release the arms and relax.

Do another wiggle worm. Shake everything out. Nobody's looking. We're looking goofy, you say you're looking at us, but we don't see you. See you can wiggle yourself as much as you want.

All right, now for the triangle pose. So, we're going to, we're going to show what Randy does first here. He's going to put his hand on the chair for support. Then he's going to separate his legs and for the triangle pose you want the the foot that is facing out to be pointed directly out, and then the foot that's on the backside to be pointed just a little bit in.

And so we're starting here with the right leg out. Put your hand on the chair or if your hand is on your thigh you're going to slide your hand down the leg and then bring the right arm out in front of you and swing it up over your ear. Exactly. And then you'll feel like you're between two sheets of glass. Try to make your body nice and flat and if it's not you can also take the back foot out a little bit more. Once you practice you'll find the right distance for you.

You should be feeling a good stretch in the whole side body. So this option that Emma is doing here is fine. The other option is to swing this arm up and around and then tuck your chin into your chest, gaze up, press into the feet for strength and lift the body up. Switch sides. If you're using that chair turn the body, so the left foot is facing forward, the left hand is on the chair.

If you're on the ground turn the left toes out, the right toes in. Bring the left hand onto the thigh or chair, your right arm up and slide yourself over. If the hand is like this you can leave it like that or you can swing it up and over the ear. So, we're up and over it like that. Perfect. Breathe deeply.

We hold a lot of tension in our intercostal muscles and if you think about how we sit all day we're collapsing those.

So when we do the triangle pose we're opening up those intercostals and helping to keep our posture nice and straight. Take one more deep breath here and then slowly come up and prepare now for the warrior pose.

The warrior pose is a powerful pose as the name implies. It's a pose where you can really tap into your inner resilience and strength. So, separate your feet a little bit wider than you did for the triangle. As you come down you want to bend into your right knee, then look down. You want your knee to be over your ankle. So if it's not you need to wiggle your feet out a little bit more, or bring them a little closer in. Once you're in position, tuck your tailbone under and then inhale, extend your arms out. Your gaze is going to be right over that right middle finger.

So, feel like you're sitting your hips down as the head lifts up. You keep making those little micro-movements. There's so much power in finding just how a little bit of a micro-movement can change the pose for you. If you're in the chair, using the chair, your arm can be extended out but likewise, see how focused Randy's eyes are as he gazes out. That's like your sword. At any point you need to come out, of course, do that.

And when you're ready, slowly come up, step your left foot forward. Now bring your right leg back. And once again make sure your feet are nice and wide. Bend into that front left knee. Look down and make sure your knee is right over the ankle. The right toes are pointed in at a 45-degree angle. Tuck your tailbone under. Extend your arms out. Gaze over that left middle finger. Keep dropping the hips down and elevating the crown of the head. Feel like you're growing into the pose, feeling the power in this pose.

Any each time we use the large muscle groups like the legs, we're bringing our minds into a point of focus. And now step your foot up to the top of your mat; if you're using the chair or you can go ahead and sit yourself down once more.

Now we're going to be coming down onto the ground. So, lift your arms up parallel with the ground. Start to sit down like you're sitting into a chair using all the muscles of the body to do it. And then slowly use your hands to lower yourself down. We're going to be doing a reclined spinal twist if you're on the ground; if you're in the chair you're going to do what Randy is doing. He's going to start by bringing his left hand onto his right knee. And then just using his hand, you can place it wherever it feels good to you; either on the arm of the chair or behind the chair, behind your back, to get a nice final twist here.

If you're on the ground you're going to lift up your right foot, place the right foot just above the left knee. Take your left hand, place it on the right knee and pull it gently over to the side. The right arm extends out and you gaze towards your right arm. Start breathing up and down the spinal column. Feeling with each breath that you're soothing your nervous system, releasing any tension in the spine.

When our spine is tense it really affects our nervous system and vice versa. When we get tuned up in our nervous system we start to get tension in the spine. That's why this is a great practice to boost our resilience. Helps us calm down the spine, calm down the nervous system. Then comes center and slide that leg out and away from you.

If you're in the chair bring your right hand on your left knee and come on over to the other side. If you're working in the down on the ground position bring the foot just above the right knee, bring the left knee over to the right. The left arm extends, and you gaze over to the left. Once again, breath long deep breaths, up and down the spine, feeling as if each breath is nourishing every little bit of your spinal column. Each breath soothing the nervous system. Sometimes we call this the "Snap, Crackle, Pop" pose, because the bones tend to find their way back into place.

Come back to center and extend the leg out. If you're lying on the ground you can give your body a big hug, and if you're sitting in that chair you can do the same thing, just wrapping your arms around you and closing the eyes and giving yourself a hug. You could be billions of places in the world right now, but you're here, nourishing your body and mind. Give yourself credit for that.

Now going to do the final relaxation pose or *shavasana*. If you're in the chair feel free to scoot back towards the backside of the chair and make any adjustments you need to be comfortable. If you're on the ground bring your feet about mat distance apart and let the toes fall out to the side. Roll the shoulder blades back and down together. Let the palms face up in an open receptive position.

If there's any tension in the neck, you can turn your head to the right and the left a couple of times. When you've released the neck tension, tuck your chin into your chest to elongate the backside of the neck and then let your neck find a neutral position. Feel that whole plane of contact between the body and the surface beneath you, all the places the body is being held. Feel the safety of that.

It's helpful to bring your inner resource to mind, that place where you feel very nourished, calm, and at ease. You can go ahead and do that.

Observe the experience of your physical body, noticing all the physical sensations that are present. Then if you'd like, you're welcome to take a few long deep breaths, breathing out any lingering tension that may be present in your body. Observe of the state of your mind, welcoming any feelings or emotions and beliefs.

Fill your heart: soft, open and alive, strong and at peace at the same time. Feel as if the heart is like the sun and it's shining love and light out to every single cell of your body. Feel this nourishing you on the deepest levels. Coming home to yourself. Resting here in the stillness that is always present inside of you. Pure consciousness. Pure awareness. Rest in this, the stillness that is your true nature. You're welcome to stay here as long as you would like.

Make sure to rest for at least five to 10 minutes before returning to your day. Thank you so much for practicing yoga with us today. *Namaste*.

Class 18

Practice 2: De-stressing with Your Breath

This class goes through several different breathing practices that you can do in your daily life. Each breath has purpose for practicing, though all can be a good way to calm yourself and refocus.

The Three-Part Yoga Breath

- To prepare for this class's first breath—the three-part yoga breath—place your right hand on your belly and your left hand on your chest. Close your eyes, and then notice where you are breathing. Observe the pattern of your breath. This is relevant because when people become stressed, they only breathe up into the very top of the lungs, or a bit into the chest. To relax, you will instead breathe consciously down into your abdomen.

- For this practice, breathe through your nose as much as possible. Take a deep breath, in through the nose, and send it down into your belly.

Expand your belly like a balloon, and then breathe up into your chest all the way up to the clavicle. As you exhale, squeeze your abdomen back in toward your spine. Take several more deep, three-part breaths like this.

- Close your eyes once more, observing the normal pattern of your breath. While inhaling, notice how long your inhalation lasts. However long that is, exhale for double that amount. If it's hard to make it to the doubled number, make your breath a little slower and steadier on the exhale. Ideally, you want the exhalation to be the same intensity from the beginning until the end.

- Doubling the exhalation helps evoke the relaxation response. This helps improve heart rate variability. Keep breathing and feeling the whole sensation of the body as the breath moves in and out.

The Energizing Breath

- This class's next breath is an energizing breath practice, which can be useful just after waking or when you need an afternoon boost. The energizing breath is also good for releasing tension.

- This breath is a forceful exhalation. The inhalation happens naturally on its own. You can put your finger under your nose to see how it feels at first. Exhale strongly, but keep the inhalation natural. Do 30 repetitions of this, with roughly one per second.

- After that, take three deep breaths, and then hold the breath for 30 seconds. While you're holding the breath, focus your attention either on your heart center or on the space between your eyebrows. While you're doing that, you can silently affirm a word or a phrase that's important to you. If you can't hold your breath for 30 seconds or don't feel comfortable doing it, feel free to replace that element with the deep three-part breaths introduced earlier.

Alternate Nostril Breathing

- This class's next breath is called alternate nostril breathing. For this, you will use your thumb and your pointer finger. The thumb will be used to block the right nostril, and the pointer finger will be used to block the left nostril.

- This exercise involves breathing in through one side of the body, holding the breath, and exhaling out of the other side. When you do this, you are moving from the left to the right hemisphere of your brain. This can help process emotions, thoughts, and other experiences that you are having. It's also very good for stimulating different aspects of neuroplasticity.

- If you don't want to hold your breath for any reason at any time, you can simply keep breathing from one side to the other. This exercise calls for you to inhale for four seconds, hold the breath, and then exhale for eight seconds. If a different pace works better for you, feel free to use that pace.

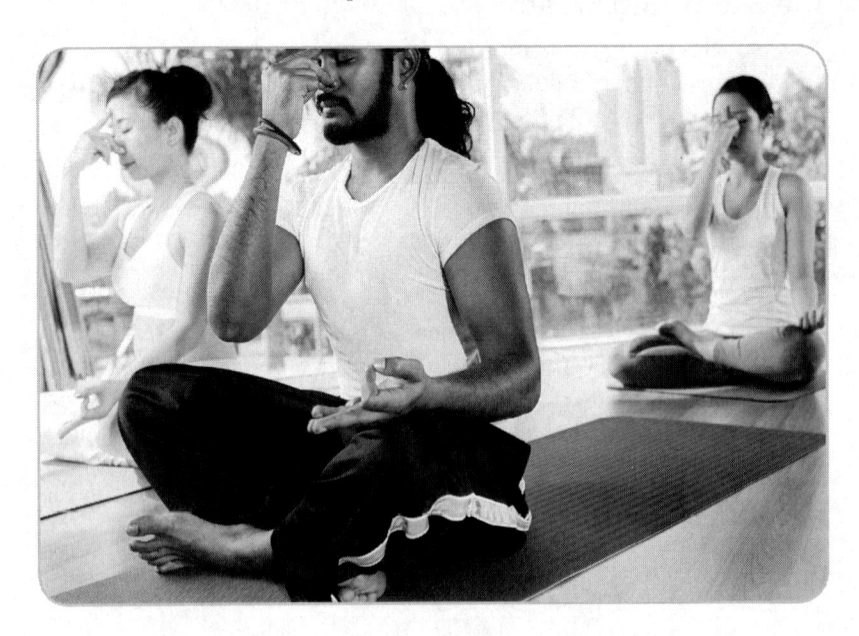

- To start, get your fingers ready. Inhale deeply through both nostrils, and then exhale completely through both nostrils. Gently block the right nostril with your thumb, and then inhale through the left nostril for four seconds. Hold your nose, blocking both nostrils. While you're holding the breath, relax the body, focusing on either the heart or the space between the eyebrows.

- Lift your thumb and exhale for eight seconds, trying to make that exhalation the same intensity throughout. Inhale for four seconds through the right nostril. Hold the breath, blocking both nostrils. Exhale through the left nostril for eight seconds, and then inhale through the left nostril.

- Gently hold the breath, blocking both nostrils, and then unblock the right nostril and exhale through it. Inhale through the right nostril for four seconds. Hold the breath, again blocking both nostrils. Exhale through the left nostril for eight seconds. Inhale through the left nostril for four seconds. Hold the nose. Exhale through the right nostril for eight seconds.

- Then, inhale through the right nostril for four seconds. Exhale and then hold the breath, blocking both nostrils. Exhale through the left nostril for eight seconds.

- Next, you can place your hand down on your knee. Keep your eyes closed and notice how your body and mind feel after practicing that breath. This is a great breath to do if you ever feel yourself feeling tense or anxious. It's a breath designed to bring balance to your body and your mind.

Meditation Preparation Breath

- This class's final breath can serve as preparation for meditation. Find a position that is comfortable. A typical meditation hand position is to bring your left hand palm up and your right hand on top of it with the thumbs touching. Then, straighten the spine.

- Picture the whole spinal column as straight. Imagine there is an elevator that goes up from the tip of your tailbone, up through your whole spine, and then out through the crown of your head. On the exhalation, that elevator goes down through the spine, through the whole body, and out through the tailbone. When inhaling, breathe up through the whole spine, connecting with the space above. Then, exhale down through the whole body. This should be performed with your eyes closed.

- Keep breathing like this, with long, steady breaths at your own pace. The mind will start to wander, so keep bringing it back to the visualization and the breath. Notice the sensation of your physical body as the breath moves up and down through the spinal column, calming and soothing your whole nervous system, signaling to your body that it has permission to relax.

- At some point, it may feel like your body doesn't want to take deep breaths anymore, and then the breath can start to become subtler. It is still rhythmic and deep, but somewhat lighter. For the next couple of minutes, let your body find its natural rhythmic breathing rate, where it is steady and constant but also peaceful and relaxed.

- If you would like to continue on with a silent meditation, focus either on your heart center or the space between your eyebrows. Continue silently affirming to yourself a word or phrase such as, "I am healthy, whole, and complete just as I am. I am here." Alternatively, you can repeat a word such as *trust*, *forgive*, *love*, or *truth*.

- Another option is to let your mind relax completely and rest in the stillness. You will notice physical sensations and changing thoughts, all on a backdrop of unchanging awareness, as well as the stillness that is present in every moment.

Class 18 Transcript

Practice 2: De-stressing with Your Breath

Hello and welcome to our class on de-stressing with the breath. Today we're going to go through several different breathing practices that you can do in your daily life. You're welcome to practice them, either one by one throughout your day, or you can do the entire class, as we're going to do today. Each breath has a little bit of a different reason why we practice. So I'll share that as we go along.

Mark is joining me here and he'll be demonstrating the breaths. So, thank you so much Mark.

So, to start out we want to think about the fact that the breath is the only function of the autonomic nervous system that we can directly affect. Therefore it is extremely important that we learn how we can effect changes in our physiology and in our mind set using the breath. In yoga we like to say that the breath reflects the mind and the mind reflects the breath. So if we're having a really stressed and tense day, if you take a moment and look at how the body's breathing, you'll notice that the breath is perhaps shallow and agitated.

However, if you're super relaxed and just lying on a beach somewhere, you can check your breath and it's probably very deep and calm and rhythmic. Likewise, you can think of a sleeping baby. A sleeping baby breaths long deep breaths into its sweet little belly, whereas a crying, screaming baby is just freaking out and you can imagine the breath, very agitated and shallow. So, we as adults are not that different than that. So the breaths we're going to do today are a great way that you can calm yourself down, just as you were calm down a baby.

The first breath we're going to do is called the three part yoga breath Absolutely anyone can do this. You've been doing it since the moment you were born, but we're just going to do more consciously. So, we'll take our right hand and place it on our bellies; the left hand is going to go on the chest.

Now before we do anything with the breath, I just want you to close your eyes for a moment and notice where you are breathing. Observe the pattern of your breath. Does your hand on your belly go up first, or does the hand on your chest go up first? Does the breath feel deep, or does it feel shallow? Typically when we get stressed we only breathe up into the very top of the lungs, or a little bit into the chest. If we want to help relax ourselves even more, we want to breathe consciously down into our abdomen.

So, now we're going to do exactly that. Breathing through your nose now as much as possible. We're going to take a deep breath, in through the nose, and you're going to send it down into your belly and you're going expand your belly like a balloon. So puff out your belly, and then breathe up into your chest all the way up to the clavicle, and then as you exhale squeeze your abdomen back in towards your spine, squeeze out all the stale air as if you're ringing out a rag, getting all the stale air out.

Then when you're done, inhaling slowly, deeply, inflating the belly when that's full, fill up the middle lungs all the way to the top. Then as you exhale feel the belly pulling in towards the spine, getting rid of all the stale air. Takes several more deep three-part breaths like this; breathing deep down into your abdomen, inflating it all the way up into the chest, up to the clavicle, and as you exhale squeezing all the stale air out of the lungs. Long full deep breaths, finding a rhythm that's right for your body. Take one more really long full deep breath.

Now you're welcome to leave your hands in position or you can place your hands down on your lap, whatever is most comfortable for you. We're going to do a very similar breath, but this time we're going to make the exhalation twice as long as the inhalation. So, if your breath last four seconds on the inhale, you're going to exhale for eight seconds. All right. So, find the rhythm that's right for you. The first time just count how long you're inhale is and then double the exhalation. So, like I said, if you're at four do eight, if you're at five do 10, like that.

All right, so like I said, leave your hands in position or you can place them on your lap, whatever's best for you. Close your eyes once more, observe the normal pattern of your breath. Now, inhaling, noticing how long your inhalation lasts. And then, however long that is, exhale for double that amount. And if it's hard to make it to the doubles number, make your breath a little slower and steadier on the exhale. Ideally, you want the exhalation to be the same intensity from the beginning till the end.

So, keep noticing how long your inhale count is, doubling the exhale count. Finding your pace. When we double the exhalation, we help evoke the relaxation response. This helps improve heart rate variability as we discuss in the lectures. Keep breathing and feeling the whole sensation of the body as the breath moves in and out.

Counting serves a dual purpose. It helps you stay on track, but it also gives your mind a point of concentration which can also help calm down the body. Take one more really full breath. And you can lower your hands down onto your lap and just notice how you're feeling after that breath.

We're going to do another breath now, which is an energizing breath practice. I like to do this breath first thing when I wake up in the morning. Sometimes I do it before I even get out of bed, I just sit up and then do the breath. Other times I'll do it before I meditate if I'm feeling sleepy and I'm afraid I'm going to fall asleep when I meditate.

This is also a really good breath to do at about three o'clock in the afternoon when I want to go for that extra cup of tea, but I know that cup of tea will keep me up at night, you can do this breath instead. It increases your oxygen count and gives you this nice boost of good, clear, crisp energy. A lot of people find it's really good for concentration and memory as well. So see how it feels to you.

So this breath is a forceful exhalation. The inhale happens naturally on its own. The breath is like this. And if you'd like, you're welcome to put your finger under your nose to see how it feels for the first couple. So, again exhaling strongly, but the inhale happens naturally, like this. Great. Yep, just like that. See you see Mark's not consciously inhaling with the breath. So that forceful exhale is helping clean out the lower lobes of the lungs.

When we're breathing very shallowly throughout our day a lot of times there's a lot of stale air that gets trapped in the lower lobes of our lungs. This breath is also really good for releasing tension, because we hold a lot of tension in our abdomens. When we do this breath the diaphragm is lifting up into the chest, which strengthens the diaphragm and abdominal muscles.

It's also really good for building core strength. You'll find the more you practice that deep exhalation will get stronger and stronger. You'll feel it in your belly. When we strengthen our respiration rates we're giving our body more chance to absorb that fresh clear oxygen and energy we need to sustain our bodies and minds.

So, this breath we're going to do 30 repetitions of what we just did, about one per second. Then we're going to take three deep breaths and we'll hold the breath for 30 seconds. While you're holding the breath, you're going to focus your attention either on your heart center or on the space between your eyebrows.

While you're doing that, you can silently affirm a word or a phrase that's important to you. For instance, if you're trying to cultivate compassion you can say that to yourself or if you have a mantra or a prayer you like to say, you're welcome to do that.

I'll keep the timing, so don't worry about that part. If you can't hold your breath for 30 seconds or you don't feel comfortable doing that, you're welcome to just take some of those deep three part breaths that we were doing at the beginning of class together.

All right, you ready? All right. So, sit with your spine nice and straight just the way Mark is, and feel the spine really long. Close your eyes. Take a long full deep breath into your belly and your chest, fill up the lungs. Exhale, settling down into the chair.

We're now going to begin the breaths, so inhale a comfortable breath and then begin. Exhale, ex, ex, ex, ex, ex, ex, ex, ex, ex, ex, ex. Keep going at a pace that is comfortable for you. You can go a little slower or faster than what Mark's doing. I'll count about 30 at his rate. And exhale completely. Inhale drawing in a nice full three part breath. Exhale completely. And now, again. Exhale.

This time you're going to inhale the breath to hold the breath. So, inhale deeply and hold the breath 30 seconds if you can. While you're holding the breath, focus on your heart or the space between your eyebrows. Pick a word that's something you're working on or a mantra and repeat that silently to that space. The more you relax your body the easier it is to hold your breath. Requires less oxygen. And gently exhale the first rounds.

Inhale deeply, exhale. Inhale another big full breath. Exhale. We're going to do two more rounds of this. So, inhale. Breath in a comfortable breath. And begin, exhale, exhale, exhale, exhale. Keep going at your own pace. And exhale completely.

Inhale, sipping in a long restorative nurturing breath. Exhale letting go of any stress or tension. Inhale deeply, exhale completely. Inhale a deep, but comfortable breath, and this time hold your breath for 30 seconds. Again, relax the body a little, so it requires less oxygen. You can feel that energy start to build in the body. That's your holding. Keep relaxing. You'll notice it gets easier. Then gently exhale. Inhale deeply, exhale fully. Inhale, and exhale.

Going to do one last round of this. Inhale a comfortable breath, and begin. Exhale, ex, ex, ex, keep going at your pace. Thirty repetitions at one per second. Gently, exhale the last one.

Inhale, fill up the belly, the chest, all the way up. Exhale. Inhale another really deep full breath. Exhale completely.

Inhale a deep, but comfortable, breath. Going to hold the breath for 30 seconds. Keep the mind focused, body relaxed. Gently exhale if you haven't already. Inhale deeply. Exhale. Inhale. Exhale. Then, before opening the eyes, observe how you're feeling after the practice.

Thank you Mark.

We're going to do one more breath, now. This next breath is called alternate nostril breathing. It takes a little bit more orientation to get this one down, but we'll make it as easy as possible. So, for this one you're going to take two fingers, your thumb and your pointer finger. We're going to be using our thumb to block the right nostril and the pointer finger to block the left nostril.

The reason we're doing this is because we're going to be breathing in through one side of the body, holding the breath, exhaling out of the other side. When we do this, we are moving from the left to the right hemisphere of our brain. And as we see through things like EMDR when we move from the left to right side of the brain it helps us process emotions, thoughts, and other experiences that we're having. It's also very good for stimulating different neuroplasticity aspects that we're working on in our resilience course.

So, as you're doing this you can visualize yourself breathing in through the whole left side of your body, holding the breath, and then exhaling out the other side of the body. So, even though you're just breathing through the nose, you kind of want to feel it on the whole side of the body that we're focusing on.

If for whatever reason you don't want to hold your breath when I am mentioning that you should retain the breath, you can just keep breathing from one side to the other.

Just as we did in the breathing practice that was improving our heart rate variability, we're going to make the exhalation double what the inhale was. So, we'll be inhaling for four seconds, holding and then exhaling for eight seconds. All right? Likewise if you have a different pace that's better for you, you're welcome to do that. What we're doing here is a general suggestion. So if it seems a little confusing, don't worry. I'm going explain it the whole way.

So, get your fingers ready. Inhale deeply through both nostrils, exhale completely through both nostrils. Gently block the right nostril with your thumb, and inhale through the left nostril for four seconds. Hold your nose, blocking both nostrils. While you're holding the breath relax the body and again you can focus on either the heart or the space between the eyebrows.

Lift your thumb, exhale for eight seconds, trying to make that exhalation very smooth in the same intensity throughout the exhale. Inhale for four seconds through the right nostril. Hold the breath blocking both nostrils.

Exhale through the left nostril. Five, six, seven, eight, inhale through the left nostril. Gently hold the breath blocking both. Exhale through the right nostril. Inhale through the right nostril for four seconds. Hold the breath blocking both nostrils. Exhale through the left for eight seconds. Inhale through for the left for four seconds. Hold the nose. Exhale through the right for eight seconds.

Inhale through the right for four seconds. Ex and then hold the breath, blocking both nostrils. Exhale through the left nostril or eight seconds. And then you can go ahead and place your hand down on your knee. Keep your eyes closed and notice how your body and mind feel after practicing that breath. It's a great breath to do if you ever feel yourself feeling tense or a little bit of anxiety or the mind ruminating. Can really help to calm down your nervous system. It's a breath designed to bring balance to your body and your mind.

We're going to do one more breath here that you're welcome to use as a meditation preparation as well. So for those of you at home who may want to do a nice meditation, silent meditation after this practice, you're welcome to keep meditating once we finish. I'll go ahead and close the class at one point, but you're welcome to keep going.

So, to do this next breath there's absolutely nothing you need to do with your body, but I'd recommend finding a position that's comfortable. A typical meditation hand position is to bring your left hand palm up and your right hand on top of it with the thumbs touching. Then straighten the spine. Go and close the eyes. And you're going to picture the whole spinal column, nice and straight, and you're going to feel like there's an elevator that goes up from the tip of your tailbone, up through your whole spine, right out the crown of your head. And on the exhalation, that elevator goes down through the spine, through the whole body, right out the tailbone connecting with the earth.

So again, inhaling, you're going to breathe up through the whole spine, connecting with the space above, exhaling down through the whole body, right out of the tailbone connecting with the earth. As we feel our body, it's a part of heaven and earth in this breath.

So, keep breathing just like this, each inhale, visualizing the breath flowing up from the earth through the spine, right out the crown of the head. And then exhaling down through the spine. Keep breathing like this, long steady breaths at your own pace.

The mind starts to wander. Keep bringing it back to the visualization and the breath. Notice the sensation of your physical body as the breath moves up and down through the spinal column, calming and soothing your whole nervous system, signaling to your body that it has permission to relax.

Some point it may feel like your body doesn't want to take those really deep breaths anymore and then the breath can start to become more subtle. Still rhythmic and deep, just a little lighter. For the next couple of minutes, letting your body find its natural rhythmic breathing rate, where its steady and constant, and at the same time peaceful and relaxed. Feeling like we're setting resetting our own rhythm here, letting the breath calm and nourish the body and mind. Finding balance inside of ourselves, no matter what is happening in the outside world.

If you would like to continue on with a silent meditation, focus either on your heart center or the space between your eyebrows. Continue silently affirming to yourself or a word or phrase, such as "I am healthy, whole and complete just as I am. I am here." Just a word like trust, forgive, love, truth. Or you can just let your mind relax completely, and rest in the stillness. Noticing physical sensations, changing thoughts, all on a backdrop of unchanging awareness. The stillness that is present every moment of everyday.

Class 19

Practice 3: Promoting Sleep

This is the sleep practice class, which you can think of as a way to prepare yourself for bed. During the first time you practice, you may want to watch the video, as an actor demonstrates the initial opening experiences. After that, you might listen to it as an audio practice, where you put it on in the background and let it guide you into a deep night's rest. This guidebook chapter provides an overview of the steps in the sleep-preparation routine.

Starting Out

- Begin by lying down. Have your blankets ready if you want to cover yourself up after the initial stretches. Find a comfortable, reclined position, and for a few moments, close the eyes and start to think about your day. Are there certain events that stand out to you from your day?

- Take a moment and think of something that might have felt challenging for you—perhaps something you said you wished you hadn't. Take a moment to consider how you would do it differently if it happened again.

- Next, bring to mind something great that happened today. If you can't think of anything great, then just think of something that went pretty well. Notice how your body feels as you consider positive events.

- Now, think of your day as a whole. Consider all the things that happened and notice what the body feels like as you start to settle. As you do this, draw your knees in toward your chest and give yourself a hug. Take a moment, curled in a ball.

Giving Thanks

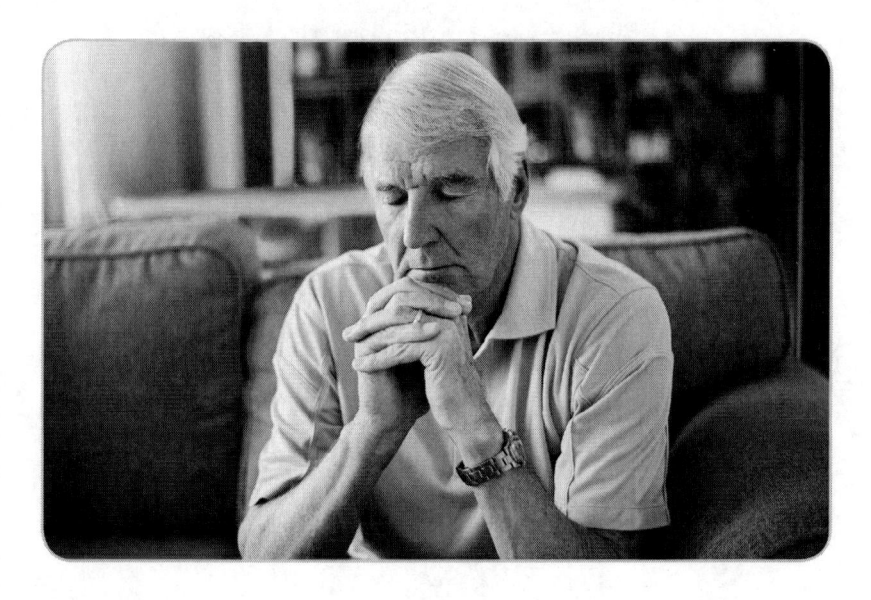

- Next, if you'd like, you can put your head down, but leave your arms wrapped around your legs. Take a moment to give thanks for your body. Think about all the things your body did today and feel gratitude toward it.

- Also give thanks to your mind. Even if there are a few things that don't seem quite right, there are actually in every moment billions of things happening right in your body and in your mind. Give thanks for those.

- Take a moment to offer any additional gratitude for whatever may have occurred today and for the people who make your life possible: your family, your friends, and your colleagues. Think of everyone who touches your day in some way. You might also express gratitude for your home, for nature, or your community.

Stretching

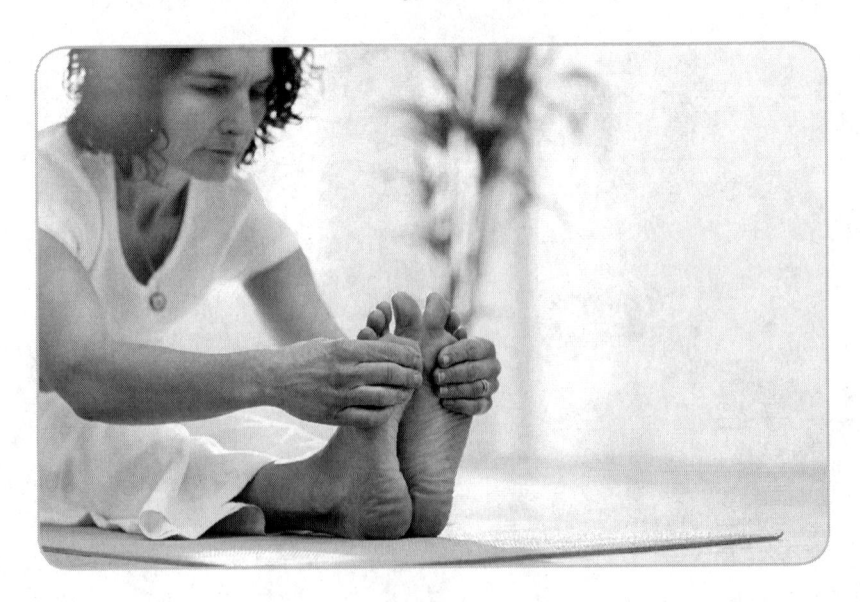

- When you're ready, stretch your legs out in front of you. Extend the arms above the head and give your body a long, full stretch. Take a couple of deep breaths, inhaling from the soles of the feet up through the whole body and out through the hands. As you exhale, breathe down through the body, out through the soles of the feet.

- Next, interlace your fingers and press your palms away from you. Flex your feet, pulling your toes back toward the body. Give the back of your body a long stretch, breathing in and out. On the exhalation, sweep the breath down through the whole body.

- Release your legs down, letting them find a comfortable resting position. If there's any tension in the lower back, you may want a bolster beneath your knees.

- For one last stretch, take your hands behind your head and interlace the fingers behind the head. You can gently pull the chin up toward the chest and turn the head to the right and the left, releasing any lingering tension in the neck. Then, place your head gently down on the pillow.

Tension and Relaxation Exercises

- Next up are the tension and relaxation exercises. Start by lifting up your right leg and squeezing your foot, calf, knee, ankle, thigh, and hamstring. Gather all the tension and then let the leg drop, just like a lead brick. After that, do the same with your left leg. Feel both of your legs. Notice the sensation: After you tense something, it tends to relax even more.

- Now, inhale, lift up both your legs, and tense your feet, ankles, calves, knees, and thighs. Tense everything in your legs and then drop. Next, lift up your hips and tense your buttocks and lower abdomen. Then, move to the lower back, tensing it and then relaxing. Drop the hips down.

- Tense your chest and lift your shoulders up toward your ears, gathering any tension in the chest and shoulders, and then releasing. Next, feel both of your arms.

- Bring the right arm into awareness. Lift the right arm up and make a fist with your right hand, tensing your hand, wrist, forearm, elbow, and upper arm. Gather all the tension that may have accumulated and then drop the arm down. Notice the difference between the right arm and left arm, and then repeat the lifting, tensing, and releasing with your left arm.

- After that, squeeze your face into a prune. Gather any tension in the face and then release. Next, extend the body, stretching out your arms and legs. Notice if there are any adjustments you'd like to make to your body. If you'd like to cover up with a blanket, this would be a good time to do so, letting the body start to find the position that you like to sleep in.

- Take a few moments to see if there's anything you could do to be more comfortable, and make those adjustments. If there's any lingering tension in the neck, you can turn the head a little to the right and the left, letting it settle eventually in the middle of the pillow. If you're a side sleeper, feel free to do the rest of the practice on your side.

Ferris Wheel Breath

- Now comes a breathing practice called the Ferris wheel breath. To begin the Ferris wheel breath, envision the entire spinal column from the tip of the tailbone all the way up to the crown of the head. Now picture a long, narrow Ferris wheel that runs up the spine and then down the back of the spine.

- Picture yourself getting on the Ferris wheel at the base of your spine, at your tailbone. On the inhalation, breathe up the Ferris wheel to the crown of your head. Notice the moment of transition at the top of the head, where the inhalation turns into an exhalation, and then breathe down the backside of the spine to your tailbone.

- Notice the moment of transition at the bottom, where the exhalation becomes an inhalation, and then breathe up the front side of the spine to the crown of the head. Again, notice the moment of transition at the top, where inhalation becomes exhalation, and then breathe down the backside of the spine to the top of the tailbone.

- Once more, notice the moment of transition from exhalation to inhalation. Continue on with the Ferris wheel breath, finding that deep, rhythmic breathing that nurtures and calms the body.

Guided Meditation

- At this point, the class transitions into a Yoga Nidra guided meditation practice. Take a moment to see if there are any additional adjustments you want to make in preparation for that practice. Then, refer to the audio or video lesson for guidance through the practice.

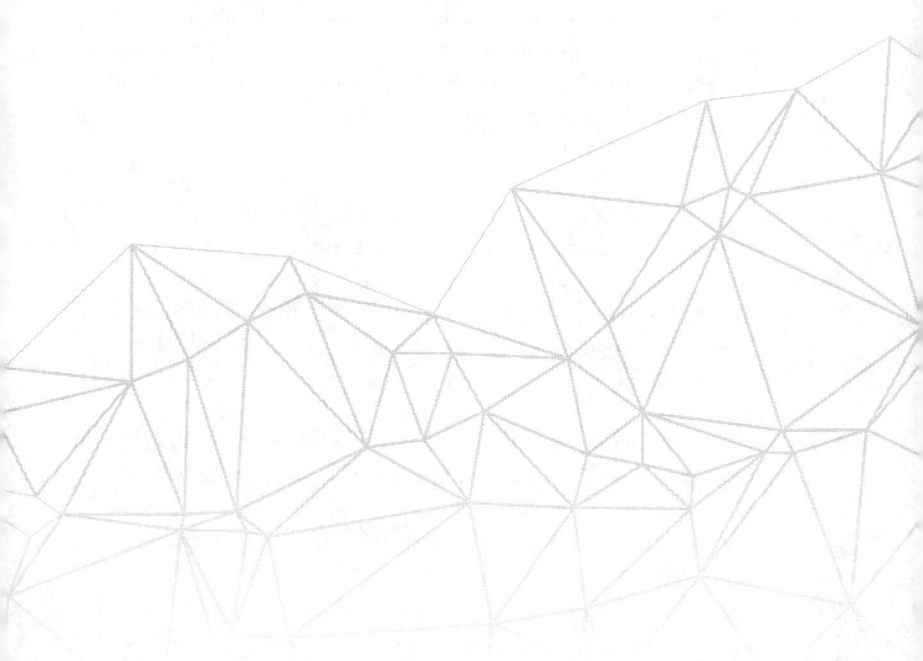

Class 19 Transcript

Practice 3: Promoting Sleep

Good evening and thank you for joining us. This is the sleep practice class, so you don't have to really think of it as a practice, but more as a way to prepare yourself for bed. During the first time you practice you may want to watch the video, and Art here demonstrated the initial opening experiences. And then after that you may want to listen to it as an audio practice, where you just put it on in the background and let it guide you into a deep night's rest. At the conclusion of the class, I will leave you in the sleeping states.

Start out lying down and to have your blankets ready if you want to cover yourself up after the initial stretches. Find a comfortable reclined position, and just for a few moments, close the eyes and start to think about your day. Are there certain events that stand out to you from your day? Take a moment and think of something that might have felt challenging for you, perhaps something you said you wished you hadn't.

Or something that happened to you, something someone else did to you perhaps. Call it to mind and notice how your body feels as you think about this. And then take a moment to consider how you would do it differently if it happened again. Try to play the experience out with a different outcome. Think of it working out coming into harmony. Even if it hasn't found harmony in your day to day real life.

And now bring to mind something great that happened today. If you can't think of anything great, then just think of something that went pretty well. Perhaps something you did that felt good. Perhaps completing a big task or spending some meaningful time with someone. Maybe you did your yoga practice today and it felt really good. Spend a few moments thinking about the things that went right today. Notice how your body feels as you consider these things that went really well.

Now think of your day as a whole. Considering all the things that happened and noticing what the body feels like as you start to settle. Think of all the things your body did today, keeping you strong healthy and alive. And as you do this draw your knees in towards your chest and give yourself a big hug. Take a moment. curled in a little ball, and then if you'd like, you can put your head down, but leave your arms wrapped around your legs and take a moment to really give thanks for your body.

Think about all the things your body did today. Give thanks to your body. Give thanks to your mind, even if there are a few things that don't seem quite right, there are actually in every moment billions of things happening right in your body and in your mind. Give thanks for those.

Take a moment to offer any additional gratitude for whatever may have occurred today or for something else in your life, for the people who make your life possible: your family, your friends, your colleagues. Think of everyone who touches your day in some way, maybe the farmer who grows the food you eat, or the people who help you in the grocery store. Everyone who touches your life in some way, give thanks. Perhaps a moment of gratitude for your home, for nature, your community.

When you're ready, you can extend your legs out in front of you. Extend the arms above the head and give your body a really long full stretch. See how long you can make the body, and here take a couple of deep breaths, inhaling from the soles of the feet up through the whole body right out the hands, and as you exhale breathe down through the body ride out the soles of the feet. Couple of deep breaths like this reversing the effects of gravity from the day.

Now you can interlace your fingers and press your palms away from you. Flex your feet pulling your toes back towards the body. Give the back side of your body a nice long stretch, breathing in and out, in through the whole body, and then on the exhale sweeping the breath down through the whole body. Now release your legs down let them find a comfortable resting position. If there's any tension in the lower back you may want a bolster beneath your knees just as Art is using here.

For one last little stretch, take your hands behind your head and interlace the fingers behind the head. You can gently pull the chin up towards the chest and turn the head a little bit to the right and the left releasing any lingering tension in the neck. Then place your head gently down on the pillow.

We'll now be moving through the tension and relaxation exercises. So, you can start lifting up your right leg, squeezing your foot, your calf, your knee, your ankles, your thigh, your hamstring, the whole right leg, tense it really, really tight. Gather all the tension and then let the leg drop, just like a lead brick, just let it drop.

Now the left leg. And now left the left leg up, tense your foot, your ankle, your calf, your knee, your thigh, and hamstring, the whole left leg is tight. Gather all the tension and then drop. Now feel both of your legs. Notice the sensation of the legs and notice the before and after, how after we tense something it tends to relax even more.

Now, inhale, lift up both your legs and tense your feet, your ankles, your calves, knees, thighs. Tense everything in your legs and then drop. Now lift up your hips and tense your buttocks, your lower abdomen. Perhaps the lower back, tense tight, tight, tight and relax. Drop the hips down.

Now, tense your chest and lift your shoulders up towards your ears, gather any tension in the chest and shoulders.

And then release. Now feel both of your arms. Bring the right arm into awareness. Lift the right arm up, make a fist with your right hand, tense a fist with your hand, your wrist, your forearm, your elbow, your upper arm, make a big muscle. Gather all the tension that may have accumulated and then drop the arm down. Notice the difference between the right and the left arm.

Now, lift up your left arm, squeeze your hand, make a fist with your hand. Some people like to keep their arm high like Art is and others like to keep their arm lower, maybe just an inch or two above the bed. Tense your whole fist, wrist, forearm, elbow, upper arm, make a big muscle. Gather all the tension and release the arm down.

Now squeeze your face into a prune. Make a funny raisin face. Gather any tension in the face, and then release. Now extend out the body, just stretching out their arms where they are, stretching out the legs, noticing if there's any other adjustments you'd like to make to your body. And if you'd like to cover up with a blanket this would be a good time to do so, letting the body start to find the position that you like to sleep in.

Taking a few moments to see if there's anything you could do to be five or 10 percent more comfortable, making those adjustments. If there's any lingering tension in the neck, you can turn the head a little to the right and the left, back and forth, letting it settle in and eventually in the middle of the pillow. Or if you're a side sleeper you're welcome to do the rest of the practice on your side.

We're going to do a breathing practice called the Ferris wheel breath, and then as we ease through that we'll finish with a guided meditation that will leave you deeply sleeping. If you have any trouble sleeping you may want to set an intention for your practice that you will sleep a long eight hours or however long you intend to rest and will awaken feeling healthy and refreshed.

To begin the Ferris wheel breath, envision the entire spinal column from the tip of the tailbone all the way up to the crown of the head. Now picture a long narrow Ferris wheel that runs up the spine and then down the back side of the spine. Picture yourself now getting on the Ferris wheel at the base of your spine at your tailbone and on the inhale, inhale breathing up the Ferris wheel right to the crown of your head. Notice that moment of transition at the top of the head where the inhale turns into an exhale and then breath down the whole backside of the spine right to your tailbone.

Noticed that moment of transition at the bottom where exhale becomes inhale and then breath up the front side of this spine, right to the crown of the head. Notice that moment of transition at the top where inhale becomes exhale, and then breathe down the backside of the spine right to the top of the tailbone, noticing that moment of transition where exhale becomes inhale. Continue on with the Ferris wheel breath, finding that deep rhythmic breathing that nurtures and calms the body.

Become very absorbed in those moments of transition where inhale becomes exhale and exhale becomes inhale, feeling how the whole body experiences this. Notice if the mind has wandered and bring it back to the Ferris wheel breath, breathing up and down the spinal column. Now let the breaths start to slow down.

Take a moment to see if there's any additional adjustments you want to make in preparation for the Yoga Nidra guided meditation practice. Once your body is found it's settling place, take a moment to feel that entire plane of contact between the body and the surface beneath you, feeling how the bed supports your body. All the places that are being supported by the mattress: the blanket and the air. Feel how the body is being held. See if you can give yourself a little more fully to that surface. Giving yourself permission to settle. The day is done. Nothing more you need to do. No one you need to be, other than exactly who you are in this moment.

Bring to mind a feeling of well-being and safety, perhaps thinking of something that brings you a sense of safety and comfort, sense of sense of well-being. Perhaps a place you love or being together with certain people who are special to you. Maybe it's being alone in meditation. Notice how as you evoke this feeling of safety and well-being the body may start to feel warm, relaxed, comfortable. Breathing may start to become easy and rhythmic. The belly and the hands are warm, relaxed. You're welcome to set that intention to have a long deep restful night's sleep. And in the morning to awaken refreshed, clear, healthy, and ready for the day. Now it's time for sleep.

Now listen to your heart. How does your heart feel in this moment? Just the physical sensation of the heart. Ask yourself the question, what do I want more than anything else in life? Whatever it is place it in a sentence in the present tense, as if it's already a fact and true. I am healthy, whole, and complete just as I am. For I am peaceful and at ease.

Letting the sound of my voice become the sound of your own voice now, as we turn our attention through the physical body, as each area of the body is named, bring your attention there and experience the sensation. You may feel something or nothing at all. Whatever you experience is absolutely perfect.

Start by becoming aware of the mouth, feeling the invisible plane of contact between the two lips, the density of the teeth, soft tongue floating in the mouth, observing any sense of taste present. Feeling the ears and sound arriving at the ears. Sound making its way from the outer ears into the inner ears. Feeling the whole body receiving the vibration of sound, the obvious sounds, the subtle sounds.

Feel the nose, the air flowing in and out of the nose, noticing the difference between the inhalation and the exhalation. One may feel a little stronger, the other a little softer. One may feel a little warmer, the other a little cooler, serving any sense of smell present.

Feel the two eyelids gently touching. Feel the eyelids, eye resting back in the head. Space behind the eyes. Observe if there's any lights or color filtering through the eyelids. Or if perhaps the mind is projecting an image of the space around you or something else. Fill the forehead, cool to alive with sensation. Feel that sensation melting back into the brain. Feel the brain becoming calm and clear, like a still pool of water and can easily see the bottom.

Feel the scalp and the place where the air touches the scalp. Feel all the sensations in the head at once, whole head feeling down into the neck and throat. Feeling down into the arms, sensation cascading down both arms, upper arms, elbows, forearms, wrists, and hands. Feel the palms of the hands and all of the fingers.

Now feeling the chest and the upper back. Feeling the sensation of the heartbeat in the chest, the subtle rhythm of life, your rhythm you've known since before the beginning. Feeling down into the abdomen and lower back, noticing any sensation in the abdomen. Feel the hips, the buttocks, and pelvis, feeling down through the upper legs into the knees, the lower legs, the ankles and feet. Feel the soles of the feet and all of the toes.

Now all parts of the body become one. Sense the sensation of your entire body at once. Whole body, its pure sensation, the feeling of being in your body, exactly who you are. Welcoming yourself just exactly as you are.

Observing the pathway of the breath now and noticing the breath as it makes its way across the nostrils and then into the throat, feeling the breath pass across the throat. Feel your chest rise and fall with each breath. Feeling your abdomen rise and fall. I see breath in and out.

Now feel the whole body breathing itself. Feel the subtle expansion that occurs in the body with each inhalation.

Feel the subtle release that occurs with each exhalation, as if your surrounded by an ocean of air and how it's like a wave from that ocean of air rises up into the chest. Exhale, that wave of air melts back into its source. That constant connection with your surroundings, that constant connection with every living being. Feel yourself as a part of the whole. Connected. Aware, also still, at peace.

Observe the mind and just notice if there are any feelings, emotions, or beliefs that may be present. What are those feel like in the body? Is there a message they're trying to share? Make a note that you know come back to it tomorrow, after a deep night's rest.

You feel the heart. Very warm, alive and filled with love. May help to think of people you love very much. Feel that love emanating out from the heart and in all directions. Infinite love doesn't even need a reason or a destination. Love that is vast and abundant. All the love she'll ever need. All the love that wants to be shared through you.

Feel that love expanding out through every cell of your body. As if, every single cell of your body was being bathed in this loving kindness, welcoming you just as you are. Loving you just exactly as you are. Feel this warmth of love. Feel that love expanding out to the space around you, filling your home and everyone and everything in it with love.

Love expanding out to your community, all the people in your life, and all the the people you know and maybe don't even know, sending them love too. Love expanding out, for nature, and all living beings. Feel this love guiding you back into stillness. This love that welcomes all, heals all as well. Creates wholeness where before, perhaps, there was separation. Feel your wholeness, the stillness that is your true nature: healthy, whole, and complete, exactly as you are. Abiding in the deep stillness of your true nature, at home in yourself.

Rest here for a deep night's sleep.

Class 20

Practice 4: Relaxing Yoga for Self-Care

This class focuses on yoga practice for self-care. The video class demonstrates these poses in chair and floor variations, and this guidebook chapter provides a summary of the activities.

If a pose or movement does not feel right to you, modify it so that it feels good or skip it. It is also a good idea to check with your doctor if you have any questions about if these practices are suitable for your body.

Breathing Practice

- This class begins with a breathing practice that also uses the arms and incorporates a gratitude element. Begin with your arms out to the sides. On a deep inhalation, extend your arms out to the sides and lift up, bringing your arms up over your head and into the prayer position. On an exhalation, draw your hands down toward the heart.

- Connect with your heart. Inhale and extend the arms up into the air, and when you exhale, extend the hands out and down. Take several more breaths. On each inhalation, think about whatever it is your body and mind need. On each exhalation, exhale, thinking of gratitude for all the blessings in life. Once finished, relax your arms toward your sides and find a comfortable resting position for your hands.

Neck Stretching

- The next part of this practice involves neck rotations to help release the tension in your neck. If you have any neck issues, don't bring your head backward when doing the neck rotation. Instead, keep it in a neutral position. If you have a healthy neck, feel free to slightly relax it backward.

- To start out, bring your chin down toward your chest and begin rolling the head to the right. Inhale, then roll the head back and exhale. Repeat this at your own pace. Eventually, you can switch directions. Throughout, listen to your body and feel the breath.

- Next, bring the head back to a neutral position. Lift your shoulders up toward your ears, gathering any tension in your shoulders. Drop the shoulders down, inhale, and lift them up again. Again, gather any tension, and then drop the shoulders. Repeat this process one more time.

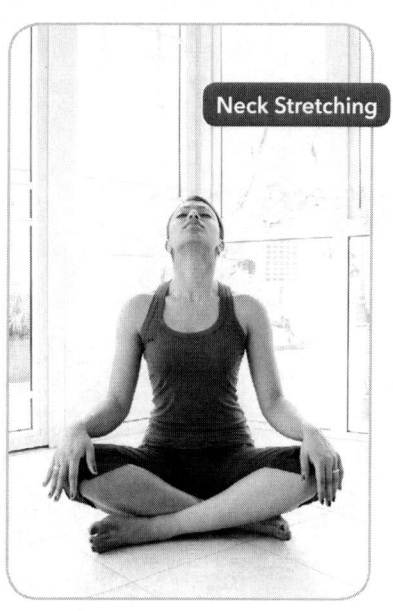

- After that, roll your shoulders forward in big rotations before going in the opposite direction. Roll your shoulder blades back together and down behind you. Next, inhale and extend your arms over your head. Stretch up, feeling as if someone is lifting your arms up.

- When you exhale, bring the arms down. At this stage, you can either interlace your hands behind you or bring them back onto a chair. Repeat this step a couple of times at your own pace before re-centering yourself.

Shoulder Stretching

- The class's next phase is a stretch for the shoulders. There are two ways to do it. The more accessible version of it is to bring the hands and elbows together, and then lift the elbows slightly up and bring the hands slightly out. Notice where you feel the best stretch, and then breathe.

- The other option is to swing your right arm over your left, interlace your hands, and lift the elbows up slightly and the hands out and away. Notice where you feel the best stretch, and then breathe.

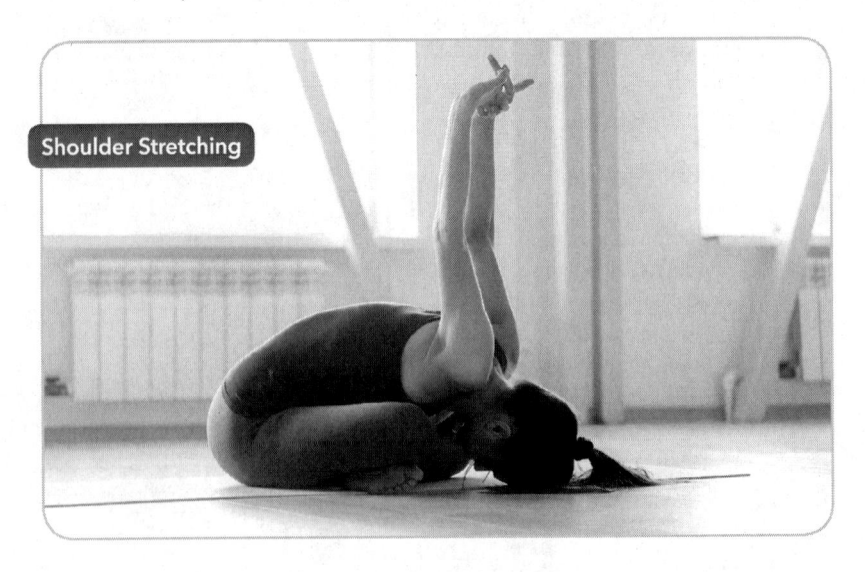

Shoulder Stretching

- After a couple of deep breaths, release the arms and switch sides. If your hands were together, you can shake your arms out for a moment before lifting them up again. If you're doing the other version, swing the left arm over the right this time. In either case, lift the elbows up and the hands slightly out and away. Then, consciously send breaths into any points of tension between the shoulder blades. When you're done, release the arms and shake them out.

Cat-Cow Pose

- Next up is the cat-cow yoga pose. One option is to place your hands on your knees. Then, roll your shoulders down and gaze at your belly button. After that, open up, bringing the head back and arching the back.

- The other option is to go onto your hands and knees, with your hands beneath your shoulders and your knees beneath your hips. The feet will be about hip-distance apart. On each inhalation, lift your head up and arch your back, and on each exhalation, tuck your head and tailbone down to stretch out the spine.

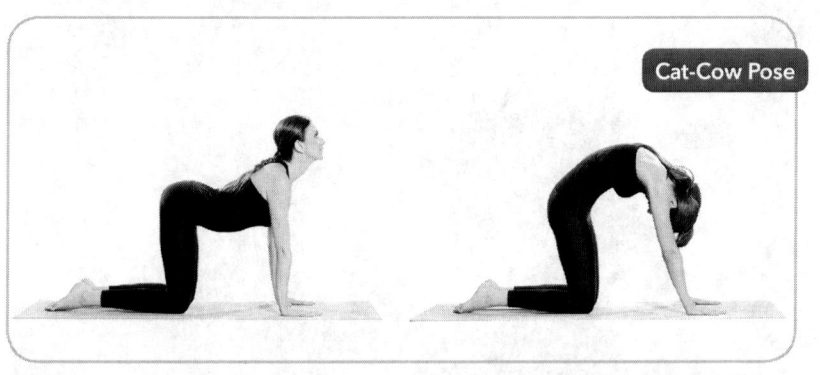

Cat-Cow Pose

Yoga involves listening to your body and finding the union between the body, breath, emotions, and spirit.

Rotations

- The class's next phase involves rotations. To do them from a seated position, leave your hands on your knees, or bring them back a bit if that feels better. Next, make big circles with your torso. Listen to your body to find the rhythm.

- The other method is to bring your hands out about as wide as your mat with your knees together. Make your hips go in a large circle. Whichever option you are doing, at some point, you may want to switch directions. When finished, come to a neutral position.

- Next, come down onto your back on the ground. Hug your knees into your chest. If you'd like, you can make some circles on the base of your spine for a lower-back massage. While hugging your legs, close your eyes and give thanks for your body.

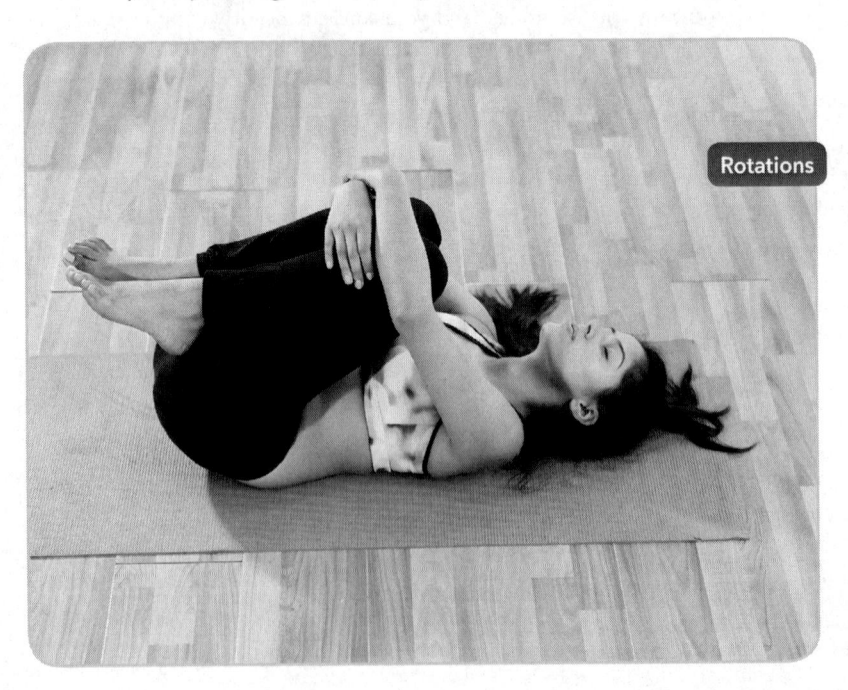

Rotations

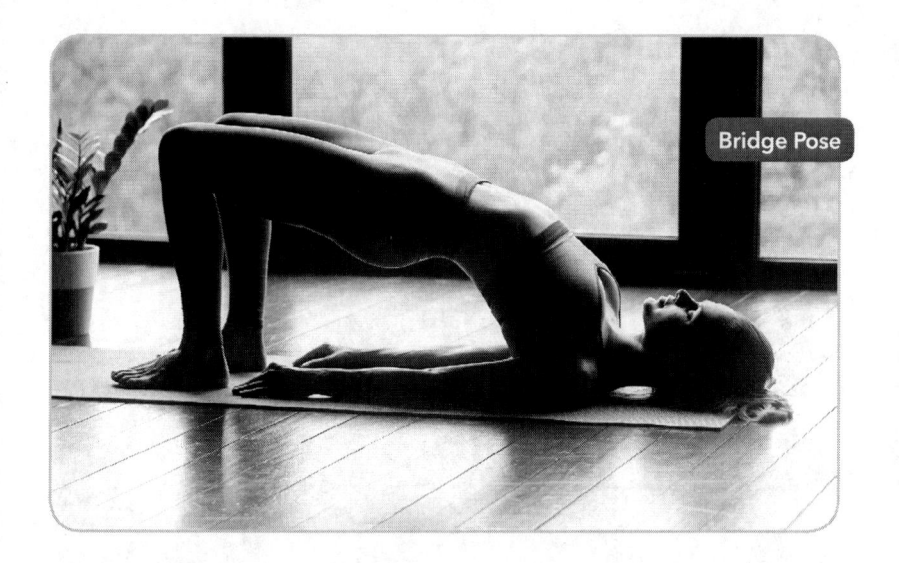

Bridge Pose

- The class's next step is preparation for the bridge pose. Place your feet roughly hip-distance apart. Bring your arms up over your head. Visualize the entire spine supported by the floor beneath you. Next, lift the tailbone very gently up off the mat, slowly lifting the hips up.

- Once you reach the farthest position that is comfortable for you, hold there for a few moments. Then, slowly place your back down on the mat until you get to the tailbone. When you get down to the tailbone, tip the pelvis forward to form a small arch in your lower back. Repeat this at your own pace, inviting your body to relax.

Shoulder Stand

- After the bridge pose comes the shoulder stand. To perform a chair variation, wiggle yourself close to the chair and place your calves on the

Shoulder Stand

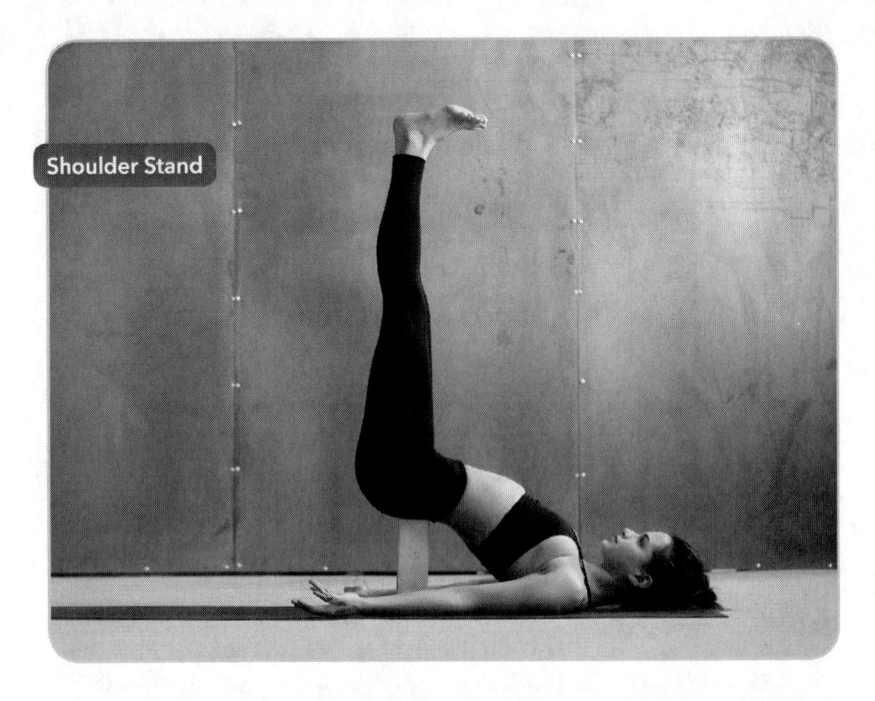

chair. To perform a variation with a block, find the height of the block that is comfortable for you, and then rest your sacrum on the block.

- Once you're in position, feel your body relax. Next, lift the right leg up, taking a couple of deep breaths. Then, bring the leg down before bringing the other leg up and slowly down. If you're doing the chair variation, leave your legs in position.

- If you're doing the other variation, you can try lifting both of your legs up for an additional experience with the pose. Keep in mind that whichever variation you choose, some days, one may feel better than the other.

- When you're done, slowly bring your legs back down. If you are using the block, you can remove it before lying down flat on your back. If you're working in the chair, you can now come down off the chair before slowly coming back into a seated position on the chair.

The Spinal Twist

- This class's next move is a spinal twist. If you're in the chair, bring your right arm behind your body. Find a comfortable position. Then, take your left hand and bring it over to the side, either on your knee or on the arm of the chair. Once you're in position, gently turn your head and gaze toward the left.

- If you're lying on the ground, bring your leg up, place it just below the knee, and then extend your leg out to the side as your head turns and gazes toward the other side. Once you're in position, take some long, deep breaths up and down the spinal column. Next, slowly come to the center.

- Switch sides and repeat the process. Once finished, re-center yourself. If you're lying down, extend the leg out in front of you.

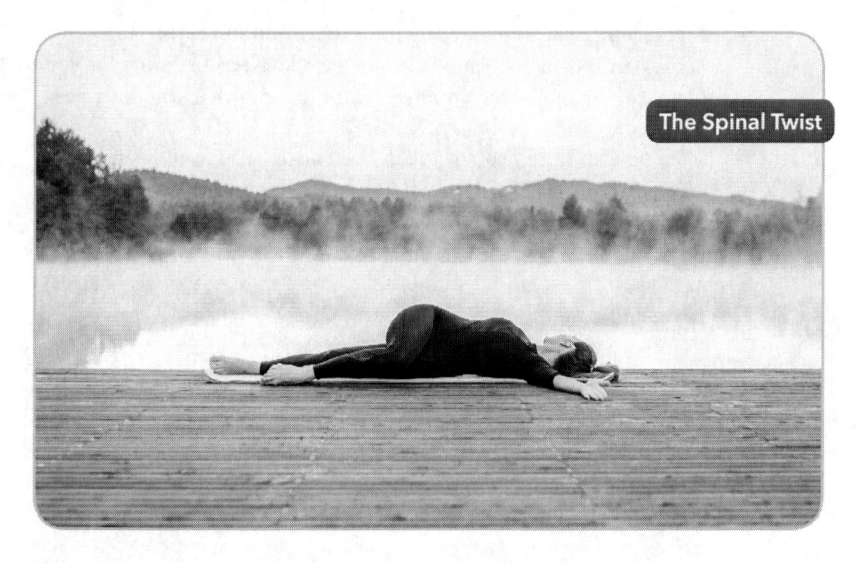

The Spinal Twist

Tension and Relaxation

- The next phase focuses on tension and relaxation, and the steps are the same whether in a chair or lying down. To begin, notice the body, and then take three deep breaths. Inhale fully before exhaling completely.

- After that, inhale again, lifting your arms and legs up. Tense your feet, calves, knees, thighs, hips, pelvis, lower back, abdomen, upper back, chest, arms, and hands. Make your face like a prune. Hold everything and drop. Next, extend out your arms and legs, and stretch your body for a moment in whatever way feels good.

The Final Relaxation Pose

- This class concludes with a final relaxation pose and a breathing exercise that will accompany that. Place your right hand on your abdomen and your left hand on your chest. Take five very conscious deep breaths. On each inhalation, think of whatever it is you need—perhaps relaxation, patience, or compassion. Breathe it in.

- As you exhale, breathe out anything that is no longer serving you—perhaps an old idea, relationship, or object. Keep breathing at your own pace, inhaling what you need and exhaling what you don't need.

- When you finish up, you can relax your arms by your sides and sit for a couple of minutes. Feel the whole plane of contact between the body and the surface beneath you. Observe the sensation of your physical body, welcoming yourself just as you are.

Class 20 Transcript

Practice 4: Relaxing Yoga for Self-Care

Welcome to your yoga practice for self-care. I'm joined today by two friends, Leslie, who is going to be demonstrating the chair variations of the poses, and Jen who will be demonstrating the floor versions of the poses. Most of the poses we're going to be doing today are fairly assessable for most people. But, of course, if anything at all doesn't feel right to you, please make the practice work for you or don't do it. It's also maybe a good idea to check with your doctor if you have any questions at all about if these practices are suitable for your body.

Keep in mind these practices are all about self-care. So, every one of the practices should be something that feels nourishing, calming, and soothing for your body. There are many different styles of yoga. This one is really about taking care of your body and giving thanks for it throughout the practice.

Going to start out with a breathing practice that also uses our arms and incorporates a gratitude practice. So begin with your arms out to the sides. On a deep inhalation extend your arms out to the sides and lift up, bringing your arms up over your head, and into the prayer position. On an exhale, draw your hands right down towards the heart.

Connect with your heart, and on an inhale extend the arms up into the air, on the exhale extend the hands out and down.

Now we'll add another component. Each inhale, think about whatever it is your body and mind need. Drive right into the heart. Connect with the heart, inhale, sending love up and exhale sending gratitude out for all the blessings in your life.

Inhaling, drawing in whatever it is you need to feel healthy and alive. Exhale right into the heart. Connect with the heart. Sense of love. Inhale, extend the arms up over your head. Exhale, sending out love and gratitude.

Keep going like this for several more breaths at your own pace. Each inhale drawing in whatever it is your body and mind need. Each exhale sending out love and gratitude for all the blessings in life and perhaps even for the challenges that are here teaching you valuable lessons. You can go as fast or as slowly as you'd like, being really conscious of the breath.

Two or three more, sipping in whatever you need, drawing it into the heart, connecting with love and kindness and breathing that out into the world with a sense of gratitude. And then relax your arms towards your sides, find a comfortable resting position for your hands.

A lot of times during busy modern lives we hold a lot of tension in our neck. So, we're going to do a couple of neck rotations now to help release the tension. If you have any neck issues don't bring your head backwards when we do the neck rotation, just keep it in a more neutral position. If you have a healthy neck you're welcome to relax it back just a little bit.

To start out bring your chin down towards your chest and begin rolling the head to the right, inhaling, rolling the head back and exhaling down the other side. You keep going at your own pace. Hanging out any place that may need a little bit of an extra stretch. Listening to your body. Remember yoga is a practice of deep listening, where we have this beautiful opportunity to listen to whatever the body needs to feel healthy and alive. You can go the other way with the neck, switching directions. Again, really listening to the body, giving it the stretch it needs, feeling the breath moving the body.

After this last one, bringing the head back to neutral. And when you do, lift your shoulders up towards your ears, gather any tension in your shoulders, anything you're holding onto from the day. And then drop the shoulders down.

Inhale, lift the shoulders up again. Gather any tension and then drop. One more. Lift the shoulders up, and then drop.

Now, roll your shoulders forward in big rotations. These are nice poses you can even do at your desk. Then go the opposite direction.

Then sit with your spine, nice and long, rolling your shoulder blades back together and down behind you. Now, inhale, extend your arms up above your head. And after you do that stretch up, feeling as if someone is lifting your arms up out of your shoulder blades. And then on the exhale, bring the arms down and then you have a choice: you can do what Jen is doing here, interlacing your hands behind you; or you can do what Leslie is doing and bring the hands back on the chair just behind you.

Breath here for a moment and then go through it a couple more times at your own pace, inhaling the arms up, feeling that nice stretch like you're growing. And then when you're ready, sweeping the arms back and down, either placing them behind you or interlacing the fingers. Finding a rhythm with the breath and the movements. Rhythm is a form of self-care. When we synchronize our movements with the breath you can find a whole new layer of resilience. And now come center.

We're going to do a nice stretch now for the shoulders. This is a great one if you've been typing a lot at a computer or carrying heavy things. These are the eagle arms. So, there's two ways to do this. Leslie is going to demonstrate the more assessable version of it by bringing the hands and elbows together, and then to get into the shoulders a little more you can lift the elbows up just slightly and bring the hands just slightly out. Notice where you feel the best stretch and then breath.

Over here Jen is going to demonstrate. You're going to swing your right arm over your left, interlace your hands and then again, lift the elbows up just slightly and the hands out and away from you. Notice where you feel the best stretch between the shoulder blades and then breathe deeply into that space.

In the practice of yoga, we say that any place where there's tension in the body is where the energy is stuck or not moving. Our breath is energy. It's our life force. So, if you want to relax a part of the body, you can take a deep inhale in and direct the breath to the place where there's tension in the body. Then as you exhale you can release the tension. Each inhale nourishing the body with that fresh clear breath, each exhale breathing out the tension. Do this for a couple of breaths here, opening up between the shoulder blades.

After a couple of deep breaths, release the arms and switch sides. If your hands were together as Leslie was doing it, just shake her arms out for a moment and then you can lift them up again just as they were. If you're doing the practice Jen is doing, swing the left arm over the right this time. And in either case lift the elbows up and the hands a little bit out in away from you. Then consciously send breaths into any points of tension between the shoulder blades. Each inhale nourishing the body, each exhale releasing tension. Every single breath we take throughout the day gives us this opportunity to absorb whatever it is we need and to release anything we don't need any longer.

Now, release the arms and shake them out a little. We're now going to do the cat-cow pose, which is honestly my favorite yoga pose. It's really simple, so most people can do it in one version or another. We're going to have Leslie over here, she's going to place her hands on her knees and then she's going to roll her shoulders down and gaze down towards her bellybutton, and then she's going to open up, bring the head back, arch the back and going back and forth like this.

Jen is going to come onto her hands and knees with her hands beneath her shoulders and her knees beneath her hips, feet are about hip distance apart. Each inhale she's going to lift her head up and arch the back, each exhale she's going to tuck her head and tailbone down and stretch out the spine. Let the breath move the body.

So, oftentimes we move in the breath follows. But through yoga we want to learn to see how we can use the breath to carry the body. This is one of the fundamental principles of resilience. The breath is our energy. It's like the wave that our body can surf on as we move through life. When we learn to move through life using the breath, we become more resilient because we always have enough energy. The breath is that life.

So, let the breath carry you. The breath also evokes the relaxation response. Keep going. You can go at whatever pace is good for you. Some people like to go really slowly, others more quickly. Whatever is right for you.

Listening to your body finding that union between the body, the breath, the emotions, and the spirit. That's what yoga means—union, to yoke the body the mind and the spirit.

Now you can bring your spine slowly to a neutral position. Now we're going to do some rotations. So, Leslie will demonstrate how to do them if you're in a seated position. You're going to leave your hands on your knees. Or if you'd like you can bring them a little farther back, whatever feels good to you. And then you're going to make big circles with your torso and just find what feels right. Again, listening to the body finding the rhythm, getting some nice mobility in the spine going one direction.

Jen is going to bring her hands out about as wide as the mat, her knees together, and she's going to make her hips go in a really big circle. So, going in one direction for a little while. Again, finding your rhythm. Find the breath first, take some long deep breaths and then let the movements flow with the breath. At some point, you may want to switch directions. That's fine, too. Again, every single pose is an invitation. Find what feels good to your body.

And then come to a neutral position.

We're now going to invite you to come down onto your back on the ground. So, preparing first here for a nice pose that should feel very nurturing. So, go ahead and lie down on your back. And before we do anything else just hug your knees into your chest. You can make some circles on the base of your spine giving the lower back a really nice massage here. And then hug your legs in and just take a moment to close the eyes and really give thanks to your body. So, thankful for the billions of things your body is doing right now for you to feel healthy and alive.

Now bring your feet down just below the hips. We're preparing for the bridge pose. So, you want your feet to be about hip distance apart. Going to bring your arms up over your head. This might be a little different than you may have done bridge pose in the past. This is a very nurturing way to do the bridge that gives an extra benefit of evoking the relaxation response, because it's really driven by the breath. It also gives a beautiful massage to the whole spinal column.

So, before you even begin the practice, close the eyes for a moment and visualize the entire spine supported by the floor beneath you, from the tip of the tailbone all the way up right out the crown of the head. Now you're going to lift the tailbone very gently up off the mat and as if you're elongating a beautiful strand of pearls you're going to lift one vertebra up off the mat at a time slowly, slowly lifting the hips up.

Once you reach the farthest position that's comfortable for you, you're going to hold there for just a few moments, feeling the soles of the feet pressing into the earth, feeling the strength of the body. And then just as slowly as you came up you're going to place a vertebra by vertebra back down on the mat until you get to the tailbone. When you get down to the tailbone you're going to tip the pelvis forward so you get a little arch in your lower back. This gives a nice compression to the adrenals and kidneys.

Remember to breath the whole time and then slowly you're going to press the lower back down into the mat and then again begin elongating that beautiful strand of pearls. This time you can move through it entirely at your own pace, holding at the top for as long as feels comfortable to you. And then after rolling down, giving that nice little arch to the lower back. Letting the breath carry the movements. Feeling the movements surfing on the wave of the breath. You know how you're caring for your spine, caring for your nervous system. Inviting your body to relax.

Do one more at your own pace. Then once you're finished you can hug your knees into your chest once more, and if you'd like make a couple of little circles. Give yourself one little nice hug. And then preparing for the next pose, which is going to be a beautiful invitation to do a variation of the shoulder stand, but a really nurturing one.

So, if you're doing Lesley's variations you're going to wiggle yourself up closer to the chair, and then you're going to place your calves on the chair. Then once you get in position you can wiggle up even a little bit more. Jen is going to demonstrate how to do the pose with a block. So, Jen if you want to go ahead and grab the block, you'll want to find the height of the block that's right for you and comfortable. Jen selected a medium height. Rest the sacrum right on the block.

Once you're here, feel your body relax. Feel how the body is supported. Then we're going to do a little bit of a variation, so, we lift the right leg up off of the chair, take a couple of deep breaths here. And then bring the leg down and then you can switch legs, bringing the other leg up. Breathing the whole time. And then slowly coming down.

Now, if you're doing the variation Leslie is doing, just leave your legs in position. If you're doing Jen's variation you can try lifting both of your legs up for a little extra experience of the pose. Keep in mind that sometimes, even if you do a variation like Jen is doing, some days you might feel better doing what Leslie's doing. Some days the best thing you can do is just give your body a nice restorative pose. Other days the body wants a little challenge and needs to move a little more. Wherever you are at, it's perfect.

Take a few more deep breaths. We spend all day on our feet. So, it's really nice to be on this restorative pose a little bit upside down. You can slowly bring your legs back down. If you have the block beneath the hips you can remove it. And then lie down flat on your back. If you're working in the chair, you can now slowly come down off the chair, taking all the time you need and slowly coming back up into a seated position on the chair. If you're lying down, you can extend your legs out in front of you.

We're now going to do a spinal twist. If you're in the chair, bring your right arm behind your body and you can find a place that feels comfortable, either on the back of the chair or on the cushion behind you. Then take your left hand and bring it over to the side, either on your knee or on the arm of the chair. Once you're in position, gently turn your head and gaze towards the left.

If you're lying on the ground, we're going to do the exact same thing. So, bring your leg up, place it just below the knee and then extend your leg out to the side as your head turns and gazes towards the other side. Once you're in position take some long deep breaths up and down the spinal column, giving a really nice breath massage to your spine. So, good for your nervous system; calms everything down. I like to do this pose before I even get out of bed in the morning.

And then slowly come center. We're going to switch sides, so whatever side you were doing, now do the opposite side. The side that your knee goes to if you're on the floor is the opposite side that your arm and head go to. Again, close the eyes and take several long full breaths up and down the spine. And come back to center, extend the leg out in front of you if you're lying down, and prepare yourself for what will be the tension and relaxation exercises.

It is oftentimes through experiencing conscious tension that we realize where we're holding tension in our bodies and are then able to release it even more fully. We're going to do this now with the entire body. So, before we do it I just want you to observe the current state of your body. Notice anywhere that you're holding tension. Oftentimes people will say to me, why are you making us tense if you want us to relax? But again, it's kind of like working with opposite emotions. The more you are consciously able to tense your body, when you relax you'll be able to relax even more fully.

So, notice the body. We're going to take three deep breaths and then we're going to tense every single muscle in the body at once. We're going to hold it for a few breaths and we're going to drop everything and relax the body. You can do this either in the chair or lying down. It's the same.

So, observe the body and then let's take these three deep breaths. Inhale fully, exhale completely. Inhale feels as if every cell of your body is breathing in. And then exhale relax. Now, inhale, lift your arms and legs up, tense your feet, your calves, knees, thighs, hips, pelvis, lower back, abdomen, upper back, chest, arms, hands, tight. Make your face like a prune. Hold everything and drop. Extend out your arms and legs and watch your body take a moment here to just stretch, whatever stretch your body needs to do. Just listen to the body and if maybe your arms want to come above your hand or you want to stretch out, do whatever feels good. Anything your body needs to feel complete.

We're going to be moving into the final relaxation and a breathing exercise that will accompany that. You can place your right hand on your abdomen and your left hand on your chest. We're going to take five very conscious deep breaths. And again, each inhale, think of whatever it is you need. Maybe it's to relax. Maybe it's patience. Maybe it's kindness or compassion. Breath it in, the deepest fullest breath.

And as you exhale, breathe out anything that is no longer serving you. Maybe it's an old idea or belief. Maybe it's a relationship. Maybe it's an object. Keep breathing at your own pace. Inhaling whatever it is you need, and as you exhale so fully breathing out whatever it is you don't need. Realize how the body has been doing this since the first moment you were born. Your breath has been carrying you always, nurturing and supporting you every step of your life.

Two more full breaths, breathing in what you need, and out what is no longer serving you. Finish up your last breath, and when you do you can relax your arms by your side, and we'll sit just for a couple of minutes in final relaxation pose.

Feel that whole plane of contact between the body and the surface beneath you. Really give yourself to that surface, letting yourself be held. Observing the sensation of your physical body, welcoming yourself just as you are. Welcoming your breath just as it is. Welcoming your mind, all your thoughts, feelings, emotions, and memories. Welcoming them all home, abiding in the deep stillness of your true nature.

It is in this moment: healthy, whole, and complete, just as you are. Rest here in the stillness for as long as you'd like.

Thank you so much for practicing with us today. *Namaste*.

Class 21

Practice 5: Practicing Mindfulness

This practice class focuses on mindfulness, which is all about paying attention on purpose. This guidebook chapter is a companion to the video or audio class, which you'll need to watch or listen to for the full experience. The chapter includes tips to prepare for the practice and considerations to be aware of as you complete the video or audio class.

Preparing for the Practice

- This class's mindfulness practice lasts about half an hour. You may want to take a few moments to gather up any creature comforts, such as a blanket, pillow, or a bolster for beneath your knees. Go ahead and start to get comfortable.

- During the practice, the instructor will guide you through different experiences. You may be very alert and aware of everything that's happening, or you might be in a space between asleep and awake, where you hear the sound of the instructor's voice without necessarily holding onto everything she says.

- Regardless of your experience, it is perfect, even if you fall asleep. Take this class as an invitation to rest and be present, welcoming yourself just as you are.

During the Practice

- From time to time, the instructor will prompt you to be aware of all five of your senses: taste, touch, smell, sight, and sound. The instructor will also prompt you to pay attention to sensations in different parts of your body, such as your chest and abdomen. They all play a role in receiving your experience of the present moment.

- You will also be prompted to notice any thoughts, feelings, emotions, or beliefs as they arise, unfold, and dissolve in your mind. This will occur once at the start of the practice and again near the end. Another section of the practice involves picturing yourself in another place and time, and paying attention to the sensations that brings.

- One section of the practice involves a specific breathing direction. You'll begin by feeling the left side of your body breathing in on an inhalation, and then breathing out through the right side of your body. You will breathe like this for a time before switching sides and directions. The mind may begin to wander during this stage, and if it does, simply refocus it on your breathing.

- Over time, the practice builds toward a state of awareness and stillness. Eventually, near the end, the instructor will ask you to welcome a deeper breath into the chest, feeling the way deep breathing brings life and vitality to your body and your mind.

- You're welcome to remain in this ending state for as long as you'd like. If you feel ready to return to the waking state, you can start to let organic movements occur, perhaps wiggling a finger or toe. Then, feel the stillness once more, and see if your thoughts, words, and deeds can arise as a reflection of the stillness.

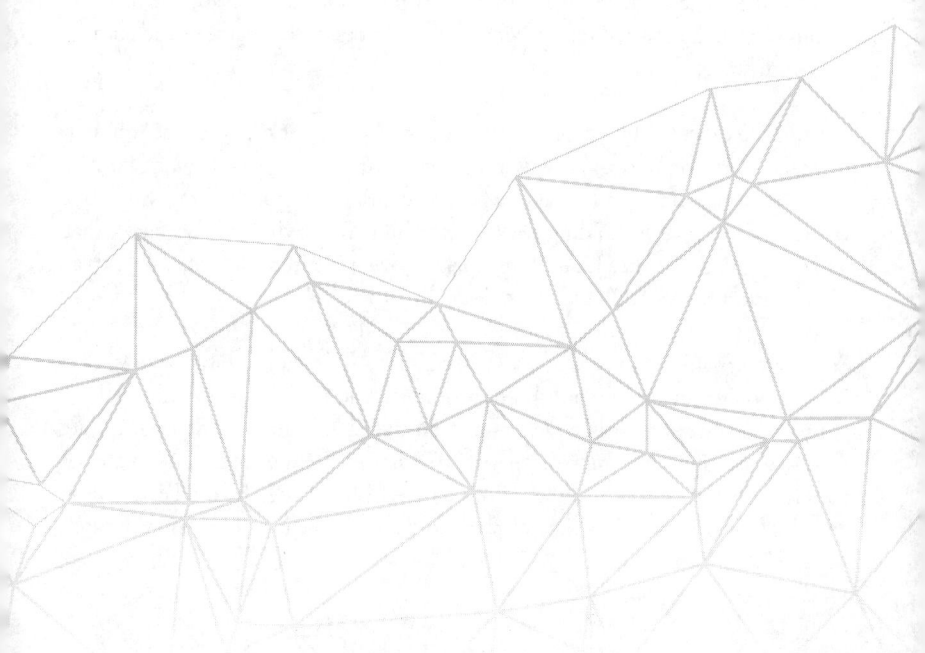

Class 21 Transcript

Practice 5: Practicing Mindfulness

Welcome to the mindfulness practice class. If you remember back to the lecture when we defined mindfulness, mindfulness is all about paying attention on purpose. Becoming aware of all the changing sensations amidst a backdrop of unchanging stillness.

I'm joined here today by Josh, who's going to be enjoying the mindfulness practice along with you. Thank you, Josh.

And today we're going to be doing about a half-hour mindfulness practice. You may want to take a few moments to gather up any creature comforts: a blanket, a pillow, or perhaps a bolster for beneath your knees. Josh, go ahead and start to get comfortable.

During the practice, I'll be guiding you through different experiences. You may be really alert and aware of everything that's happening or you might be in a space between asleep and awake, where you hear the sound of my voice but you're not necessarily holding on to everything I'm saying. Please know that whatever you experience is absolutely perfect, even if you fall asleep. Take this as an invitation to rest and be present, welcoming yourself just as you are.

So, make any final adjustments you need to be fully comfortable. Know that if at any point during the mindfulness practice you feel like you need to adjust your body, you're more than welcome to do that. Now close your eyes and start to just sense the room and the space around you. Feeling that whole plane of contact between the body and the floor or the surface beneath you. Feeling how your body is being held by that surface, noticing the feeling of heaviness against the floor, the chair. Feel the touch of your clothing or the blanket on your skin, the soft pillow.

Feeling the temperature of the air on your skin. Observe any sounds around you. Observing, first, the obvious sounds, sound of the voice, then tuning into more subtle sounds. Notice if there is any sense of taste present, perhaps from your last meal or toothpaste or something else. Notice if there are any smells present. Even if the eyes are closed, is there an image present in your awareness?

Let the five senses be wide open now; observing, witnessing, being aware: touch, taste, smell, sight, and sound. All five senses receiving your present moment experience.

Observing now, what is present? If only this moment were present in your physical body, what is the physical sensation of your body? Notice the temperature of the body, any places in your body where your attention is drawn.

Observe your mind. Noticing any thoughts, feelings, emotions, or beliefs as they arise, unfold, and dissolve.

We'll be checking in again with this at the end of the practice. Just observe your present moment state as we dive into the mindfulness meditation.

Become aware of your mouth, feeling that invisible plane of contact between the two lips. Observing the feeling of the mouth, the teeth, the tongue. Temperature of the mouth. Observing the feeling and sensation in your jaw. Is there any tension present in your jaw? If so, go straight into it. See if you can find at the epicenter of tension in your jaw.

Where does the tension and a sense of spaciousness begin?

Feeling the ears, outside architecture of the ears. Sound making its way from outer ears into inner ears. Feeling the nose, sensation of air in the nose. Feeling the eyes, space behind the eyes. Feel the forehead and the scalp. All the sensations of the head.

Feel sensation now moving down the left arm. Sensation cascading down from the left neck and shoulder, down all the way through the left arm into the left hand. Feeling the left pinky, ring finger, middle finger, pointer finger, thumb. Feel the palm of the left hand.

Now, shifting over to the right side from the right side of the neck, down through the right shoulder. Sensation cascading down the right arm into the right hand. Feeling the whole right hand: the pinky finger, ring finger, middle finger, pointer finger, right thumb. Feel the palm of the right hand.

And then feeling your way back up the arm into the chest. Become aware of the sensation inside your chest,

observing all the sensations present, how the rib cage expounds on releases with each breath. Feel the pulsation of the heart in the chest. Tuning into that rhythm of the heart. Can you find a single place in your entire body that doesn't feel the sensation of the heartbeat? Feel the heart beat in the palms of the hands.

Another location where your attention is naturally drawn, feel the sensation in the abdomen, observing any sensation of fullness or perhaps a little bit of hunger. The sensation of the hips, the pelvis. Feel sensation cascading down the left leg, all the way from the top of the left leg down through the knee and lower leg to the ankle and the foot. Feel the left foot, all of the toes, and the sole of the left foot. Feeling the whole left leg.

Crossing over the midline of the body and feeling the sensation of the right leg. The top of the legs, sensation cascading down through the knee, the lower leg, the right ankle, and foot. Feel the toes and the sole of the right foot.

Then feeling the whole body at once, sensing the sensation of your entire body, the whole body filled with sensation. Notice how even though the body is very still, it's also full of life. Feel the stillness in the body. Feel the life: heart beating, lungs breathing, billions of cells performing their functions. Body is still, and yet fully and completely alive.

Now ask yourself the question: who is aware of the physical body? Become aware of this, observing self, aware of a body and yet also aware, unchanging witness. Bringing your attention now to the breath, feeling the whole left side of the body breathing on an inhale, filling the whole left side of the body with air, and then on the exhale feel as if you're breathing out the whole right side of your body, as if a wave of air was moving out the right side of the body. Then that wave of air moves back in through the right side of the body on the inhalation and on the exhale that wave of air melts out through the left side of your body.

Keep breathing like this. Each inhale feels as if a wave moves from the left side of the body, and then on the exhale that wave of air melts out the right side of the body. And that wave of air comes back in through the right side of the body. And now, the left side of the body. Continue on like this at your own pace, observing the changing sensations in the physical body as the breath moves in and through you.

Observe if the mind may start to wander and bring it back to breathing, from one side of the body to the other. Now release consciousness around the breathing and ask yourself: who is observing the breath? Turn the observer on itself, and witness the unchanging part of you. Aware of a body, aware of a breath, and yet also aware of this, the silent witness.

Now, as if you were the witness of your mind, like a scientist studying your mind, observe. Are there any feelings or emotions that are present? What feelings or emotions are present in this moment? Once you identify one, observe where you feel it in your physical body. What is the physical sensation like of this feeling or emotion? Watch it as if you're witnessing a movie, while also staying tuned into the physical sensations that are present. Where on your body do you feel this emotion? Is that sensation like for you?

Now, observe any thoughts or memories or beliefs that may be present. What is here? Perhaps a belief about yourself or the world around you. Perhaps some memories associated with that belief. Witness the belief as an object in your awareness. The thought arises, notice the moment it arises, grows and unfolds, and then how it starts to dissolve as you place your attention upon it, eventually disappears.

From this witnessing state of awareness watch your thoughts for a few moments, noticing as one arises and comes into awareness, unfolds and tells its story and then dissolves back into its home ground of stillness. Where does the thought come from? Where does the thought go when it leaves? Notice thoughts unfolding and dissolving on a backdrop of unchanging stillness. The blank movie screen upon which all of life is projected. You are the one who is aware.

Observe the experience of your entire body and mind, now; welcoming your body and mind exactly as they are.

If only this moment were present, because only this moment is present. What is here? What is the full totality of being you? Feel that unique experience of being precisely who you are in this moment, welcoming yourself so fully.

And now, picture yourself doing something that you do in your life. You may want to picture yourself at home with your family. You may want to picture yourself doing what you do for your work or perhaps doing something you enjoy, like working in your garden or running in a race. Select something that leaps to your attention. Once you select it, observe the experience of being you in that moment, when you are running that race or working in your garden, at work or at home. Pick your scene and then observe the physical experience of being in that moment.

What does your body feel like while you're doing that activity? What are all of the physical sensations present in your body? How might they change as you move through the experience. Imagine yourself going all the way through the experience present in your mind. Notice how you feel. Notice the breath and any emotions that may come up. Notice any beliefs that may arise.

Notice yourself as you complete this experience. How will you feel then? Then notice the whole totality of what you're feeling as you participate in this moment. Ask yourself the question: who is aware of this experience?

Consider yourself the one who is aware, aware of your physical body, aware of your breath, aware of your feelings, emotions and beliefs. Also, aware of this awareness.

Feel yourself so fully connected to this state of awareness that any sense of separation starts to dissolve. Feel yourself as the unchanging witness, the stillness, the home ground from which all sensation and emotion arises and then melts back into. Settle back into this, a deep ground of being: the wholeness, silence, pure consciousness.

Rest in this: your true nature; healthy, whole, and complete. Exactly as you are. Here you are: timeless, infinite, and vast, connected to the whole and yet untouched by any of it. Something arises into the foreground of your attention.

Observe it. Feel it in your body, then let it melt back into that stillness. At home in yourself, complete.

And now, let the five senses begin to start to open up once more, staying fully connected to this state of awareness.

Pure consciousness. Not going away from it. Just letting yourself start to open up to this sensorial experience of this moment. Feeling in the caress of the air on your skin. Noticing sounds, smells, or tastes around you, in you.

Do you wake up in the world or does the world wake up in you? Slowly allowing yourself to welcome a deeper breath into the chest, feeling the way deep breathing brings life and vitality to your body and your mind.

You're welcome to remain here for as long as you'd like. If you feel ready to return to the waking state, you can start to let a little bit of organic movements start to occur, perhaps wiggling a finger or toe and then feeling stillness once more. Perhaps a stretch is ready to happen. Whatever it is don't go away from the stillness. See if your thoughts, words, and deeds can arise as a reflection of the stillness, a part of the whole never separating from this, pure consciousness, your true nature, always here. Changing sensations on a backdrop pure, untouched peace.

Thank you so much for practicing today. *Namaste*.

Class 22

Practice 6: Evoking the Relaxation Response

This class's practices are oriented toward triggering your parasympathetic nervous system by using the relaxation response. This is an essential piece of being a resilient person. The video lesson demonstrates different versions of the poses involved, and this guidebook chapter is a summary of those movements. If a particular movement doesn't feel right for you, find a version that does feel good or skip the activity.

Starting Out

- This class begins with a breathing practice. Begin in a comfortable seated position, either on the floor or in a chair. Make your spine straight. You can start by putting your right hand on your belly and your left hand on your chest. Inhale for four seconds, and then exhale for eight seconds. Feel free to change the timing to make it feel better, but make sure your exhalations are twice as long as your inhalations. Repeat this several times at your own pace, keeping your mind focused on the breath.

- Next comes alternate nostril breathing, which is an excellent practice for alleviating anxiety or integrating challenging emotions. This class's variation is different from the one in the practice class on breathing.

- You will use your thumb and pointer finger. Take a deep inhalation through both nostrils, and then block your right nostril with your thumb. Inhale for four seconds, block both nostrils, and then lift the thumb and exhale through the right nostril for eight seconds. Repeat this process, alternating nostrils, for several repetitions.

Preparation for Physical Movements

- After that comes preparation for the physical movements. Bring your left arm out to the side and bring your right ear down toward your right shoulder. Here, you will begin stretching the neck. Extend the arm, moving it slightly from the front to the back. You can also bring your chin down if desired.

- While you're moving, breathe fully into the body, directing your breath to any points of tension. Then, switch sides, extending your right arm out and bringing your left ear down toward your left shoulder. Move the arm, head, or neck to find the place where you get the most stretch, and then consciously breathe into the body.

- For the next move, if you're sitting in a chair, you can place your left forearm down on the chair. Then, lift your right arm up and over your ear. If that's not possible, come as far up as you can. If you're doing the floor variation, you can bring your forearm down onto the ground, inhale, and then lift your right arm up and over your head. Take several long, deep breaths, feeling the sensations in your body and observing what is present in the pose.

- Re-center and then switch over to your other side. Place your right forearm on the arm of the chair or on the ground, and lift your left arm up and over your ear. Again, take long, deep breaths, enjoying this opportunity to alleviate tension in the body.

- Come back to center, and then place your hands on your knees. Roll your shoulders down and gaze down at your belly button. On an inhalation, lift up and arch your back. If you have a healthy neck, you can relax your head back. If not, keep your chin in a neutral position.

- Moving at your own pace, roll the shoulders down, gazing toward the belly button, and then come back up while inhaling. Repeat by exhaling on a downward roll. When you've done this as much as you like, return to a neutral position.

Stretching the Legs and Lower Back

- The next step is a stretch for the backside of the legs and the lower back. Start by extending your left leg. If you're in the chair, make your

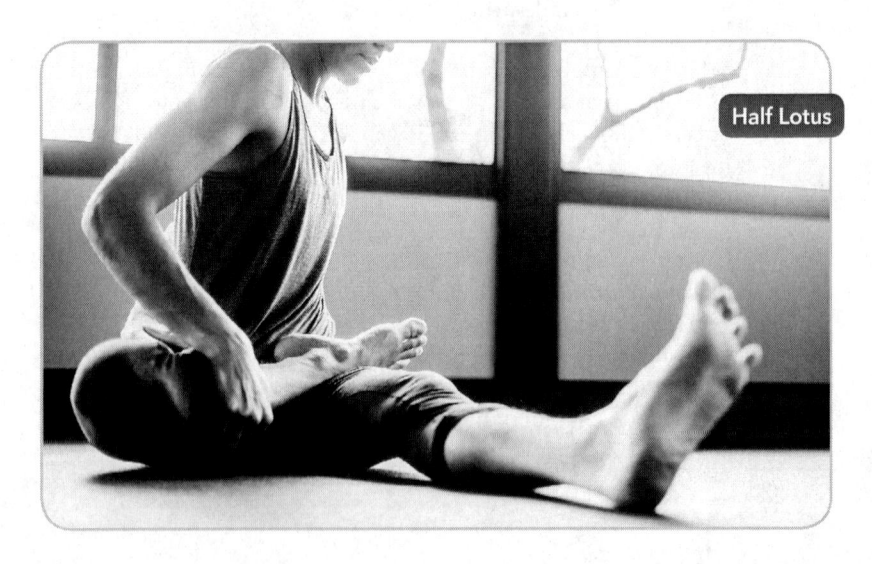

Half Lotus

way down onto the ground. An accessible variation is to bring the foot to the inside of your thigh. Another option, if you're more flexible, is to bring your foot into the half lotus pose. Avoid the half lotus if you have any knee issues.

- Once you're ready, inhale and lift your arms up into the air, and then exhale and bring the arms out and down. Draw your fingertips up the leg and the side of your body, inhaling. Exhale while extending out and down. Keep going for one or two more repetitions, feeling the body unfold into the pose.

- When you are prepared, slowly come back up and repeat this process, reversing the directions to target the other side of the body. Once you are done with this movement, you can stay down in a forward fold.

- Next, make some space around the points of tension in the body and release the body into that space. Consciously direct your breath to draw in calm energy and exhale any tension or stress. After that, inhale and stretch your body once more, extending your arms straight up as you bring your legs out. Finally, release.

> Through the practice of yoga, you build your resilience by seeing how the things you do can have an effect on your body. In each moment, you have the opportunity to create the relaxation response.

Five-Pointed Star or Tortoise Pose

- The next part of the class has two pose options: the five-pointed star or the tortoise. To perform the five-pointed star pose, bring the soles of your feet together and relax the knees out to the side. Bring your feet a little farther out away from the body, and then interlace your fingers around the toes. You can then bring your torso and head down over that star, tucking the head in even to the soles of the feet. If you

Tortoise Pose

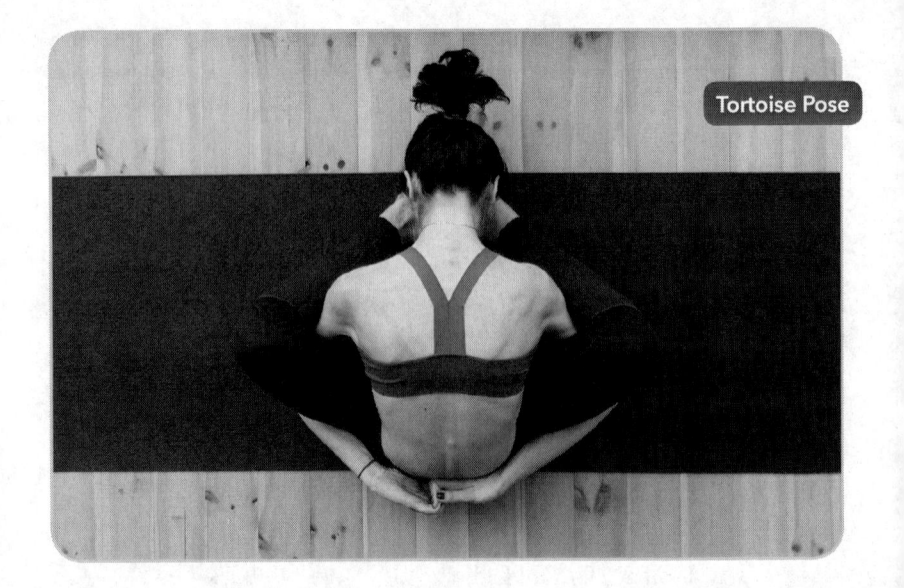

need to, you can wiggle the feet out a little farther, finding the place that feels best for your body.

- To perform the tortoise, bring the soles of the feet together, fairly far out from the body, and then thread your arms beneath your thighs and bring your head down toward the soles of your feet. Once you're in position, take some deep breaths, inviting your body to relax.

- Next, take the arms out slowly, eventually extending your legs out in front of you. Once your legs are out in front of you, take a moment to give your legs a massage, which is good for releasing tension.

The Full Seated Forward Fold

- The next step is preparation for a full seated forward fold. Root yourself firmly on the mat. Then, straighten the spine. Inhale, extending the arms up above your head. Once again, exhale, extending out and down. Flow through this several more times at your own pace. When you are done, lift out of the pose slowly on an inhalation.

The Pigeon Pose

- This class now turns to two different variations of the pigeon pose. The first is an accessible version. For this version, bring your left foot just above the knee. Make sure the foot is not on the knee, as that could put pressure on the knee. Then, your knee will come out to the side.

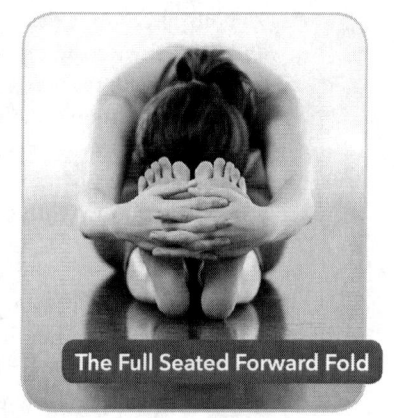

- If this is not an option for you, you can also place your foot on the ground. Otherwise, bring it up into position, and then use your elbow to gently push out the left knee. Keep your torso centered as you slowly come over the legs.

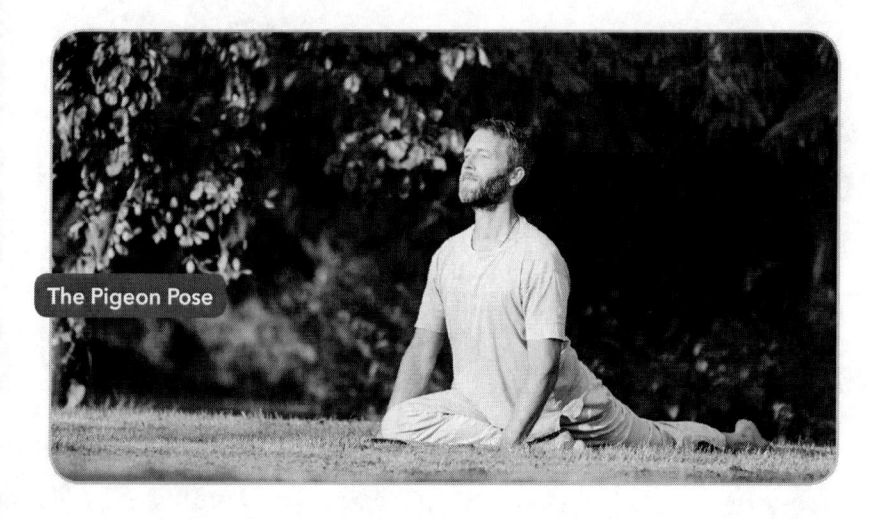

The Full Seated Forward Fold

The Pigeon Pose

- The other version is the full pigeon pose. To do this, bring your left shin parallel with the top of the mat, and then bring your right leg behind you with the toes pointed backward. Straighten the spine, and then walk your hands out. Stretching this pose to the max takes a lot of flexibility, so do whatever feels good to you. While in the pigeon pose, breathe deeply into the body. Then, slowly come up out of the pose and perform it with your other side, again breathing deeply.

- When you're ready, slowly come up and then over onto your abdomen, making a pillow with your hands. Put your right hand on top and your right cheek on that hand. Bring your big toes to touch behind you, and then relax your legs and wiggle your hips from side to side. This helps release some tension in the lower back.

The Cobra Pose

- This class's next pose is the cobra pose. Bring the palms of your hands beneath your shoulders, fingertips in line with the edge of

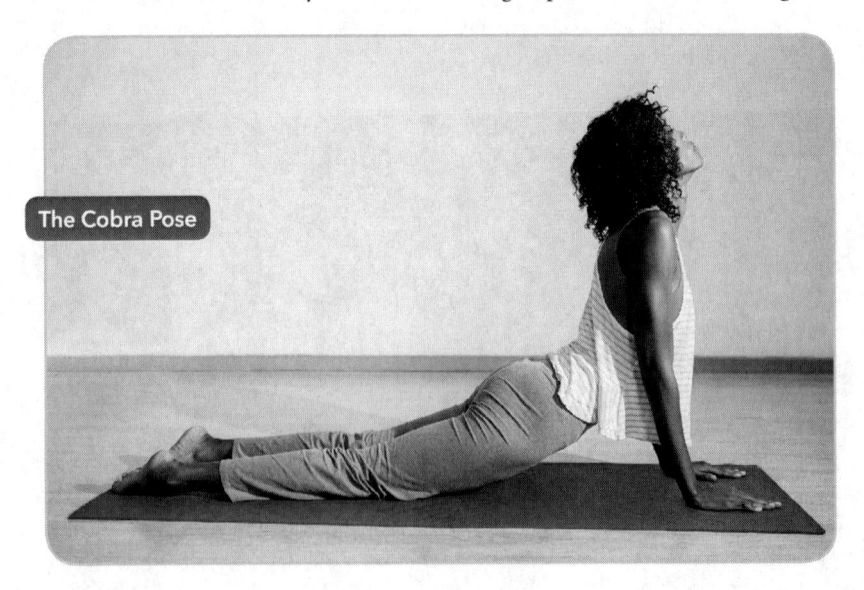

The Cobra Pose

your shoulders. Bring the legs together behind you and your forehead down onto the mat. Slowly lift your forehead up off the mat. You can keep the elbows pinned in toward the rib cage to make the movement more challenging.

- Once you're in position, breathe deeply. Roll your shoulders back and down away from your ears. Then, slowly come up one more time, giving compression to the lower back.

- Slowly roll down out of the pose. This time, once your head reaches the ground, make another pillow, using the left hand to support the left cheek this time. Your big toes should be touching behind you. If there's any tension in the hips, you can shake them out.

Super Person Pose

- The class's next activity is the super person pose. Extend your arms out in front of you. When you're ready, lift your arms and legs up off the ground. See how little of your body you can leave on the floor. Remember to breathe.

- When your body has had enough, slowly roll down. Hold for a moment. On an inhalation, lift the body again. This time, you can bend your knees and swing your arms slowly out behind you. An

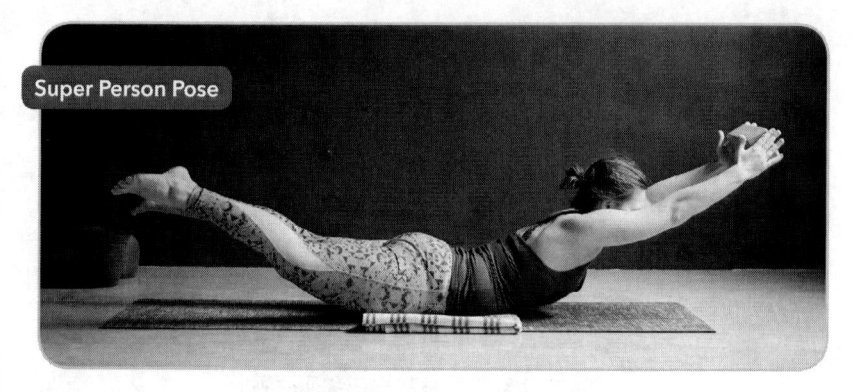

Super Person Pose

option is to catch your feet or ankles with your hands, but if you can't do this, just reach back in that direction.

- Once you're up, lift your head up and breathe deeply. Then, slowly come down. Place your hands beneath your shoulders and press back into the child's pose.

The Child's Pose

- There are several ways you can do the child's pose. One option is to do it with your knees out as wide as your mat, with your toes touching behind you. Extend your arms out, with your torso down between the knees. Another option is to do it with the knees together and the hands brought back by the ankles. Different bodies feel different in this pose, so do what feels good to you.

- Consciously turn your attention inward. Take some long, deep breaths, feeling the breath nourishing the body. Then you can start to come back over onto your back for the final relaxation or *shavasana* pose.

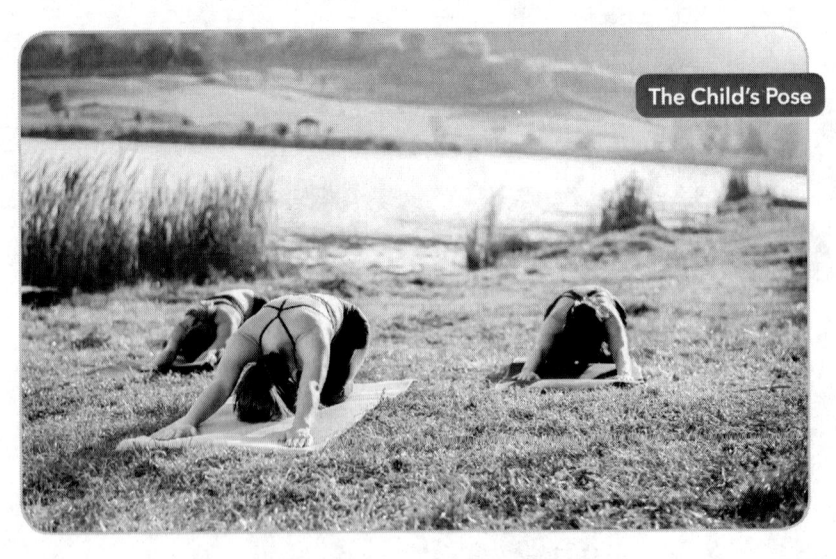

The Child's Pose

The *Shavasana* Pose

- Once you come down, you can hug your knees in toward your chest, giving yourself a hug. You can make some circles to the right and the left. Rhythmic movements are very soothing for the body.

- When you're ready, extend the legs out and notice if your body needs any sort of extra stretch. Do whatever makes your body feel good the way it is, allowing you to stay where you are.

- Once you have found your position, let the legs come out about as wide as the mat and let the toes fall out to the sides. Lift your shoulders up toward your ears, then roll them back and down, placing the shoulder blades flat on the mat. The palms should be open, facing up in a receptive position. If there's any tension in the back of your neck, you can inhale. When you exhale, roll the head to the right and then back and forth a couple of times.

- Next, center your head, tucking your chin a bit into your chest. Place the back of your neck down on the mat. Feel all the places the body is supported. Now, feel as if you are breathing the breath in from the soles of your feet up through your legs, up through your torso, and through the crown of your head. On the exhalation, breathe down through the body and through the soles of the feet.

- Take several breaths like this, feeling how the breath can move energy and sensation in the body. These long, full body breaths are like an opportunity to sweep through any tension that may have accumulated. When your body feels ready to rest in stillness, let the breath find its normal, natural rhythm. Allow yourself to relax here in *shavasana*, the final relaxation pose, for as long as you'd like.

Class 22 Transcript

Practice 6: Evoking the Relaxation Response

Hello and welcome to our practice class on invoking the relaxation response. All of the practices we're going to be doing today are practices oriented towards triggering your parasympathetic nervous system by using the relaxation response. This is an essential piece of being a resilient person.

When we are put in stressful circumstances we need to learn to trigger that relaxation response. So, think of all the poses and practices we do today as things that you can also apply in your daily life when you start to feel stressed. For instance, we're about to begin with some breathing exercises. These are perfect to do in the middle of your day when you just need to calm down a little.

So, to get started I'd like to introduce you to Kate, and also to Heidi, they're going to be demonstrating different variations of some of these poses. You're welcome as always to find the level that feels right to you. And of course, an essential piece of resilience is knowing when not to do something. If something doesn't feel right, for whatever reason, please don't do it or find a version that feels right for your body.

Let's start out in a comfortable seated position, either on the floor or in a chair. Make your spine nice and straight.

We're going to do a breathing exercise to start calming us down and easing us into the practice. You can start by putting your right hand on your belly and your left hand on your chest. We're going to be inhaling for four seconds and exhaling for eight seconds. We'll do several of these.

So, before we start just notice how you're feeling right now before we begin the practice. Observe the state of the mind and the body. Observe the natural state of your breath. Now inhale for four seconds: one, two, three, four. Exhale for eight seconds: five, six, seven, eight. Inhale for four seconds. Exhale for eight seconds. Keep going at your own pace. If you feel better inhaling for a little longer, just double what the exhalation is.

Notice where the mind is, keep it focused on the breath. The full body sensation of the inhale and the exhale. Take one more very full deep breath. Then as you release you can lower your hands down. Notice how just a couple of breaths may have changed states of your body.

Next, we're going to do alternate nostril breathing, which is an excellent practice for alleviating anxiety or integrating challenging emotions. We'll do it a little bit differently than we do in the practice breathing class. But this time we're not going to hold the breath.

So, use your thumb and pointer finger. We'll start out by taking a deep inhalation through both nostrils, then you're going to block your right nostril with your thumb and inhale through the left. One, two, three, four. Block both nostrils, hold just for a moment, and then exhale out the right nostril lifting the thumb for eight seconds. Five, six, seven, eight. Inhale through the right for four seconds. Hold the nose just for a moment. Exhale on the left for eight seconds. Inhale through the left nostril for four seconds. Hold the nose blocking both nostrils, now lift your thumb, exhale on the right for eight seconds.

Now, inhale through the right for four seconds. Hold the nose just for a moment, lift your pointer finger, exhale on the left for eight seconds. One more on each side. Inhale through the left for four seconds. Hold the nose blocking both nostrils. Exhale on the right for eight seconds. Inhale on the right for four seconds. Hold the nose, exhale on the left for eight seconds. Release the hand down onto your lap and take several long deep breaths and inhaling through the whole body, exhaling out through the whole body.

Now, we'll prepare for the physical movements. Bring your left arm out to the side and bring your right ear down towards your right shoulder. We're going to start stretching through the neck here. So, extend the arm out and you can move it a little from the front to the back. And if you'd like you can bring your chin down a little bit too. Really stretch out the neck. This is a really nice practice to do if you're working at a desk a lot, or you feel like you're holding a lot of tension in the shoulders. It's a great way to counter that movement.

While you're moving, breathe fully into the body directing your breath to any points of tension. And then come center, switch sides, extend your right arm out to the right, and bring your left ear down towards your left shoulder. Once again move the arm in the head or the neck a little bit to find the place where you get the most stretch, and then consciously breath into the body; feeling as if each breath is nourishing any places in the body that are harboring tension. Inhale breathing in calm relaxing energy, each exhale breathing out any tension. Now come back to center.

For this next one, if you're sitting in the chair like Kate, you can place your forearm down on the chair, then you're going to lift your right arm up and over your ear. If that's not possible just come as far up as you can. If you're doing the floor variation, you can bring your forearm down onto the ground, inhale, lift your right arm up and over your head.

We hold a lot of tension between our intercostal muscles between each of our ribs. So, when you're in a position like this it's a really great chance to breathe deeply into all those places where you may have tension. Each inhale really expand the rib cage, each exhale push out all the stale air, opening up all those muscles on the side body. Take two or three more long deep breaths, being fully present, feeling the sensations in your body observing what is present in the pose.

And come back up to center and switch sides over to your other side, either placing your right forearm on the arm of the chair or on the ground, and lifting your left arm up and over your ear. Breathe deeply into the whole side body, feeling like that side body is like the arc of a rainbow and you're really opening up that arc, breathing deeply. Two or three more full breaths, enjoying this beautiful opportunity to alleviate tension in the body. Come back to center.

Now place your hands on your knees. Roll your shoulders down, gaze down at your belly button. And then on an inhalation lift up and arch your back. If you have a healthy neck you can relax your head back. If not, don't bring your head back like that, just keep your chin in a neutral position.

Now moving at your own pace, rolling the shoulders down, gazing down towards the belly button, inhaling up, exhaling down, inhaling up. Keep going and your own pace. If there's any place that you want to hang out because your body has a little more tension go ahead and do that. Listening to your body in each moment. Every pose an invitation to explore more deeply. This is a great pose to do if you're sitting on a plane or in the car for a long time; while you're stopped of course. Do one more, really enjoying the stretch. When you're finished come back to a neutral position.

We're now going to do a stretch for the backside of our legs and our lower back. So, start by extending out your left leg. If you're in the chair, make your way down onto the ground. An accessible variation is to do what Kate is doing here by just bringing the foot inside of the inside of your thigh there. Another option, if you're more flexible, is to bring your foot into the half lotus as Heidi is doing. If you have any knee issues at all, please do not do the half lotus. This is only if it feels good to your body.

Then once you're ready, inhale, lift your arms up into the air. Exhale, extend the arms out and down. And then draw your fingertips up the leg, up the side body, inhaling up, lifting up. Exhaling, extending out and down. Keep going like this for one or two more times. Feeling the body unfold into the pose.

Sometimes, if we force ourselves into a position we create more tension. When you ease into it, doing something like this, you let your body relax and release into the pose. So, this time go ahead and move down into the pose.

And hold here. You can bring your head down any amount, and also moving with the torso forward.

Once again, if you find any places of tension in the body you can make a little space around the tension and then invite your body to relax into that space. Keep making space around the tension, relax into that space. And as always, nourish your body with some deep full breaths, each inhale sending the breath down into any points of tension, each exhale sending the breath out releasing the tension.

Now, slowly come up. You can go ahead and switch sides, extending your right leg out, bringing in the left leg in, either inside of the thigh or you can bring it up into the half lotus. Once more, inhale, lift your arms up, stretch your arms up and feel as if somebody's come along and is pulling your arms up away from you know, lifting the rib cage out from the waist. Exhale, extending out and down, and then drawing the finger tips up the legs, up the side body, flowing with grace and strength. You bring several more times like this at your own pace, inhaling up, exhaling down. Feeling that easefulness, the kindness with which you're treating your body. When you're ready you're welcome to stay down in the forward fold.

Once you're in position make some space around the points of tension in the body and release the body into that space. Make space around the tension, release into that space. Consciously direct your breath, like a tool that you're using, breathing in calm clear energy, exhaling out any tension or stress.

Through the practice of yoga, we build our resilience by seeing how the things we do can have an effect on our body. In each moment, we have the opportunity to create the relaxation response. We just need the tools to do it.

These are the tools.

Now, inhale, come up, stretch your body up once more, extend those arms straight up as you bring your legs out. And then release.

And now, we're going to do either the five-pointed star pose or the tortoise. So, Kate here is going to do the five-pointed star pose, bringing the soles of your feet together and relax the knees out to the side. You want to bring your feet a little farther out away from the body and then interlace your fingers around the toes. You can then bring your torso and head down over that star, tucking the head in even to the soles of the feet. If you need to you can wiggle the feet out a little farther, finding the place that feels best for your body.

Heidi is going to demonstrate the tortoise us by bringing the soles of the feet together, fairly far out from the body, and then threading her arms beneath her thighs and bringing her head down into the soles of her feet. Once you're in position take some really deep breaths here. Each inhale expanding the body, nourishing the body with a breath, each exhale releasing tension.

Every breath a choice. Every breath an opportunity. Invite your body to relax. It may relax or it might not, but let the invitation be there. Stay very tuned into the sensations in your body, cultivating mindfulness of the body. So, notice what parts of your body feel tuned up, notice which parts feel spacious and expansive. This pose always feels like tucking into a cocoon, always feels really nourishing and restorative to go inside and find that internal energy and strength again.

Now, like the butterfly unfolding out of your cocoon, taking the arms out slowly, and eventually extending your legs out in front of you. Once your legs are out in front of you take a moment to give your legs a little massage, rubbing the thighs, the knees, even the feet a little bit. Massage so good for releasing tension and evoking the relaxation response. We can even take our fingers and really dig into any points of tension in the muscles, helping to release whatever's present.

Now, we'll prepare for a full seated forward fold. You want to take your hands under your hips and remove any flesh from beneath the sit bones to get your sit bones really firmly rooted down on the mat. Then straighten the spine, make your spine really nice and long. Inhale, extend the arms up above your head. And once again, exhale, extend out and down and then flow through this several more times, inhaling up and exhaling down, at your own pace.

Each breath observing sensation in the body as the breath moves up and through the body. Now as you exhale the body unfolds. Listen to your body for the moment, where it's ready to take the pose and then settle in to the forward fold. So, you're in position, you can hold onto the outsides of your feet or your shins. Whatever feels good to you.

Now, on an inhalation, slowly lift up out of the pose. Notice how your body's feeling now and then prepare for the pigeon pose. We'll be doing two different variations of the pigeon pose. The first is an assessable version. Over here Kate's going to demonstrate. She's going to bring her left foot either up into this position here, where the foot is just above the knee. Make sure the foot's not on the knee, because that could put pressure on the knee. And then her knee will come out to the side. If this is not an option for you, you can also place your foot on the ground similar to how we had it in the other pose. Otherwise, bring it up into position and then Kate's going to use her elbow to gently push out, just gently push out her left knee and then she'll keep her torso centered as she slowly comes over the legs any amount.

Heidi is going to do the full pigeon pose. To do this she's going to bring her shin, her left shin, parallel with the top of the mat and then she's going to bring her right leg back behind her with the toes pointed backwards. She'll stand up straight first, to straighten the spine and then she'll walk her hands out away from her. Heidi is very flexible, so don't feel badly if you can't come all the way down into the pose. Do whatever feels good to you.

In yoga, we learn that every part of our body holds onto emotions in different ways. The more we cultivate mindfulness you'll start to see that when you feel nervous, perhaps your arms cross in front of your chest or something else. What's interesting is that a lot of people hold grief in their hips. So, when we're doing this pose I'm just going to invite you to notice what emotions come up for you. It might be grief or it might not, might be something else, and that's fine, too. Just to become conscious of how different parts of our body may harvest different emotions when we come into these certain poses.

While you're here breath deeply into the body and then slowly come up out of the pose and go ahead and switch sides. Again, either placing the right foot just below the left knee, closer to the body or bringing it onto the floor. And then, as Heidi's doing, bringing the right leg parallel with the top of the mat. Inhale, lift up through the torso. Exhale, come over. Come down any amount.

Once you're down, breathing deeply, each inhale nourishing the hips and lower back with fresh, clear, clean oxygenated breath. Exhale, breathing out the tension. Every single inhale we have the opportunity to breathe in whatever we need. Could be more strength, more resilience. Could mean more healing for our bodies. Could be patience or kindness. Each exhale we can breathe out what is no longer serving us.

Then when you're ready, slowly come up, and you're going to come over onto your abdomen, making a pillow with your hands and whatever hands on top, put that same cheek on top. So, if your right hands on top put your right cheek on it. Bring your big toes to touch behind you, and then relax your legs and wiggle your hips a little bit side to side. This helps release some tension in the lower back.

We're now going to do the cobra pose, so bring the palms of your hands beneath your shoulders, fingertips in line with the edge of your shoulders. Bring the legs together behind you, the forehead down onto the mat, and then very slowly you're going to lift the forehead up off the mat. You're going to lift up, very slowly, you can keep the elbows penned into the rib cage. So, Kate is coming up a gentle amount. And Heidi is coming up a little further.

You may notice that when you do this pose with the elbows penned in that the body might shake a little. It's a lot harder to do it that way and that's natural.

Once you're in position, breathe deeply. Roll your shoulders back and down away from your ears. And then slowly rolling down, we're going to come up one more time, with that grace just as you came into the first pose. When you're ready slowly lifting up, once again, giving that nice compression to the lower back. In this pose we're really strengthening our lower back and we're also giving a nice little compression to the adrenals and kidneys. Every yoga poses like a little massage for some part of the body.

Slowly roll down out of the pose. This time, once your head reaches the ground, make a pillow the other direction, placing the left hand on top and placing your left cheek gently on your hands. Big toes touching behind you. If there's any tension in the hips you can shake them out a little bit. Feel how the earth below you supports the body and just let go of anything you're holding onto into the earth.

Now, we have two amazing women here so they're going to be doing this super women pose. But if you're a man you can do the superman pose or whatever kind of super person you'd like to be. So, extend your arms out in front of you. And when you're ready, lift your arms and legs up off the ground lift everything up. See how little of your body you can leave on the floor lift up like you could fly here. Remembers to breath.

When your body says enough slowly roll down. Hold for a moment down. And on an inhalation left the body back.

And this time you can bend your knees and swing your arms slowly out behind you. If you can catch a hold of your feet or your ankles. And if you can't reach your feet or ankles that's okay, you can just reach back in that direction.

Once you're up, lift your head up, breathe deeply hear, deep into the valley, giving the whole abdomen a nice massage. Also, getting that compression in the lower back. And then slowly come down. Place your hands beneath your shoulders and press back into the child's pose.

There are several ways you can do the child's pose. Kate is going to do it with her knees out as wide as her mat and her toes touching behind her. Her arms extended out with her torso down between the knees. Heidi over here is going to do it with the knees together and then she's going to bring her hands back by her ankles. Different bodies feel different in this pose, so do what feels really good to you.

While you're here, once again you're going into that cocoon, that internal place of nourishment. So, consciously turn your attention inwards, take some long deep breaths, feeling the breath nourishing the body. Giving yourself what you need to feel complete. Being aware of your body, all the changing sensations.

Then you can start to come back over onto your back for the final relaxation or *shavasana* pose. Take your time. Once you come down you can hug your knees in towards your chest, give yourself a little hug. You can make some circles to the right and the left. Rhythmic movements are very soothing for the body.

And then, when you're ready extend the legs out and notice if your body needs any sort of extra stretch, maybe arms extended or a little twist. Whatever might feel good for you. Maybe your body feels good the way it is and you can just stay where you are.

Once you found your position let the legs come out about as wide as the mat and let the toes fall out to the sides. Lift your shoulders up towards your ears roll them back and down, placing the shoulder blades flat on the mat, the palms are open, facing up in a receptive position. If there's any tension in the back side of your neck, you can inhale, and on an exhale, roll the head to the right and then back and forth a couple times. Every pose an opportunity to calm and nourish the body.

And bring your head center, tuck your chin a little bit into your chest and place the back side of the neck down on the mat. Feel all the places the body is supported. Now, feel as if you are breathing the breath in from the soles of your feet up through your legs, up through your torso, right out the crown of your head. And on the exhale breath down through the body, right out the soles of the feet.

Take several breaths like this, feeling how the breath can move energy and sensation in the body. These long full body breaths are like an opportunity to sweep through any tension that may have accumulated. When your body feels ready to rest in stillness, let the breath find its normal natural rhythm, and let yourself relax here in *shavasana*, the final relaxation pose, for as long as you'd like.

Going to finish the class here, but please take your time. Thank you so much for practicing today. *Namaste*.

Class 23

Practice 7: Finding Safety with Yoga Nidra

This practice class on Yoga Nidra invites you to go on a journey to find safety inside of yourself, no matter what is occurring in your outside world. The video lesson provides demonstrations of the movements, starting from a reclined position or sitting in a chair. You may also want to use a blanket if you are chilly, and a pillow or bolster beneath your knees so that you can rest throughout the practice. This guidebook chapter consists of a summary of the steps of the class.

Starting Out

- Once you've settled, start by feeling the body. What is the present moment experience of your body? What is it that you're bringing with you into your practice? Feel your whole body. Notice how, as you continue to settle in, the body is almost like a waterfall. It should start to feel supported as the settling process continues to unfold.

- If it's helpful, you can take a few long, deep breaths, letting each breath draw you even more fully into the present moment. Observe what is present in your mind.

- Next, allow an inner resource to arise. Find an internal space of well-being: a place where you feel comfortable and safe. This can be a real place, such as a place in nature, a place from your childhood, or your home. It can also be a totally imaginary place. Feel this as an internal place, not dependent on the outside world.

- As you open up to this place of safety, let your five senses open up as well. What do you see, hear, and smell? What tastes allow you to feel comfort and safety? What makes your body comfortable and warm? Welcome any sensations that help you feel safe, calm, nourished, and at peace, and focus on how your body feels when you experience a sense of well-being.

- Next, set an intention for your practice. Perhaps your intention is to find inner peace that can hold you no matter what is occurring in daily life. Invite in questions: What is it that I truly want more than anything else in life? What is my heart's deepest desire?

- Whatever the answer is, affirm it in a sentence in the present tense, as if it's already a fact. An example is this: "I am peaceful and complete just as I am." This can feel like home and promote stillness.

Attention to the Body

- The next phase of the class involves moving attention through the physical body. Whatever you experience from a given part is absolutely perfect.

- First, feel your mouth and all of the textures and sensations within. Do the same for your ears, and then feel your way across your face to your nose. After that, feel your eyes, eyelids, forehead, and skull.

Eventually, feel the entire head as a pure sensation, also paying attention to your neck and throat.

- Move down into the shoulders. Ask yourself: What is the sensation of the shoulders? Is there any tension present? If so, see if you can find the epicenter of tension in the shoulders. It may be where you thought it was, or it may disappear when you search for it.

- Next, feel your way down through the arms, reaching the palms of your hands, fingers, and thumbs. Feel your way back up the arms and into your chest, covering the ribs, lungs, heart, and the center of the chest.

- Come down to your abdomen and lower back. Notice the sensation of the abdomen and lower back, and how that might change as you move down into the hips and the pelvis. Feel your way through the legs, all the way down into the ankles and feet. Feel the soles of your feet and your toes.

- Finally, feel the symphony of sensation in your whole body. See if it's possible to welcome the body just as you are. Observe if a feeling of safety and comfort arises.

- You may also notice some judgments about the body, physical pain, or something else that doesn't feel welcome. Notice what that feels like. Ask yourself: Where did they come from? What do they want and need to feel safe?

- Welcome your body and any feelings that are still present of judgment or doubt about the body. Gather up all the feelings and opinions you may have ever had, as if you're giving them all a hug, letting them know it's safe to be who you are in this moment. It's possible to feel this without changing anything at all about your body.

- Affirm to yourself: "My body is a safe place to be. I feel healthy, whole, and complete just as I am." Do this even if it doesn't yet feel entirely true. Feel as if it's in the process of becoming a reality. Alternatively, perhaps it is already true, and you've developed a willingness to accept that belief.

Attention to the Breath

- Next, bring your attention to the breath, feeling how its rhythm brings a sense of safety and comfort. Feel how the breath is bringing you balance, life, and opportunity for harmony. Each inhalation and exhalation provides a chance to connect more fully with yourself.

- On each inhalation, feel the world becoming you. On each exhalation, feel a part of the whole. Notice the sense of safety that comes from feeling a part of the whole, where separation starts to dissolve. You have a body and a mind, but at the same time, you are a part of the whole. Feel the safety and the comfort of being part of nature and humanity.

Attention to the Mind

- After that, observe the mind. Notice what safety feels like. Think of the sense of safety that you may have experienced at one point of your life or are experiencing now. Ask yourself: What is safety? What does that mean to me? When I think of safety, where do I feel it in the body?

- Let this experience of safety unfold. Notice if any sense of separation from safety starts to arise. Feel that, asking yourself: Where do I separate from a sense of safety? Where do I go away from that home ground of stillness within? How can I feel safe amidst even this?

- Allow the answer to arise, knowing the body is always trying to find safety and harmony. Give it credit for this. Also give yourself credit for how every moment of life, your body has been working hard for you to feel safe and at home in your skin and in your mind. Commit to yourself to do things that will increase the chances for this peace and safety to be your constant experience.

- Whenever separation arises, invite the question: How can I come home to myself so that I never go away? Let yourself draw back into stillness, silence, and the center of your being. Come back home to your true nature, a place where you are always safe, resting, and feeling a sense of well-being and stillness.

- Imagine yourself abiding in the stillness as you go about your day—doing things at home, eating, sleeping, working, preparing a meal, resting, relaxing, and playing. Do this while resting in stillness, staying connected to the peace that is your true nature.

- Commit to a heartfelt intention to stay connected to the peace that is always present inside of you. Intend that all of your thoughts, words, and deeds arise as a reflection of this stillness. Know that every potential lives in you. Feel inspired to bring it to life in the way only you can.

- Remain here for as long as you'd like. Once you're ready to come back to your day, start taking some deeper breaths or moving the body slightly. Take all the time you need to transition to wakefulness, staying connected to the stillness and embodying your true nature.

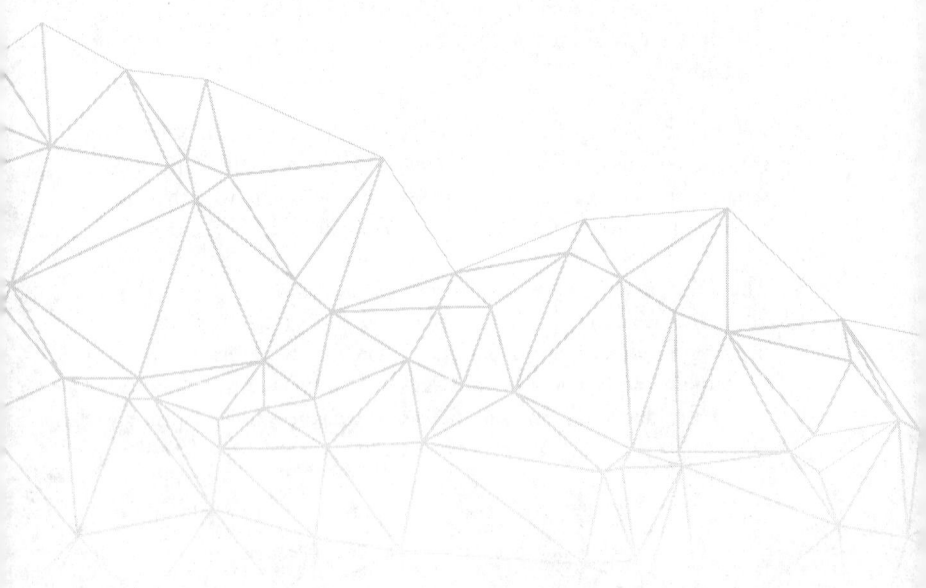

Class 23 Transcript

Practice 7: Finding Safety with Yoga Nidra

Welcome to your Yoga Nidra practice class. Today, I'll be inviting you to go on a journey to find safety inside of yourself no matter what is occurring in your outside world. Take a moment to adjust your body, either reclined like Jane is here, or sitting in a chair the way that Tammy. If you're chilly at all you may want to cover the body with a warm blanket. Use a pillow or bolster beneath your knees so that you can really rest in the practice.

Once you've adjusted your body notice if there's any additional changes you'd like to make to be five or 10 percent more comfortable. Know that if at any point in the practice you don't feel relaxed or comfortable, you can always adjust your body, rolling on your side or changing your position in any way that's helpful for you.

Once you've settled, start by feeling the body. What is the present moment experience of your body? What is it that you're bringing with you today into your practice? Feel your whole body, and notice how as you continue to settle into the surface beneath you how the body is almost like a waterfall, how it starts to feel supported and that settling process continues to unfold. It's like a waterfall down onto the mat or onto the chair.

If it's helpful you can take a few long, deep breaths, letting each breath draw you even more fully into the present moment. Observe what is present in your mind. Know that the invitation is present to work with whatever's here during the Yoga Nidra. This is your journey. Let it nurture you. Let it serve you wherever you are in your life today.

Now, allow an inner resource to arise. Find an internal space of well-being; a place where you feel comfortable and safe, where you feel like you can really be yourself. This can be a real place: perhaps a place in nature; a favorite place from your childhood; Could be your home; a place you enjoy going on vacation; or it can be a totally imaginary place. You can bring in any elements that help you feel a sense of calm, nourished safety. Feel this as an internal place, not dependent on the outside world.

As you open up to this place of safety, let your five senses open up as well. What do you see? Notice any colors, textures, shapes, images? Notice any sounds that evoke a sense of well-being for you? What smells help you feel a sense of well-being, comfort? What tastes allow you to feel that comfort and safety; perhaps something from childhood that someone you love made or something you love to make? Your special delight. Taste of a favorite fruit.

Feeling the skin. What makes your body feel comfortable and safe? Perhaps a warm blanket. A favorite sweater. Maybe the feeling of a gentle breeze on the skin. Five Senses wide open, welcoming anything that sensorially helps you feel safe, calm, nourished and at peace. Creating your own internal resource, a place where you can always come home to inside of you. If there's anything else that would be helpful to draw into this experience, go ahead and do that.

What does the body feel like when you experience a sense of well-being? What's the physical experience of feeling safe and comfortable? Let it open up; know that you can return to this inner resource at any time, both during the Yoga Nidra and in your daily life.

Now set an intention for your practice today. Perhaps your intention is to find inner peace, a peace that can hold you no matter what is occurring in daily life. And then feeling down even deeper into the heart and inviting in the question: What is it that I truly want more than anything else in life? What is my heart's deepest desire? Whatever it is, affirm it in a sentence in the present tense, as if it's already a fact. I am peaceful and complete just as I am. Feel how this can feel like home; the home in your heart, the home in your true nature. Just stillness, pure consciousness, stillness from which life arises. The stillness life melts back into.

Now, begin to move attention through the physical body. As I name each area of the body, bring your attention there and experience the sensation. You may feel something or nothing at all. Whatever your experience is absolutely perfect. Feel the mouth and all of the textures and sensations in the mouth. Feeling the ears. Feeling pure sensation of the ears. Feeling your way across the face over to your nose. What is the sensation of your nose?

Feeling your eyes. Eyelids and behind the eyes. The eyes themselves. Feel the forehead, the skull. What is the physical sensation inside the head? Feel the whole head as pure sensation, feeling your way how the head may feel different than the neck. Feeling the sensation of the neck, throat.

Notice if sensation changes again as you move down into the shoulders. What is the sensation of the shoulders? Is there any tension present? If so go into it? See if you can find the epicenter of tension in the shoulders. Is it actually there when you go to look for it? Or does it disappear when you got close?

Feeling out, away from the tension and noticing where tension unfolds into a feeling of spaciousness. Feeling your way down your arms, both arms as pure sensation. Feeling down into the palms of the hands, down into the fingers and thumbs. Feeling your way up your arms and over into your chest. Feeling the ribs, the lungs, the heart, the center of the chest.

Coming down to your abdomen and the lower back. What's the sensation of the abdomen and lower back, and how that might change as you move down into the hips and the pelvis? Feeling your way down through the legs, all the way down the legs into the ankles and feet. Feel the soles of the feet and toes. And all parts of the body become one. Feel the symphony of sensation in your whole body. The whole body, alive with sensation.

See if it's possible to welcome the body just as you are. Observe if a feeling of safety and comfort arise, so you stop trying to fix and change the body and just really welcome it, just as you are, feeling if you've befriended your body, perhaps for the first time, coming home to your body, feeling your body as a safe place to live. Create and rest.

Notice if anything arises. Some judgements you may still have about the body or physical pain or something else that arises that doesn't feel welcomed. Notice what that feels like? What does it feel like when you think of the body as aging or having some sort of problem; not being good enough or healthy enough? Where do you feel that in the body when those types of experiences arise? Let yourself feel those, too. Where did they come from? What do they want and need to feel safe?

Welcome your body and welcome any feelings that are still present of judgment or doubt about the body. Welcome all of this at the same time, gathering up all the feelings and opinions you may have ever had, as if you're giving them all a hug, letting them know it's safe to be who you are in this moment. It's safe to be yourself, your authentic self. What if it's possible to feel peaceful and healthy in the body just as it is, even with all its quirks and imperfections? It's possible to feel this without changing anything at all about your body.

Affirm to yourself: My body is a safe place to be. I feel healthy, whole, and complete just as I am; even if it doesn't feel entirely true, yet. Feel as if it's in the process of becoming a reality. Or maybe it's already true, it's just a willingness to accept that belief.

Bringing your attention now to your breath, feeling how the rhythm of the breath brings a sense of safety and comfort. Feel how the breath is bringing you balance, life, and opportunity for harmony. Each inhale, each exhale a chance to connect more fully with yourself. As you breath in a deep inhale, feel that breath nourishing every cell of your body. And as you exhale, feel yourself as a part of the whole. Each inhale feel how the world becomes you. Each exhale feel how you are a part of the whole.

Staying so tuned in with this. Each inhale feeling the world becoming you. Each exhale feeling a part of the whole. Notice the sense of safety that comes from feeling a part of the whole, where separation starts to dissolve. We realize the interconnectedness between ourselves and the world around us. Yes, you have a body and a mind. At the same time you are a part of the whole. Feel the safety and the comfort in this. Part of nature. Part of humanity.

Now observe the mind. Notice what does safety feel like? You think of the sense of safety that you may have experienced at one point of your life or are experiencing now. What is safety? What does that mean to you? What arises in the body as you unfold a sense of safety? What parts of your body experience safety? When you think of safety, where do you feel it in the body?

Let this experience of safety unfold. Notice if at any point in time any sense of separation from safety starts to arise, perhaps something that feels unsafe, maybe thought, maybe a memory. Feel that. Where do you separate from a sense of safety? Where do you go away from that home ground of stillness within? Notice that. Ask yourself how can I feel safe amidst even this? How can I feel safe even amidst what may bring me fear or may make me feel separate? Or not good enough? Allow the answer to arise, knowing the body is always trying to find safety and harmony. Give it credit for this.

Give yourself credit for how every moment of life your body has been working hard for you to feel safe and at home in your skin, in your mind; how your body and mind are always seeking equilibrium. How deeply they strive for balance and peace. You commit to yourself to do things that will increase the chances for this peace and safety to be your constant experience.

Anytime separation arises invite the question: How can I come home to myself, so that I never go away? I can abide in this deeper state of stillness and equanimity. Let yourself draw back into this stillness, the silence, the center of your being. It's already here. There's nothing to achieve. Dropped back from the foreground movements and rest in your true nature. Pure consciousness, pure being. Like a river of stillness, you're falling back into, letting it carry you all the way home. Home to yourself. Home to your true nature, a place where you are always safe, always resting, well-being.

Feel this: presence permeates everything; the stillness from which sensations and thoughts arise unfold and then dissolve back into. Feel that your true nature is holding you always in the warmest embrace, accepting you just as you are. Dissolving separation, inspiring you to thrive in life, able to meet, greet, welcome, and respond to whatever happens in your daily life.

Imagine yourself abiding in the stillness as you go about your day doing all the things you do. Your acting at home, eating, sleeping, working, preparing a meal, resting, relaxing, playing, all the while resting in stillness, staying connected to the peace that is your true nature.

Make a very sincere heartfelt intention to stay connected to this, this peace that is always present inside of you. So that all your thoughts, words, and deeds arise as a reflection of this silence, stillness. So, that your very presence brings a sense of peace to the world around you. Brings a joy to the world around you. Brings harmony to the world around you. Know that every potential lives in you. Feel inspired to bring it to life in the way only you can.

Welcome to remain here for as long as you'd like. If you're ready to come back to your day, evening you're welcome just start taking some deeper breaths, or moving the body a little. Taking all the time you need to transition to wakefulness, staying connected to the stillness, embodying your true nature.

Thank you so much for joining us for the practice today. *Namaste*.

Class 24

Your Hero's Journey

This class draws the course to a close by bringing themes from throughout the course together. It begins by returning to the Resilience Self-Evaluation Tool. Additionally, the video and audio lessons contain a guided mindfulness meditation practice based on the hero's journey. A recap of the hero's journey is provided in this guidebook chapter. This is a class you may come back to many times to move through the hero's journey again as you uncover deeper layers of meaning present in your life.

Evaluating Your Resilience

- If you haven't done so yet, use the Resilience Self-Evaluation Tool. This tool will measure your resilience in eight different categories. Even if you have already taken the evaluation, it's a good idea to take it again, as some of your answers may have changed now that you've worked your way through the course. As you take the evaluation and look through your results, keep in mind that it's normal to feel more resilient in some areas than others.

- The purpose of this tool is twofold. It allows you to realize the ways in which you are very resilient already so that you can harness those skills. It also allows you to uncover areas in which resilience comes less naturally to you, so that you can find ways to amp up your resilience in those areas.

- Once you're done with the evaluation, take some time to reflect on your results. Where are your strengths? Which areas are more difficult for you? Do your results surprise you? Look at each category in isolation, and really think about how each one has manifested in your life.

- It's helpful to do this self-evaluation in your areas of weakness as well as in your areas of strength. By harnessing your strengths, you could very well uncover some skills that you could transfer to other categories as well. For instance, if you have a very proactive worldview but struggle with equanimity, your ability to find options in the practical world could be applied to your emotional world, too, perhaps through recognizing that you also have options in how you respond to the uncomfortable emotions that you experience.

Recap of the Hero's Journey

As a reminder and as a companion to the guided meditation in the audio/video lesson, here is a recap of the steps of the hero's journey:

1. The Ordinary World.

2. The Call to Adventure.

3. The Refusal of the Call.

4. Meeting the Mentor.

5. Crossing the Threshold.

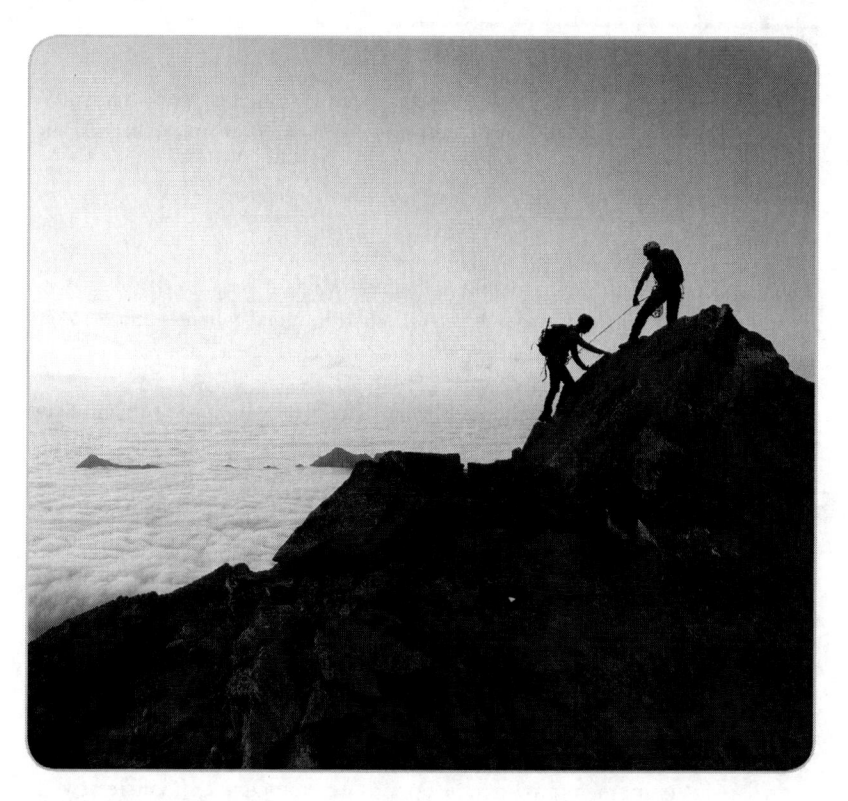

6. Tests, Allies, and Enemies.

7. The Approach to the Inmost Cave.

8. The Ordeal, Death, and Rebirth.

9. The Reward.

10. The Road Back.

11. Resurrection.

12. The Return with the Elixir.

Bringing Everything Together

- There are many different ways to measure resilience. Now that you've had the chance to look at your resilience from both an intellectual and experiential angle, take some time to continue exploring what brings you resilience. After all, this is your hero's journey.

- Remember, no two people are the same, meaning you are your own benchmark. Some people might feel resilient because they leveraged their difficulties to reach their top performance, whereas others might feel resilient because they survived an incredible hardship.

- Others may define their resilience by how they have been able to draw strength from their challenges in order to achieve their life's mission. Still others may measure their resilience by how they respond the next time they find themselves in a truly challenging situation. Just as you change over time, it's normal for your definition of resilience to change over time, too.

- Resilience is something that everyone already has. You have already made it through 100 percent of your hardest days, and that in itself shows resilience. It's not a question of whether you have resilience, but rather a question of how you use it.

- Every moment provides the opportunity to practice and increase your resilience, including how you respond to stress, how you perceive adversity, and how you care for yourself during the good times so that you're ready when things get hard. These everyday choices determine how well you are able to withstand difficulties, bounce back from adversity, and learn from each and every experience.

- Ultimately, resilience comes down to what you choose to give your personal power to. You will have challenges, and you will have people who disappoint or hurt you. It's healthy to acknowledge those experiences and how they impact you, but you don't have to give them your power. Instead, you can gain power, wisdom, and insight from the experiences.

- Your problems are your path. No matter what you've experienced, nothing can take away your power to choose how you respond to the changing circumstances of life. This reality is the true heart of resilience.

Activities

- Complete the Resilience Self-Evaluation Tool, on page 182, and respond to the questions at the end of the tool.

- Complete the Hero's Journey guided meditation as many times as is helpful for you.

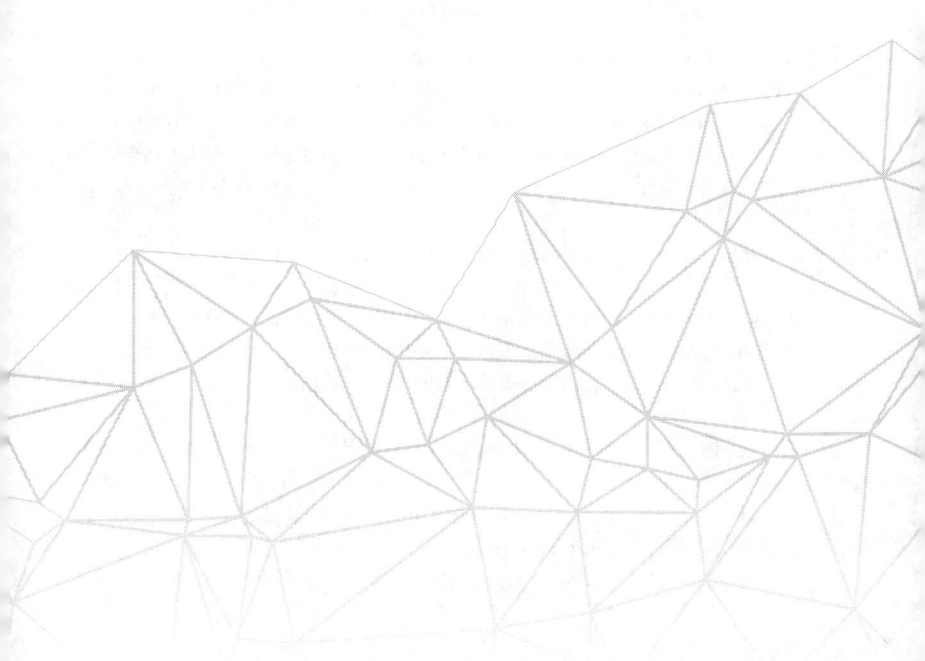

Class 24 Transcript

Your Hero's Journey

Really, every one of us is on our own hero's journey—learning, struggling, persisting, growing—venturing through life's trials and tribulations, but also through its beauty and its rewards. Imagine making it through it all without resilience. It's impossible. What would happen if every time we fell down, we just didn't get back up? Resilience is essential to navigating life successfully and reaching our fullest potential. It really is one of the most important skills we can master. We've spent the last 23 classes flooding you with inspirational stories, knowledge, and practice opportunities to support your own resilience, and now it's time to put everything together.

As I said way back in class one, the best way to use this course is to make it your own, and this class is going to be an opportunity to do just that. Think of this class as a practice class for your whole being—body and mind. This is where you can take all of the information from each individual class and apply it to your own unique life, and from both an intellectual and an experiential perspective.

We're going to start by talking briefly about how to use the self-evaluation tool in your guidebook. Then I am going to share a hero's journey guided mindfulness meditation practice with you to help you explore your experience. This is a class you may come back to many times to move through that hero's journey again as you uncover deeper layers of meaning present in your own life.

Oftentimes the only difference between people who want to change, but don't, and people who want to change, and do it, are that the people who actually change have a plan for how they're going to do so. This class is your chance to put what you've learned into action.

Let's start our evaluation from an intellectual perspective. If you haven't done so yet, take the resilience self-evaluation tool, which can be found in your guidebook. This tool will measure your resilience in the eight different categories I walked you through back in class one. And even if you have already taken the evaluation, it's a good idea to take it again, as some of your answers may have changed now that you've worked your way through the course. As you take the evaluation and look through your results, keep in mind that it's normal to feel more resilient in some areas than others, just as it is normal for us to excel at certain subjects or activities more than others.

The purpose of this tool is twofold. It allows you to realize the ways in which you are very resilient already, so that you can harness those skills, and it allows you to uncover areas in which resilience comes less naturally to you, so that you can find ways to amp-up your resilience in those areas, making you even more prepared to take on life's challenges.

Once you're done with the evaluation, take some time to reflect on your results. Where are your strengths? Which areas are more difficult for you? Do your results surprise you? Look at each category in isolation, and really think about how each one has manifested in your life.

It's helpful to do this self-evaluation in your areas of weakness, but also in your areas of strength. By harnessing your strengths, you could very well uncover some skills that you could transfer to other categories as well. For instance, let's say you have a very proactive worldview, but you struggle with equanimity. Your ability to find options in the practical world could be applied to your emotional world, too, perhaps through recognizing that you also have options in how you respond to the uncomfortable emotions that you experience.

For those of you looking for even further exploration, we've included a list of reflection questions in your guidebook for you to work through. You'll find the questions directly after the evaluation tool itself.

Now we're going to explore the hero's journey through resilience on an experiential level. If you think back to the second class in this series, you'll recall our discussion of the 12 steps of the hero's journey. Well, for the next 20 minutes or so I'm going to guide you through each of these 12 Steps as you have your own experience. You are welcome to choose an experience from your past or a current hero's journey you are on to explore during the guided meditation. You are welcome to do this meditation many times to gain new insights into your journey.

Take a moment now to find a comfortable position. You're welcome to sit in a chair or a sofa, or you are welcome to lie down if that is more comfortable for you, but if you want to do this on a cognitive level you might not want to lie down. You could tend to fall asleep if you are reclined. So, pick what's best for your body and for your experience.

Take a couple minutes, and pause if necessary, to prepare for the practice. Start out feeling the whole body in this moment. Notice all the places your body is supported; opening up to the space around you. What is your present moment experience? Feel a sense of well-being and safety, calling upon your inner resource if that is helpful for you to evoke that feeling of security knowing that you'll be able to go more deeply into the practice if you're feeling a sense of well-being. Know that this is your journey. You can make it whatever you want.

Now, call to mind an experience in your life that's been challenging for you, a journey where you've been called to question your beliefs about the world; a journey that's transformed you or is transforming you in some way. And start, once you select a place, start thinking about all of the ways that you've felt before the journey began in your ordinary world, the life you had before the call to adventure.

Think about the way you spent your time, the people in your life, in your home and community. What did you perceive as your strengths during this time? What were your core values? What were your challenges? Feel yourself as that person before the journey began. Feeling the sensation of the body being that person about to be transformed, but not there yet.

Notice the assumptions that you might have had about life. Notice your perceptions, picturing yourself so fully in this life, opening up to what it looked like: perhaps the music you listened to, or the activities you did in your day to day, the place you lived and worked. Picture yourself heading through that life and then suddenly you encounter your call to adventure. This could be some sort of long-term feeling that life needed to change that suddenly comes to a head. Or, it could be something sudden, like an accident or an injury, or some sudden experience that changes your life profoundly.

What does your body feel like when you first encounter this call to adventure? Do you feel shocked? Perhaps afraid? Maybe nervous, but inspired? Welcome whatever is present in you as you start realizing that your life is never going to be the same again. Suddenly, your circumstances have changed. Notice what it feels like in the body as you realize you can never go back to the life you had before. What does it feel like in your body as you start to realize that your life will never be the same again?

What's present in your body? What's present in your mind? What beliefs may feel challenged or affirmed? As you feel into all of this start to notice, are you ready for the journey ahead? Or do you feel a sense of resistance? Perhaps, a refusal of the call, a desire to crawl back into your old life and just have everything be just as it was. Notice what happens in your body as you stand at this threshold and not really want to cross. What is that resistance in you? Where do you feel that resistance in your body?

Listen to that resistance for a little while, here. What are you afraid of? Are you afraid you might lose something from the past? Are you afraid of not knowing what the future holds? Are you afraid of the unknown? Perhaps, sadness is present, a sense of loss or grief. Welcome whatever is present. Perhaps a feeling you don't deserve to change. Notice what holds you back from going on your way. Observe the obstacles as they arise. Notice how the body and the heart feel as you stare down these obstacles, knowing you can't go back, but are also afraid to move forward.

Now, notice yourself meeting a mentor, a person or some form of wisdom that comes into your life. Perhaps a teacher or a guide, a person that has the capability to see in you what you can't see in yourself just yet. Someone who holds keys to wisdom and truth that you need for your journey ahead. Notice what's present in the body as you encounter this person or wisdom. What does it feel like to discover someone who had the ability to help show you the way or send you on your way? What do they offer you that helps create a bridge from that feeling of fear of moving forward into a sense of inner-strength that will empower you to move forward?

Feel the connection with this teacher or guide. Feel what they liberate inside of you, how they point you to the truths inside of you; how they give you just enough that you prepare for what's next. Observe the feeling of gaining just enough inner-strength to know that you can take that first step forward across the threshold into the unknown. Notice what emotions arise as you begin to head into the future, out of the life you lived, and into the unknown, a journey that will reveal many challenges and also many strengths. Really feel what is present in you. What is the physical sensation of taking that step, the step that you've been afraid to take?

What is the feeling? What is the feeling of that inner- knowing that you have to take the step, that you can't stay in the middle anymore? Notice that moment when the courage inside of you to move forward becomes greater than the fear of staying where you are. And with that, feel yourself stepping across the threshold fully embarking on your journey.

And now you set out on your way, moving out into the world. Moving out into the unknown knowing the challenges will be here to teach you the lessons you need to learn, but not even being able to fully see those challenges yet. What is the first test or challenges you encounter? What does it feel like inside of you when you encounter this challenge? What comes to support you as you head into it? Perhaps an ally, a friend who appears along the way, an unexpected person or teacher. What role do they play? What is their part of the story?

You may encounter an enemy along the way, someone you feel called to fight. Can you fight without disturbing your inner-peace? Can you leave the ego behind, and approach it with a sense of confidence, grace, and ease? Prepared for the battle. Perhaps nervous, yes, perhaps afraid, but also knowing there is no other choice. You have to fight this fight. There is no moving forward until you do.

So, you take these steps finding your wisdom, your tools, your strength along the way. What are those tools? What unique lessons do you find that empower you to continue on? Set a practice, set a value, a bit of wisdom, perhaps another person helps give you strength in a way that you don't have it, but then helps you find that same strength inside of you.

Notice this journey you're walking as you approach the inmost cave, the place where you know you will encounter the proverbial dragon. The fight that must be fought in order to move on. What is the experience of that like for you, as you take those steps towards the cave, as you enter into the darkness not knowing what is there? But also, feeling the call to go in, the undeniable call to have to face your darkness so completely.

What tools do you need as you approach that innermost cave? What are you discovering about yourself as you go into the darkness? Notice what emotions and beliefs arise as you do this. Notice the feeling of your body. And now, in the midst of the darkness, there lies the biggest challenge yet, the proverbial dragon. Whatever it is for you, the ordeal you must face, the ordeal your life depends upon and perhaps the life of many others.

Feel yourself entering into the battle with this: the darkness at the core of your fear. The darkness that has kept you trapped, the darkness that inside your unique gifts and wisdom reside. Approach this as if your life depended upon it, because it does. What is there here? What is there to fear really? What do you call upon as you fight this battle? Can you stay connected to stillness, your inherent wholeness, in the midst of it?

Notice, if, perhaps, at some points it feels like you can't go on, that it is impossible, that your death is eminent. There is no way you can tackle this challenge. What does it feel like when you're afraid that this might be it? Observe the body. Notice what you must call upon as you take this last step, this step where you must slay the proverbial dragon, where you must die as your former self, to become the person that you are meant to be in this life.

Feel that rising up of your potential. The rebirth that comes when you surrender your former self to become the person you are destined to be. Feel the vulnerability, but also the strength that arises as you slay the dragon, as you find your way to the center of that darkness where the darkness melts away, and all that is left is the lesson, the core of truth that resided at the center of the darkness, the one you would have never found had you never entered the cave.

Feel yourself seizing the sword, getting your reward: that wisdom, that truth that you earned through the battle. Feel how you can welcome it even more fully because of how hard you had to fight to get it. Feel yourself absorbing this reward. Absorbing freedom from the dragon that had kept you enslaved for so long. Sense into this freedom as you start to explore it. What does it feel like as you realize the darkness was just an illusion? What does it feel like to tap into that inner-strength that may have been there the whole time, but you just couldn't see it? What does it feel like to really earn your truth? Embrace your truth. Know that you deserve it.

As you begin walking the road back home, notice what is present in you. As you think of the journey you've just been on, and yet the future that awaits, what are the experiences happening inside of you? As you walk back the road you just came on, what do you see? How does the world look different? And as you begin to approach your former life, notice how a sense of excitement and enthusiasm may arise. A sense of knowing what you did not know.

Excitement about the potential of this.

But then, as you start coming back to your life and getting closer again, notice how everything is different, how everyone and everything you left behind may still be the same, but you are different. Notice how these two worlds may feel unreconciled. Feel the struggle within yourself, how you have to fully let go of the person you were before to embrace the person you are meant to be. Feel this is perhaps the biggest challenge yet—the full melting away of the former self. You feel how the world around you reacts as that happens, how the people and situations in your life may want to hold you to being that other person. Feel the strength it takes to fully embody the person you were meant to be, the one you are now.

Feel this reconciliation as a resurrection, a rising up from the darkness, to merge the past with the present, so that you are uniquely prepared to walk into the future, empowered, inspired, filled with the wisdom you never knew was possible when you first began. Feel yourself embodying that unique wisdom. Your highest potential.

As you return into life with this elixir, feel how your path unfolds before you, how suddenly the right people are drawn to you. Feel how opportunities unfold with grace and ease. How yes, you will have to show up and work very hard, perhaps harder then you've ever worked before. But now, you are in alignment with your destiny: empowered, strong, and free; free to be the person you truly are, full of love, full of light, uniquely you. Prepared to walk the path that only you can walk, in only the way you can walk it. No one else can do it but you.

And feel how you embodying your authentic truth liberates those around you to do the same; how finding your unique harmony empowers other to find their harmony. Feel the world around you coming into harmony as you bring your unique gifts to life. As you embark on this journey, one hero's journey ends, and another begins. Set forth into this with a renewed sense of knowledge, knowing you will find your way, exactly as you just did, new and different. Evolving, stronger, full of grace, supported every single step of your way.

May you have everything you need in each moment. Thank you so much.

There are so many different ways to measure resilience. Now that you've had the chance to look at your resilience from both an intellectual and experiential angle, take some time to continue exploring what brings you resilience. After all, this is your hero's journey.

Remember, no two people are the same, meaning you are your own benchmark. Some people might feel resilient because they've leveraged their difficulties to reach their top performance, whereas others might feel resilient because they survived an incredible hardship. Others may define their resilience by how they have been able to draw strength from their challenges in order to achieve their life's mission. Still others may measure their resilience by how they respond next time they find themselves in a truly challenging situation. Just as you change over time, it's normal for your definition of resilience to change over time, too.

Resilience is something that all of us already have. Every single person watching or listening to me now has already made it through 100 percent of their hardest days, and that in itself shows resilience. It's not a question of whether you have resilience, but rather, how do you use it? Every moment provides us with the opportunity to practice and increase our resilience—how we respond to stress, how we perceive adversity, and how we care for ourselves during the good times so that we're ready when things get hard. It's these everyday choices that determine how well we will be able to withstand our difficulties, bounce back from adversity, and learn from each and every experience.

What does resilience look like in your life? What do you want resilience to look like in your life? Ultimately resilience comes down to what we choose to give our personal power to. We all have challenges. We all have people who have disappointed or hurt us. It's healthy to acknowledge those experiences and how they impacted us, but we don't have to give them our power. Instead, we can gain power, wisdom, and insight from the experience.

Remember, our problems are our path. No matter what we've experienced, nothing can take away our power to choose how we respond to the changing circumstances of life, and this reality is the true heart of resilience. This is your life. This is your hero's journey. This is your time to recognize the truth that you always know the perfect way to respond, no matter what you experience in life. This is your time to rise with grace and strength to live at your fullest potential.

Thank you so much for being a part of our hero's journey. Just as you learn when you share something with other people, I have learned an incredible amount sharing this course with you. I would love to hear about your story and your hero's journey. You are welcome to reach out to me through social media or my website to share your stories or get involved in the wonderful programs we are bringing to life in the world. We are grateful for the opportunity to have shared this and hope it brings tremendous meaning to your life and the lives you touch with your own special gifts. Thank you.

Resilience Self-Evaluation Tool

Resilience—the ability to withstand difficulties, bounce back from adversity, and learn from your experiences—is the key to thriving in life. This quick assessment will tell you where you stand across eight different measures of resilience. Select one answer for each question below to find out in which categories you are the most resilient and in which categories you have the opportunity to boost your resilience even more.

1. I have a life purpose.
    - ☐ Strongly Agree
    - ☐ Agree
    - ☐ Unsure
    - ☐ Disagree
    - ☐ Strongly Disagree

2. I have core values that are meaningful to me (i.e., I know what my values are, why they are my values, and have made sure they are true to me rather than simply passed down to me).
    - ☐ Strongly Agree
    - ☐ Agree
    - ☐ Unsure
    - ☐ Disagree
    - ☐ Strongly Disagree

3. I have strategies for sticking to my core values.
    - ☐ Strongly Agree
    - ☐ Agree

- ☐ Unsure
- ☐ Disagree
- ☐ Strongly Disagree

4. I feel determined to live out my purpose, even during difficult times.
- ☐ Strongly Agree
- ☐ Agree
- ☐ Unsure
- ☐ Disagree
- ☐ Strongly Disagree

5. When I'm feeling sad, scared, or vulnerable, I tend to hide it or suppress it.
- ☐ Strongly Agree
- ☐ Agree
- ☐ Unsure
- ☐ Disagree
- ☐ Strongly Disagree

6. I am able to identify the emotions I'm feeling.
- ☐ Strongly Agree
- ☐ Agree
- ☐ Unsure
- ☐ Disagree
- ☐ Strongly Disagree

7. I engage in practices that encourage a mind-body connection, such as deep breathing, body scans, yoga, relaxing exercise, Yoga Nidra, meditation, or tai chi.
- ☐ Strongly Agree
- ☐ Agree
- ☐ Unsure
- ☐ Disagree
- ☐ Strongly Disagree

8. I have a short temper and/or tend to feel overwhelmed by my emotions.
- ☐ Strongly Agree
- ☐ Agree
- ☐ Unsure
- ☐ Disagree
- ☐ Strongly Disagree

9. I notice early on when I start to feel stressed.
- ☐ Strongly Agree
- ☐ Agree
- ☐ Unsure
- ☐ Disagree
- ☐ Strongly Disagree

10. When I'm stressed, I cope by smoking, drinking, using drugs, overeating or undereating, gambling, or engaging in abusive or unhealthy sex habits.
- ☐ Strongly Agree
- ☐ Agree
- ☐ Unsure
- ☐ Disagree
- ☐ Strongly Disagree

11. When I'm stressed, I use stress management tools, such as exercise, deep breathing, humor, and spiritual practice.
- ☐ Strongly Agree
- ☐ Agree
- ☐ Unsure
- ☐ Disagree
- ☐ Strongly Disagree

12. I have a steady sense of hope, faith, and/or optimism in my life.
- ☐ Strongly Agree

☐ Agree
☐ Unsure
☐ Disagree
☐ Strongly Disagree

13. I tend to neglect my physical needs (such as sleep, eating healthy, exercise, and so on).
☐ Strongly Agree
☐ Agree
☐ Unsure
☐ Disagree
☐ Strongly Disagree

14. I regularly take care of my emotional needs (by checking in with myself, talking to someone I trust, allowing myself to express feelings, and/or other methods).
☐ Strongly Agree
☐ Agree
☐ Unsure
☐ Disagree
☐ Strongly Disagree

15. I have a good balance of mental stimulation and mental breaks in my life.
☐ Strongly Agree
☐ Agree
☐ Unsure
☐ Disagree
☐ Strongly Disagree

16. It is important to me to take care of myself.
☐ Strongly Agree
☐ Agree
☐ Unsure

☐ Disagree
☐ Strongly Disagree

17. Deep down, I like myself and recognize my inherent worth.
☐ Strongly Agree
☐ Agree
☐ Unsure
☐ Disagree
☐ Strongly Disagree

18. I question my ability to accomplish tasks and reach my goals.
☐ Strongly Agree
☐ Agree
☐ Unsure
☐ Disagree
☐ Strongly Disagree

19. I am compassionate with myself.
☐ Strongly Agree
☐ Agree
☐ Unsure
☐ Disagree
☐ Strongly Disagree

20. I feel envious or jealous of others.
☐ Strongly Agree
☐ Agree
☐ Unsure
☐ Disagree
☐ Strongly Disagree

21. I am a trustworthy person.
- ☐ Strongly Agree
- ☐ Agree
- ☐ Unsure
- ☐ Disagree
- ☐ Strongly Disagree

22. I have a support system of people I trust who I know will be there if/when I need help. (This can include friends, family members, a therapist, a teacher, and so on.)
- ☐ Strongly Agree
- ☐ Agree
- ☐ Unsure
- ☐ Disagree
- ☐ Strongly Disagree

23. I am apprehensive to reach out to people when I need help.
- ☐ Strongly Agree
- ☐ Agree
- ☐ Unsure
- ☐ Disagree
- ☐ Strongly Disagree

24. I regularly give back. (Examples include volunteering, helping/supporting people in my life, donating to causes, and so on.)
- ☐ Strongly Agree
- ☐ Agree
- ☐ Unsure
- ☐ Disagree
- ☐ Strongly Disagree

25. I easily adapt to change.
- ☐ Strongly Agree
- ☐ Agree
- ☐ Unsure
- ☐ Disagree
- ☐ Strongly Disagree

26. I naturally see failure as an opportunity for growth.
- ☐ Strongly Agree
- ☐ Agree
- ☐ Unsure
- ☐ Disagree
- ☐ Strongly Disagree

27. I feel gratitude in my life.
- ☐ Strongly Agree
- ☐ Agree
- ☐ Unsure
- ☐ Disagree
- ☐ Strongly Disagree

28. It is difficult for me to see the perspectives of other people.
- ☐ Strongly Agree
- ☐ Agree
- ☐ Unsure
- ☐ Disagree
- ☐ Strongly Disagree

29. I believe challenges can make me stronger.
- ☐ Strongly Agree
- ☐ Agree
- ☐ Unsure

☐ Disagree
☐ Strongly Disagree

30. I find meaning in adverse circumstances.
☐ Strongly Agree
☐ Agree
☐ Unsure
☐ Disagree
☐ Strongly Disagree

31. I feel stuck in the traumas and problems of my past.
☐ Strongly Agree
☐ Agree
☐ Unsure
☐ Disagree
☐ Strongly Disagree

32. I have strong sources of inspiration in my life. (This can include love, people, teachers, heroes, books, nature, stories, spiritual/religious teachings, and so on.)
☐ Strongly Agree
☐ Agree
☐ Unsure
☐ Disagree
☐ Strongly Disagree

Scoring

Below you will see a scoring chart that depicts the eight categories of resilience. Each question you answered above is listed in this scoring chart in its corresponding category. Next to each question number, you will see point values ranging from 0 to 4, which correspond with each possible answer for that question. SA stands for Strongly Agree, A stands for Agree, U stands for Unsure, D stands for Disagree, and SD stands for Strongly Disagree.

Use the scoring chart to see how many points you earned for each question. You might want to circle or mark your answers in the scoring chart if it helps you keep track of your answers. Write down the number of points you earned for each question in the My Points column.

At the bottom of each category, you will total your points by adding your point values for the four questions you answered in that category. Your total point value will range from 0 to 16 points for each category.

Category	Question	Point Values					My Points
Core Values and Purpose	1	SA: 4	A: 3	U: 2	D: 1	SD: 0	___
	2	SA: 4	A: 3	U: 2	D: 1	SD: 0	___
	3	SA: 4	A: 3	U: 2	D: 1	SD: 0	___
	4	SA: 4	A: 3	U: 2	D: 1	SD: 0	___
						TOTAL POINTS	
Equanimity	5	SA: 0	A: 1	U: 2	D: 3	SD: 4	___
	6	SA: 4	A: 3	U: 2	D: 1	SD: 0	___
	7	SA: 4	A: 3	U: 2	D: 1	SD: 0	___
	8	SA: 0	A: 1	U: 2	D: 3	SD: 4	___
						TOTAL POINTS	
Healthy Coping Skills	9	SA: 4	A: 3	U: 2	D: 1	SD: 0	___
	10	SA: 0	A: 1	U: 2	D: 3	SD: 4	___
	11	SA: 4	A: 3	U: 2	D: 1	SD: 0	___
	12	SA: 4	A: 3	U: 2	D: 1	SD: 0	___
						TOTAL POINTS	

Category	#						
Self-Care	13	SA: 0	A: 1	U: 2	D: 3	SD: 4	___
	14	SA: 4	A: 3	U: 2	D: 1	SD: 0	___
	15	SA: 4	A: 3	U: 2	D: 1	SD: 0	___
	16	SA: 4	A: 3	U: 2	D: 1	SD: 0	___
						TOTAL POINTS	
Positive Sense of Self	17	SA: 4	A: 3	U: 2	D: 1	SD: 0	___
	18	SA: 0	A: 1	U: 2	D: 3	SD: 4	___
	19	SA: 4	A: 3	U: 2	D: 1	SD: 0	___
	20	SA: 0	A: 1	U: 2	D: 3	SD: 4	___
						TOTAL POINTS	
Support and Connection with Others	21	SA: 4	A: 3	U: 2	D: 1	SD: 0	___
	22	SA: 4	A: 3	U: 2	D: 1	SD: 0	___
	23	SA: 0	A: 1	U: 2	D: 3	SD: 4	___
	24	SA: 4	A: 3	U: 2	D: 1	SD: 0	___
						TOTAL POINTS	
Proactive Worldview	25	SA: 4	A: 3	U: 2	D: 1	SD: 0	___
	26	SA: 4	A: 3	U: 2	D: 1	SD: 0	___
	27	SA: 4	A: 3	U: 2	D: 1	SD: 0	___
	28	SA: 0	A: 1	U: 2	D: 3	SD: 4	___
						TOTAL POINTS	
Finding Meaning in Adversity	29	SA: 4	A: 3	U: 2	D: 1	SD: 0	___
	30	SA: 4	A: 3	U: 2	D: 1	SD: 0	___
	31	SA: 0	A: 1	U: 2	D: 3	SD: 4	___
	32	SA: 4	A: 3	U: 2	D: 1	SD: 0	___
						TOTAL POINTS	

Plot Your Results

Each resilience category has its own line on the graph below. For each category, plot your total point value (the bolded box from the corresponding category in the scoring chart) on the line. Then, connect your dots around the circle to see a comprehensive view of your resilience totals.

Scores range from 0 (low resilience) to 16 (high resilience) in each category.

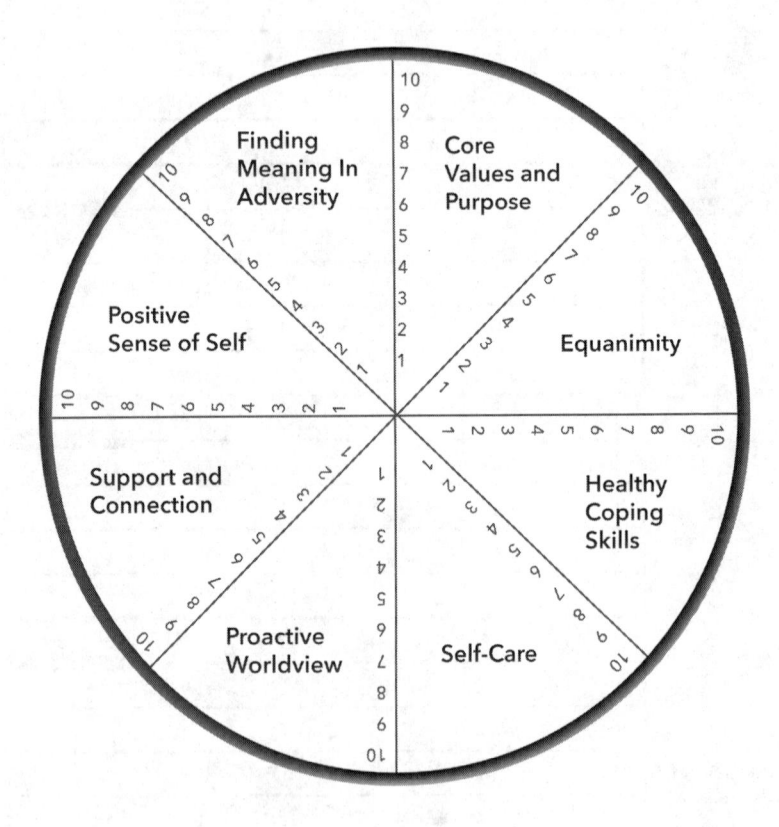

448 | BUILDING YOUR RESILIENCE: FINDING MEANING IN ADVERSITY

Description of Resilience Categories

Core Values and Purpose: Having an overarching purpose that guides you in life, and that is supported by core values that are meaningful to you. Having determination and sticking to your life purpose and core values, even when times get rough.

Equanimity: Welcoming your entire experience—the good and the bad. Accepting and allowing yourself to feel all emotions, including uncomfortable ones like fear and sadness. Regulating your emotions. Maintaining a healthy connection between body and mind.

Healthy Coping Skills: Having a set of healthy coping skills (such as exercise, humor, and deep breathing) and avoiding unhealthy coping mechanisms (such as smoking, drinking, drug use, gambling, and unhealthy sex habits). Recognizing when you are stressed and using healthy coping skills quickly in response to stress. Maintaining a sense of hope, faith, and/or optimism in your life.

Self-Care: Maintaining your energy reserves by regularly taking care of your physical, emotional, and mental needs. Whereas coping skills involve taking care of yourself in response to stress, self-care is routinely taking care of your needs in order to buffer you from life's challenges.

Positive Sense of Self: Recognizing your inherent worth as a person, but also not seeing yourself as better than others. Having self-compassion, trusting your ability to accomplish tasks and reach your goals, and feeling the desire to celebrate others' successes as opposed to feeling jealous or envious of them.

Support and Connection with Others: Knowing you have people you can reach out to for support (such as friends, family, and professionals), and reaching out to them when you need help. Having people in your life whom you can trust and engaging in altruistic behaviors (such as volunteer work, giving time to friends/family/strangers in need, and donating to good causes).

Proactive Worldview: Having psychological flexibility, easily adapting to change, feeling like you have options, seeing failure as an opportunity for growth rather than as an inherent flaw in yourself, having gratitude, and being able to see beyond your own perspective.

Finding Meaning in Adversity: Believing that challenges can make you stronger, finding wisdom in life's challenges, proactively seeking to find meaning in adversity, and taking the time to heal from past hardship and trauma.

Questions for Reflection

After completing the self-evaluation, answer the following questions for each resilience category:

- Does this category play a role in your life?

- If so, how has it been helpful?

- If not, what is standing in the way? For example, consider how this category was modeled for you during your upbringing, or what beliefs you have about it, such as the thought that self-care is self indulgent or that showing emotions is weak.

- What are your strengths in this category?

- What are your weaknesses in this category?

- Where on the wheel do your protective factors come into play? Your protective factors are things like family support, wealth, religion, a well-paying job, or having an education.

- Where on the wheel do you find vulnerabilities or triggers? This could be a tendency to use unhealthy coping mechanisms, difficulty regulating your emotions, or an unprocessed past.

- Find a takeaway. What is something you're doing in terms of this category that has helped support your resilience, and what can you do to maintain that? Alternatively, what is something in terms of this category that has not supported your resilience, and what can you do to change that?

Finding a Support Network

Support Resources

If you or someone you know feels unsafe in a relationship, you can call the National Domestic Violence Hotline at 1-800-799-7233. You can learn more about what abuse looks like in relationships here: http://www.thehotline.org.

If you or someone you know are looking for support following sexual assault, you can call the National Sexual Assault Hotline at 1-800-656-4673. You can learn more about sexual assault here: https://www.rainn.org/.

If you or someone you know is involved in human trafficking, you can call the National Human Trafficking Hotline at 1-888-373-7888, or learn more here: https://humantraffickinghotline.org/.

If you or someone you know has suicidal thoughts or intentions, you can call the National Suicide Prevention Hotline at 1-800-273-8255, or learn more here: https://suicidepreventionlifeline.org/.

If you or someone you know is looking for substance abuse treatment or mental health services, you can call the Substance Abuse and Mental Health Services Administration at 1-877-726-4727, or learn more here: https://www.samhsa.gov/find-help.

If you or someone you know has or might have an eating disorder, you can call the National Eating Disorders Association at 1-800-931-2237, or learn more here: https://www.nationaleatingdisorders.org/.

Tools for Finding a Therapist

To find a therapist for PTSD, you can use this website: https://www.ptsd.va.gov/public/treatment/therapy-med/finding-a-therapist.asp.

To find a therapist who uses the Pacifica mental health app, you can use this website: https://www.thinkpacifica.com/find-a-therapist/.

The article "How to Find the Right Therapist" by Marissa Miller is also a helpful resource, which you can find at this website: https://www.nytimes.com/2017/07/17/smarter-living/how-to-find-the-right-therapist.html.

Bibliography and Additional Resources

Anik, L., L. Aknin, M. Norton, and E. Dunn. "Feeling Good About Giving: The Benefits (and Costs) of Self-Interested Charitable Behavior." Harvard Business School Marketing Unit Working Paper no. 10-012 (2009).

Babbel, S. "Post Traumatic Stress Disorder After 9/11 and Katrina." *Psychology Today*, 2011. Retrieved from https://www.psychologytoday.com/us/blog/somatic-psychology/201109/post-traumatic-stress-disorder-after-911-and-katrina.

Bear, S. Y. *Standing in the Light: A Lakota Way of Seeing*. University of Nebraska Press, 1996.

Beck, J. "Hard Feelings: Science's Struggle to Define Emotions." *The Atlantic*, 2015. Retrieved from https://www.theatlantic.com/health/archive/2015/02/hard-feelings-sciences-struggle-to-define-emotions/385711/.

Becker-Asano, C., and I. Wachsmuth. "Affective Computing with Primary and Secondary Emotions in a Virtual Human." *Autonomous Agents and Multi-Agent Systems* 20, no. 32 (2010).

Birkholm, M. The Women's Empowerment Initiative. Yoga International. Retrieved from www.yogainternational.com/empowerment.

———. "Creating an Inner Resource." Class 3 in *iRest: Integrative Restoration Yoga Nidra for Deep Relaxation*. The Great Courses. The Teaching Company LLC, 2018.

Bowers, M. E., and R. Yehuda. "Intergenerational Transmission of Stress in Humans." *Neuropsychopharmacology* 41 (2016).

Braga, L. L., M. F. Mello, and J. P. Fiks. "Transgenerational Transmission of Trauma and Resilience: A Qualitative Study with Brazilian Offspring of Holocaust Survivors." *BMC Psychiatry* 12 (2012).

Bremner, D. "Traumatic Stress: Effects on the Brain." *Dialogues in Clinical Neuroscience* 8, no. 4 (2006). Les Laboratoires Servier. Retrieved from www.ncbi.nlm.nih.gov/pmc/articles/PMC3181836/.

Brown, B. *I Thought It Was Just Me (But It Isn't): Making the Journey from "What Will People Think?" to "I Am Enough."* Penguin Group LLC, 2007.

———. "Shame Shields: The Armor We Use to Protect Ourselves and Why It Doesn't Serve Us." Digital seminar presentation. PESI. 2017.

Campbell, J. *The Hero With a Thousand Faces*. New World Library, 2008.

Campos, M. "Heart Rate Variability: A New Way to Track Well-Being." Harvard Health Publishing, 2017. Retrieved from https://www.health.harvard.edu/blog/heart-rate-variability-new-way-track-well-2017112212789.

Chödrön, P. *Tonglen: The Path of Transformation*. Vajradhatu Publications, 2001.

Coghlan, A. "The Brain Starts to Eat Itself after Chronic Sleep Deprivation." New Scientist, 2017. Retrived from https://www.newscientist.com/article/2132258-the-brain-starts-to-eat-itself-after-chronic-sleep-deprivation/.

Cohn, M. A., B. L. Fredrickson, S. L. Brown, J. A. Mikels, and A. M. Conway. "Happiness Unpacked: Positive Emotions Increase Life Satisfaction by Building Resilience." *Emotion* 9, no. 3 (2009).

De Jonge, P. "How Roger Federer Upgraded His Game." *The New York Times*, 2017. Retrieved from https://www.nytimes.com/interactive/2017/08/24/magazine/usopen-federer-nadal-backhand-wonder-year.html.

Dimidjian, S., B. V. Kleiber, and Z. V. Segal. "Mindfulness-Based Cognitive Therapy." *Cognitive and Behavioral Theories in Clinical Practice*. Guilford Press, 2009.

Ducharme, J. "5 Places Where People Live the Longest and Healthiest Lives." TIME Health, 2018. Retrieved from http://time.com/5160475/blue-zones-healthy-long-lives/.

Duckworth, A. L. "Grit: The Power of Passion and Perseverance." TED Talks Education, 2013. Retrieved from https://www.ted.com/talks/angela_lee_duckworth_grit_the_power_of_passion_and_perseverance#t-320930.

Dunn, E., L. Aknin, and M. Norton. "Spending Money on Others Promotes Happiness." *Science* (2008).

Ekman, P. "An Argument for Basic Emotions." *Cognition and Emotion* 6, no. 3–4 (1992).

Epel, E. "Can Meditation Slow Rate of Cellular Aging? Cognitive Stress, Mindfulness, and Telomeres." *Annals of the New York Academy of Sciences* (2009). Retrieved from www.ncbi.nlm.nih.gov/pmc/articles/PMC3057175/.

Eyre, C., and S. Grimberg. *American Experience: We Shall Remain*. Television series. United States: PBS, 2009.

Falke, K. and J. Goldberg. *Struggle Well: Thriving in the Aftermath of Trauma*. Lioncrest Publishing, 2018.

Frankl, V. E. *Man's Search for Meaning*. Simon and Schuster, 1985.

Gallegos, D. "Research Finds Volunteering Can Be Good for Your Health." *The Wall Street Journal*, 2018. Retrieved from https://www.wsj.com/articles/research-finds-volunteering-can-be-good-for-your-health-1524449280.

Hall, D. Kordich, and J. Pearson. "Resilience—Giving Children the Skills to Bounce Back." Reaching IN … Reaching OUT Project, 2003.

Hammond, C. "Impacts of Lifelong Learning upon Emotional Resilience, Psychological and Mental Health: Fieldwork Evidence." *Oxford Review of Education* 30, no. 4 (2007).

Hanson, R., and R. Mendius. *Buddha's Brain: The Practical Neuroscience of Happiness, Love, and Wisdom*. New Harbinger Publications, 2009.

Harvard Health. "How Stress Affects Seniors, and How to Manage It." Harvard Health Publishing, 2016. Retrieved from www.health.harvard.edu/aging/how-stress-affects-seniors-and-how-to-manage-it.

———. "Understanding the Stress Response." Harvard Health Publishing, 2011. Retrieved from www.health.harvard.edu/staying-healthy/understanding-the-stress-response.

Hayes, S. C., J. B. Luoma, F. W. Bond, A. Masuda, and J. Lillis. "Acceptance and Commitment Therapy: Model, Processes and Outcomes." *Behaviour Research and Therapy* 44, no. 1 (2006).

Hedrick, J. D. *Harriet Beecher Stowe: A Life*. Oxford University Press, 1995.

Holiday, R. *The Obstacle Is the Way: The Timeless Art of Turning Trials into Triumph*. Penguin, 2014.

Holz, G. *Secrets of Aboriginal Healing: A Physicist's Journey with a Remote Australian Tribe*. Inner Traditions/Bear, 2013.

Hölzel, B. K., S. W. Lazar, T. Gard, Z. Schuman-Olivier, D. R. Vago, and U. Ott. "How Does Mindfulness Meditation Work? Proposing Mechanisms of Action from a Conceptual and Neural Perspective." *Perspectives on Psychological Science* 6, no. 6 (2011).

Hosie, R. "How Sleep Deprivation Affects Your Brain." Independent, 2017. Retrieved from https://www.independent.co.uk/life-style/health-and-families/sleep-deprivation-how-affects-your-brain-tiredness-insomnia-a7809756.html.

Hsu, M. H., T. L. Ju, C. H. Yen, and C. M. Chang. "Knowledge Sharing Behavior in Virtual Communities: The Relationship between Trust, Self-Efficacy, and Outcome Expectations." *International Journal of Human-Computer Studies* 65, no. 2 (2007).

Huffington, A. *The Sleep Revolution: Transforming Your Life, One Night at a Time*. Harmony, 2016.

Keller, A., K. Litzelman, L. E. Wisk, T. Maddox, E. R. Cheng, P. D. Creswell, and W. P. Witt. "Does the Perception That Stress Affects Health Matter? The Association with Health and Mortality." *Health Psychology* 31, no. 5 (2012).

Keye, M. D., and A. M. Pidgeon. "An Investigation of the Relationship between Resilience, Mindfulness, and Academic Self-Efficacy." *Open Journal of Social Sciences* 1, no. 6 (2013).

Killian, K. D. "Helping till it Hurts? A Multimethod Study of Compassion Fatigue, Burnout, and Self-Care in Clinicians Working with Trauma Survivors." *Traumatology* 14, no. 2 (2008).

Lama, D., and D. Tutu. *The Book of Joy*. Random House, 2016.

Lawrence, D. H. *"Psychoanalysis and the Unconscious"* and *"Fantasia of the Unconscious."* Cambridge University Press, 2004.

Lentz, T. L., et al. "Human Nervous System." *Encyclopædia Britannica*, 2017. Retrieved from www.britannica.com/science/human-nervous-system.

Levine, P. A. *Waking the Tiger: Healing Trauma—The Innate Capacity to Transform Overhwleming Experiences*. North Atlantic Books, 1997.

Lynch, T., J. Sykes-Kennedy, and T. Kennedy. *Dancing Light: The Spiritual Side of Being Through The Eyes of a Modern Yoga Master*. Power Living Media, 2015.

McCall, T. *Yoga As Medicine: The Yogic Prescription for Health and Healing*. Bantam, 2007.

McGonigal, K. "How to Make Stress Your Friend." TEDGlobal, 2013. Retrieved from https://www.ted.com/talks/kelly_mcgonigal_how_to_make_stress_your_friend?utm_source=tedcomshare&utm_medium=email&utm_campaign=tedspread#t-367810.

Mednick, S. C., and M. Ehrman. *Take a Nap! Change Your Life*. Workman Publishing, 2006.

Meier, S. and A. Stutzer. "Is Volunteering Rewarding in Itself?" *Economica* 75 (2008).

Miller, R. *Yoga Nidra: A Meditative Practice for Deep Relaxation and Healing*. ReadHowYouWant, 2010.

———. *The iRest Program for Healing PTSD: A Proven-Effective Approach to Using Yoga Nidra Meditation and Deep Relaxation Techniques to Overcome Trauma*. New Harbinger Publications, 2015.

Mineo, L. "Good Genes Are Nice, but Joy Is Better." *The Harvard Gazette*, 2017. Retrieved from https://news.harvard.edu/gazette/story/2017/04/over-nearly-80-years-harvard-study-has-been-showing-how-to-live-a-healthy-and-happy-life/.

Mitchell, M. "Dr. Herbert Benson's Relaxation Response." *Psychology Today*, 2013. Retrieved from https://www.psychologytoday.com/us/blog/heart-and-soul-healing/201303/dr-herbert-benson-s-relaxation-response.

Mitsuhashi, Y. "Japan May Have Worked Out the Secret Formula for a Happy Life." *The Huffington Post*, 2018. Retrieved from https://www.huffingtonpost.com/entry/japan-ikigai-happiness_us_5ac3545ae4b00fa46f85fc70.

Morgan, M., and R. Alexander. *Mutant Message Down Under*. Thorsons, 1995.

Neale, L. *The Power of Ceremony: Restoring the Sacred in Our Selves, Our Families, Our Communities*. Eagle Spirit Press, 2011.

Nerburn, K., ed. *The Wisdom of the Native Americans: Including The Soul of an Indian and Other Writings of Ohiyesa and the Great Speeches of Red Jacket, Chief Joseph, and Chief Seattle*. New World Library, 2010.

Paddock, C. *Alcohol Disrupts Body's Sleep Regulator*. Medical News Today, 2014. Retrieved from https://www.medicalnewstoday.com/articles/286827.php.

Paul, M. "How Traumatic Memories Hide in the Brain, and How to Retrieve Them." Northwestern Now, 2015. Retrieved from https://news.northwestern.edu/stories/2015/08/traumatic-memories-hide-retrieve-them.

Pearson, J., and D. Kordich. *Reaching IN ... Reaching OUT Resiliency Guidebook*. First Folio Resource Group, Inc., 2006.

Pellissier, H. *How Stress Affects Your Child*. Great Schools, 2016. Retrieved from www.greatschools.org/gk/articles/how-stress-affects-your-child/.

Poulin, M. J., S. L. Brown, A. J. Dillard, and D. M. Smith. "Giving to Others and the Association between Stress and Mortality." *American Journal of Public Health* 103, no. 9 (2013).

ReShel, A. *The Science Behind Yoga*. Video file. UpLift, 2016. Retrieved from https://upliftconnect.com/the-science-behind-yoga/?utm_source=facebook&utm_medium=link&utm_campaign=uplift.

Reynolds, E. "Truth Is, Everyone Lies All the Time." The Conversation, 2012. Retrieved from http://theconversation.com/truth-is-everyone-lies-all-the-time-6749.

Richie, C. *Trail of Tears—A Native American Documentary Collection*. DVD. United States: Mill Creek Entertainment, 2010.

Sandberg, S., and A. Grant. *Option B: Facing Adversity, Building Resilience, and Finding Joy*. Ebury Publishing, 2017.

Schwerdtfeger, K. L., R. E. Larzelere, D. Werner, C. Peters, and M. Oliver. "Intergenerational Transmission of Trauma: The Mediating Role of Parenting Styles on Toddlers' DSM-Related Symptoms." *Journal of Aggression, Maltreatment & Trauma* 22, no. 2 (2013).

Segal, Z. V., J. M. G. Williams, and J. D. Teasdale. *Mindfulness-Based Cognitive Therapy for Depression*. New York: Guilford Press, 2002.

Shapiro, F. *Getting Past Your Past: Take Control of Your Life with Self-Help Techniques from EMDR Therapy*. Rodale, 2012.

Siegel, D. J., and T. P. Bryson. *The Whole-Brain Child: 12 Revolutionary Strategies to Nurture Your Child's Developing Mind*. Random House Digital, Inc., 2011.

Silverman, L. "7 Reasons Why Baths Are Great for Your Health." *Town & Country*, 2018. Retrieved from https://www.townandcountrymag.com/style/beauty-products/a18673205/hot-baths-benefits/.

Sivananda, S. *Bliss Divine*. Divine Life Society of South Africa, 1990.

———. *Thought Power*. Youcanprint, 2018.

Smith, E. "The Benefits of Optimism Are Real." *The Atlantic*, 2013 Retrieved from https://www.theatlantic.com/health/archive/2013/03/the-benefits-of-optimism-are-real/273306/.

Storoni, M. *The Science of Breathing*. Video file. UpLift TV, 2018. Retrieved from https://uplift.tv/2018/the-science-of-breathing/.

Takeuchi, H., Y. Taki, H. Hashizume, K. Asano, M. Asano, Y. Sassa, S. Yokota, Y. Kotozaki, R. Nouchi, and R. Kawashima. "The Impact of Television Viewing on Brain Structures: Cross-Sectional and Longitudinal Analyses." *Cerebral Cortex* 25, no. 5 (2015).

UHN staff. "4 GABA Deficiency Symptoms You Can Identify Yourself." University Health News Daily, 2013. Retrieved from https://universityhealthnews.com/daily/depression/4-gaba-deficiency-symptoms-you-can-identify-yourself/.

Vaiva, G., V. Boss, F. Ducrocq, M. Fontaine, P. Devos, A. Brunet, P. Laffargue, M. Goudemand, and P. Thomas. "Relationship between Posttrauma GABA Plasma Levels and PTSD at 1-Year Follow-Up." *American Journal of Psychiatry* 163, no. 8 (2006).

Van der Kolk, B. *The Body Keeps the Score*. New York: Viking, 2014.

Vogler, C. *The Writer's Journey*. Studio City, CA: Michael Wiese Productions, 2007.

Willcox, G. "The Feeling Wheel: A Tool for Expanding Awareness of Emotions and Increasing Spontaneity and Intimacy." *Transactional Analysis Journal* 12, no. 4 (1982).

Additional Resources

American Psychological Association. "Stress: The Different Kinds of Stress." Retrieved from http://www.apa.org/helpcenter/stress-kinds.aspx.

Boulder Crest Retreat Center. *Warrior PATHH Student Guide.*

Centers for Disease Control and Prevention. "About the CDC-Kaiser ACE Study." Retrieved from https://www.cdc.gov/violenceprevention/acestudy/about.html.

Cleveland Clinic. "Stress." Retrieved from https://my.clevelandclinic.org/health/articles/11874-stress.

Feel That. Retrieved from www.feelthat.ca.

HealthBarn USA. Retrieved from www.healthbarnusa.com.

HeartMath. Retrieved from https://www.heartmath.com/.

National Heart, Lung, and Blood Institute. "Why Is Sleep Important?" Retrieved from https://www.nhlbi.nih.gov/node/4605.

Palmo, J. *Tenzin Palmo—Tonglen Meditation.* Video file. Retrieved from https://www.youtube.com/watch?v=GZOaaHN6DQY.

———. *Video Teachings.* Video files. Retrieved from http://tenzinpalmo.com/jetsunma-tenzin-palmo/teaching-resources/video/.

Stress Management Society. "How Stress Affects Us." Retrieved from www.stress.org.uk/how-it-affects-us/.

Substance Abuse and Mental Health Services Administration. "Risk and Protective Factors." Retrieved from https://www.samhsa.gov/capt/practicing-effective-prevention/prevention-behavioral-health/risk-protective-factors.

Vivyan, C. "Unhelpful Thinking Habits." Getselfhelp.co.uk. Retrieved from https://www.getselfhelp.co.uk/unhelpful.htm.

What is Epigenetics. "Epigenetics: Fundamentals." Retrieved from https://www.whatisepigenetics.com/fundamentals/.

Other Great Courses Relevant to Resilience

Cognitive Behavioral Therapy: Techniques for Retraining Your Brain, taught by Jason M. Satterfield, PhD. Available at: https://www.thegreatcourses.com/courses/cognitive-behavioral-therapy-techniques-for-retraining-your-brain.html or on The Great Courses Plus.

iRest: Integrative Yoga Nidra for Deep Relaxation, taught by Molly Birkholm. Available at: https://www.thegreatcourses.com/courses/irest-integrative-restoration-yoga-nidra-for-deep-relaxation.html or on The Great Courses Plus.

Masters of Mindfulness: Transforming Your Mind and Body, taught by multiple instructors. Available at: https://www.thegreatcourses.com/courses/masters-of-mindfulness-transforming-your-mind-and-body.html or on The Great Courses Plus.

Image Credits

GoodLifeStudio/Getty Images.	6
KidStock/Getty Images.	8
mattjeacock/DigitalVision Vectors/Getty Images.	9
Tatyana Tomsickova Photography/Getty Images.	42
Hill Street Studios/Getty Images.	45
JGI/Jamie Grill/Getty Images.	61
fizkes/Getty Images.	65
Caiaimage/Martin Barraud/Getty Images.	81
Tom Werner/Getty Images.	84
FatCamera/Getty Images.	100
Peter Lourenco/Getty Images.	103
Colin Anderson/Getty Images.	118
Inti St Clair/Getty Images.	122
Steve Smith/Getty Images.	144
Michael H/Getty Images.	159
petrenkod/Getty Images.	163
R.Tsubin/Getty Images.	164
MangoStar_Studio/Getty Image.	178
Maskot/Getty Image.	181
Michael Joven / EyeEm/Getty Images.	198
Alistair Berg/Getty Images.	203
Didi_Lavchieva/Getty Images.	220
Lifesavers, Inc.	236
Joana Lopes / EyeEm/Getty Images.	255
asiseeit/Getty Images.	259
FG Trade/E+/Getty Images.	273
Bastian Weltjen/Getty Images.	279
Westend61/Getty Images.	295
SilviaJansen/E+/Getty Images.	313
MmeEmil/E+/Getty Images.	314
altmodern/Getty Images.	315
fizkes/Getty Images.	316
Oleh_Slobodeniuk/E+/Getty Images.	318
DragonImages/Getty Images.	319
MangoStar_Studio/Getty Images.	321
FatCamera/E+/Getty Images.	322
DragonImages/Getty Images.	338
Tinpixels/E+/Getty Images.	351
Dean Mitchell/E+/Getty Images.	352
JuriahMosin/Getty Images.	365
fizkes/Getty Images.	366
rilueda/Getty Images.	367
triloks/Getty Images.	368
fizkes/Getty Images.	369
fizkes/Getty Images.	370
AzmanL/E+/Getty Images.	371
RyanJLane/Getty Images.	394
undrey/Getty Images.	396
Erin_Elizabeth/E+/Getty Images.	397
laflor/Getty Images.	397
Wavebreakmedia/Getty Images.	398
Koldunov/Getty Images.	399
bluecinema/E+/Getty Images.	400
Buena Vista Images/Getty Images.	425

Notes

Notes

Notes

Notes

Notes

Notes

Notes